the picture
of health

the picture
of health
medical ethics and
the movies

edited by

henri colt, silvia quadrelli,

and

lester d. friedman

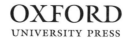

OXFORD

UNIVERSITY PRESS

OXFORD
UNIVERSITY PRESS

Published in the United States of America by Oxford University Press, Inc.,
198 Madison Avenue, New York, NY, 10016
United States of America

Oxford University Press, Inc., publishes works that further
Oxford University's objective of excellence
in research, scholarship, and education

Oxford is a registered trade mark of Oxford University Press in the
UK and in certain other countries

Library of Congress Cataloging-in-Publication Data

The picture of health : medical ethics and the movies / edited by Henri Colt,
Silvia Quadrelli, and Lester Friedman.
    p. cm.
 ISBN 978-0-19-973536-5 (alk. paper)
 1. Medicine in motion pictures. 2. Medical ethics. I. Colt, Henri G. II. Quadrelli, Silvia.
III. Friedman, Lester D.
 PN1995.9.M44P53 2011
 791.43'653—dc22   2010034548

978-0-19-973536-5
1 3 5 7 9 10 8 6 4 2

Typeset in Dante MT
Printed on acid-free paper
Printed in the United States of America

preface

In the Wachowski Brothers' science fiction epic, *The Matrix* (1999), Morpheus (Laurence Fishburn) offers Neo (Keanu Reeves) a critical choice: take the blue pill "the story ends. You wake up in your bed and you believe whatever you want to believe," or the red pill "you stay in Wonderland, and I show you how deep the rabbit hole goes." Using film to teach medical ethics is like swallowing the red pill. Abstract concepts and ideas can be extracted from film, debated, and discussed. Viewers can relate with or alienate themselves from the actors, the plot, or the context. They can address the issues portrayed in the film and identify others that may not be fully developed. Regardless of their level of expertise and experience, viewers can voice opinions, argue contradictory positions, display their emotions, and justify their perspectives based on external evidence, their personal experiences, and what actually happens in the fictional narrative of the cinematographic experience.

From an educator's standpoint, film provides a multilayered nucleus from which significant learning can take place: it also makes available a myriad of scenes and scenarios that can be dissected, critiqued, and used as examples to highlight moral dilemmas. Not only can films teach us *how* to restrain ourselves from doing what we know,[1] or think we know, is wrong, but they can portray situations that might confuse us and thus prompt reflection on the *why* we do what we do (or don't do). Movies can thus be used to help health care providers develop skills in the human dimensions of medical practice. They promote enthusiasm for learning, highlight themes, enhance discussion and reflection, and sometimes, help illustrate specific teaching points on clinical topics, social and health care policy issues, cultural differences, and science.[2–4]

This is cinemeducation, and, as stated in the preface of Alexander, Lenahan, and Pavlov's book on the subject,[5] if you are not already using film in your curriculum, we are confident that you will be after reading this book. Films with a solid plot and coherent story often work more dramatically and engagingly than a printed case description.[6] Visual images impart important information that simply cannot be duplicated in the written case history, which usually presents the facts and often ignores the broader context of an ethical situation; equally important, film narratives put a human face on an abstract ethical issue, taking it from the realm of the theoretical and placing it firmly within the realm of the personal. Thus, film can be effectively used as an experiential exercise, as part of problem-solving sessions, or as a metaphor to clarify or dramatically magnify perspectives about a disease process or health care–related issue. Even a discussion of how cinematographic techniques reinforce the emotional, psychological, and intellectual impact of film—the use of flashbacks, special sequencing, framing, lighting, or animation, can dramatically illustrate social behaviors, values, and ethical principles that contribute to learning and knowledge retention. While using film enhances the intrinsic value of the educational process, and both learning and teaching should be inherently fun and satisfying, it would be incorrect to presume that simply showing a film suffices to teach medical ethics, or that the integration of film could replace thoughtful reading and analysis of essential texts. Unless educators want to entice their students to reflect de novo about a subject, reading pertinent course material prior to viewing a film is a prerequisite for a more enlightening and enriching discussion.

We designed this book to give readers specific tools to use in the classroom or the auditorium. Short scenes, with their specific DVD time sequences, are described and serve as a springboard for discussions of a particular ethics issue. Authors return to the scene and integrate their analysis into a brief commentary about the film itself. While it may not be necessary for readers, or their students, to view the entire film prior to integrating the scene into a teaching session or lecture, it is certainly preferable to do so before using the short clip in the classroom. That way, the teacher obtains a firmer grasp of how the scene fits into the overall narrative flow, as well as its place within the various characters' situation at that particular moment in the movie. Much like a particular section you might take out of a novel to illustrate a specific ethical dilemma, it remains important for instructors to know what comes before and after that scene to fully appreciate its significance.

We choose to use short scenes because our electronic age differs dramatically from any era that preceded it. Today, media saturates every level of our daily environment. Young people, in particular, dwell in a world dominated by an onslaught of visual images; they inhabit a dynamic, high-speed, rapidly changing, and sensitive environment stuffed with information acquisition and powerful emotional impact. They customarily receive, process, interpret, and react to visual images, be they on movie, television, or computer screens, Blackberries, and cell phones. As such, short scenes, often characterized by powerful emotions, can effectively help illustrate or intensify a particular point. Additionally, the use of short scenes allows a broader use of film in the context of conventional courses without altering traditional class schedules. Scenes can be carefully chosen based on the educator's learning objectives and tailored to the educator's style and personality.

The analysis of a selected scene usually constitutes the central, strategic component of any film-based educational approach.[7,8] Some educators, however, may choose to play an entire movie, advising students to view the film with an eye for reflecting on larger concepts.[9] Quite exceptionally, full-length film has been used solely to provide the audience with an artistic and aesthetic experience that they would otherwise have missed, with no specific intent to afford talking points or to illustrate ethical or clinical dilemmas.[10,11] In contrast, in a manner similar to discussions that follow the reading of a complete short story or novel, the viewing of a film in its entirety provides a group with the opportunity to respond affectively, cognitively, comprehensively, and collectively to the narratives viewed on screen,[12] resulting, at times, in a deeper understanding of the issues being portrayed.

This book aims to supplement core texts and other readings in medical ethics. A large number of scenes, therefore, have been selected based on their value to illustrate ethical dilemmas or motivate discussions. Films were selected on the basis of their power for evocative, visually based, cinematic imagination, and a particular author's desire or experience using that film in a teaching setting. We preferred using easily accessible feature films rather than documentaries or animated films produced specifically as teaching tools with explicit didactic foci. In addition, often times, in popular, as well as in lesser known or even commercially unsuccessful films, authors may actually address what the viewer might first think is a side issue of the film itself but discover to be an important component of the overall narrative.

Our goal throughout this book was to harness the powerfully seductive, emotional, and attention-driving intensity of film to provide educators, and any viewer interested in health care professions and ethics, with a collection of films that illustrate some of the more common issues appearing in medical practice and under discussion in ethics courses. Sometimes, the entire context of a film is relevant to one's interpretation of the scene. Other times, the scene has an intrinsic value that is quite independent from the rest of the film. While we provide time sequences for scenes in order to facilitate their retrieval and bookmarking on modern DVD formats, they will not always be absolutely accurate depending on the DVD and DVD player being used. We leave to the discretion of the viewer how much or how little of each scene needs to be shown in order to succinctly comment on the ethics issue they wish to address.

As a springboard for discussion, a short essay accompanies each selected scene. These essays stress many of the more relevant theoretical and practical issues pertaining to the situation or dilemma illustrated in the scene. They are not intended to replace the rich existing literature about ethics theory; nor do we presume that the scene can be used only to address that particular teaching point. We did our best to assure that both the scene and the essay are engaging, and that the information provided will help viewers enhance their knowledge and understanding of ethics, as well as link ethical principles, theories, and abstract concepts to the concrete situations illustrated in the film. Our goal was to provide both professionals and a general readership with a collection of precise, accessible examples of how film can be applied to help illustrate, learn, and teach medical ethics. Chapters are constructed so that the reader can choose a film or an ethics issue. While educators can use the essays to help stimulate classroom discussions about a film or a medical ethics issue, interested readers can easily move from essay to essay based on their intellectual curiosity. Material from this book can be thus accessed by a general readership interested in the use and understanding of film, as well as for illustrating various aspects of situational ethics in hospitals and universities, and for lectures or classroom teaching of humanities in medicine, film and cinematography, clinical medicine, philosophy, psychology, and ethics.

This anthology of essays encompasses a broad range of relationships between medical practice, health care and social policy, professionalism, illness, medical ethics, and film. The abundance of topics and possible perspectives, therefore, warranted that this book bring together an eclectic group of internationally recognized scholars and practitioners from diverse disciplines including medical ethics, clinical medicine, philosophy, psychology, media and communication studies, medical humanities, public health, business, theology, law, cultural studies, political science, women's studies, English, psychology, and health care education. Each author has experience using film in his or her teaching of medical ethics or other course materials. Each essay in *The Picture of Health: Medical Ethics and the Movies* is based on a scene extracted from a specific film in order to define, illustrate, and discuss a specific medical ethics issue. While each essay contains enough material to make it valuable as a resource and guide, essays are not so technically overloaded as to overwhelm readers, either in how they utilize film, or in the intellectualization of medical ethics. Although we provided creative license to authors in regards to the manner with which they presented their perspectives, we maintained a similar structure so that readers may easily understand the issues being addressed in their clinical, philosophical, scientific, and cinematographic context.

The book is divided into three parts. Part I includes a series of personal reflections whereby authors discuss specifically how they have incorporated film into their respective teaching careers. In the first essay, renowned ethicist and philosopher Al Jonsen reflects on how *Frankenstein* gave rise to medical ethics. In the second essay, medical ethicist and physician Peter Dans reflects on more than 40 years teaching ethics in the hospital and classroom setting. Johanna Shapiro, professor of humanities addresses the educational use of film in the third essay, while in the fourth, Professors Stephen Crawford and Henri Colt reflect on how a scene from *City of Angels* (1998) prompted exploration of "the dark room of their souls" while they address guilt, compassion, and the power of forgiveness in the health care professions.

The second part of this book is the longest, containing 80 essays in eight sections of ten essays, each section categorized according to the type of ethics issue they illustrate: Autonomy, justice, and informed consent; professionalism; communication and provider-patient relationships; health care policy and social responsibility; rights, responsibilities and research; reproduction, genetics, and sexuality; end-of-life and right to die; other ethical issues in medical specialties.

Part III is comprised of a filmography listing the titles of 140 films not used in this volume, but that contain powerful scenes that might be integrated into ethics lectures or training curricula. This list is by no means complete, but provided only to guide readers toward possible additional resources.

With the introduction of any innovative teaching method, some part of the academic community, especially in biological sciences, requests proof of the effectiveness of that new technique before advocating or even supporting its widespread application. Educators, except for the most conservative ones, have long ago learned that the measurement of success in teaching remains an elusive, controversial, and at the least quite ambiguous goal. As stated by Fenstermacher,[13] we should not confuse quality teaching with *successful teaching*, one that produces learning as is understood exclusively in its achievement sense. Quality teaching pertains to *what* is taught and *how* it is taught. Content must be appropriate, proper, and aimed at some worthy purpose. The methods employed must be morally defensible and grounded in shared conceptions of reasonableness.

We submit that acquiring a taste for the aesthetic provides an additional dimension to medical learning, and that even when morality is at issue, reason is an ideal tool for understanding. There is a place in this context for art, including that most powerful medium, film, that mobilizes all of our human resources for action: reason, intuition, instinctive responses, emotion and affectivity, and a need to find and provide answers. Scenes from films can encourage students to see various sides of an ethical dilemma. They contribute to classroom activities by providing an accessible point of reference that personalizes the more arcane philosophical commentaries that often characterize health care ethics debates. By introducing such provocative narrative experiences into the educational setting, the ethics teacher stimulates students to integrate abstract principles with concrete situations, a methodology that encourages students to combine theory and practice into an organic whole.[14] If we add to this a careful selection of insightful readings, and a vivid, professional, interactive, student-centered, and objectives-guided discussion of the contents of a film potentially guided by the essays in this book, we are certain that the enhanced quality of our teaching of ethics will benefit colleagues, students, and other professionals interested in this fascinating field of human behavior and psychology.

In closing, we would like to thank the diligent and always helpful contributors to this volume. Not only have they enlightened us with their knowledge and expertise, but they engendered among us fresh interests and a desire to explore new horizons. They have unselfishly shared their perspectives, trials, and tribulations using film to teach medical ethics to health care professionals, medical students, attorneys, communication and media professionals, and students of humanities studies in both the classroom and the workplace. Reading, and occasionally revising their essays, has been, for the editors, an extraordinarily enriching experience. We trust that it will be so for you as well.

REFERENCES

1. Tong, R. 2002. Teaching bioethics in the new millennium: Holding theories accountable to actual practices and real people. *Journal of Medicine and Philosophy* 27: 417–432.

2. Carroll, N. 1985. The power of movies. *Daedalus* 114: 79–103.

3. Lepicard, E., and Fridman, K. 2003. Medicine, cinema and culture: a workshop in medical humanities for clinical years. *Medical Education* 37: 1039–1040.

4. Wolkenstein, A.S. 2002. Application of movies helpful for teaching. *Family Medicine* 34: 563–564.

5. Alexander, M., Lenahan, P., Pavlov, A. (Eds.). 2005. *Cinemeducation*, p. xiv. London: Radcliffe Publishing.

6. Champoux, J.E. 1999. Film as a teaching resource. *Journal of Management Inquiry* 8(2): 240–251.

7. Blasco, P.G., Moreto, G., Roncoletta, A.F., Levites, M.R., and Janaudis, M.A. 2006. Using movie clips to foster learners' reflection: Improving education in the affective domain. *Family Medicine* 38: 94–96.

8. Alexander, M., Hall, M.N., and Pettice, Y.J. 1994. Cinemeducation: An innovative approach to teaching psychosocial medical care. *Family Medicine* 26: 430–433.

9. Weber, C.M., and Silk, H. 2007. Movies and medicine: An elective using film to reflect on the patient, family, and illness. *Family Medicine* 39: 317–319.

10. Quadrelli, S., Colt, H.G., and Semeniuk, G. 2009. Appreciation of the aesthetic: A new dimension for a Medicine and movies program. *Family Medicine* 41(5): 316–318.

11. Salinsky, J. 2005. Half a day at the movies: film studies in the VTS course. *British Journal of General Practice* 55: 806–809.

12. Sondheimer, A. 2000. The life stories of children and adolescents using commercial films as teaching aids. *Academic Psychiatry* 24: 214–224.

13. Fenstermacher, G., and Richardson, V. 2005. On making determinations of quality teaching. *Teachers College Record* 107(1): 186–213. Retrieved from http://www-personal. umich.edu/~gfenster/teaqual14ss.PDF (p 7).

14. Friedman, L.D. 1995. See me, hear me: Using film in health-care classes. *Journal of Medical Humanities* 16(4): 223–226.

acknowledgments

We heartfully thank Nazanin Zamanian Rohani M.D., for her diligence, patience, hard work, and good humor while assisting us with this work.

caveats

The use of movies and scenes from movies for teaching purposes appears to be protected under the Fair Use Doctrine, as codified in Title 17, Section 107 of the U.S. Copyright Code. This allows for copywritten material to be used for non-profit educational purposes. Readers are encouraged to use original DVDs, book-marking selected scenes, for classroom teaching. Any questions regarding possible infringement should be addressed to institutional legal services or local copyright attorneys.

contents

part three
professionalism

part four
communication and provider–patient relationships

part five
health care policy and social responsibility

part six
rights, responsibilities, and research

part nine
other ethical issues in medical specialties

about the editors

Henri Colt, MD, is professor of pulmonary and critical care medicine at the University of California, Irvine. He is an internationally recognized expert and opinion leader in the development and dissemination of novel technologies for lung cancer diagnosis and interventional palliative procedures. During his career, he has lectured widely on ethics and humanities issues in the context of medical practice, social injustice, humanitarian aid, and education, including the use of simulation and role playing. He has held numerous leadership positions in international and national societies, has more than 130 original research publications in various fields, and has authored or coauthored many books, book chapters, review articles, and commentaries. The recipient of several honorary society memberships, as well as national and international awards from Japan, South America, Australia, and the United States, Dr. Colt has a long experience incorporating film and other media into lectures pertaining to pulmonary medicine, cultural diversity, medical ethics, religion, and end-of-life care.

Silvia Quadrelli MD, MEd, PhD, is director of the pulmonary and critical care section of the British Hospital in Buenos Aires, Argentina. She is an internationally recognized authority in the area of humanitarian assistance, and has devoted more than 30 years of her life to the global combat against poverty and injustice. In 2010, Dr. Quadrelli received the prestigious Medal of the Bicentennial from the City of Buenos Aires, as a "woman who has helped shape modern society." In addition to her background in medicine and teaching, she holds degrees in bioethics and university political sciences. She has designed several medicine and movies programs for the University of Buenos Aires, and lectures widely in South America and abroad on medical ethics, philosophy, and medicine.

Lester D. Friedman, PhD, is currently professor and chair of the media and society program at Hobart and William Smith Colleges. Prior to this appointment, he was a member of the medical humanities program in the Feingold School of Medicine (Northwestern University) and the medical humanities and bioethics program at Upstate Medical Center (Syracuse), as well as the radio, TV, and film department at Northwestern University and the art media studies department at Syracuse University. A internationally recognized expert in cinema and medical humanities, with a particular emphasis on health care and media studies, he has authored or coauthored more than 15 books, two screenplays, and numerous peer-reviewed manuscripts. In particular, he is the editor of *Cultural Sutures* (Duke University Press), the first comprehensive book to explore the intimate connections between the cultures of medicine and media.

contributors

Dan Aalbers, Doctor of Philosophy (ABD). York University, Toronto, Ontario, Canada

Armand H. Matheny Antommaria, **MD, PhD.** Assistant Professor, Division of Pediatric Inpatient Medicine, University of Utah School of Medicine, Salt Lake City, Utah

Robert M. Arnold, MD. Associate Director for Education, Center for Bioethics and Health Law, University of Pittsburgh, Pennsylvania

Cristiane Avancini Alves, PhD in Legal Science. Scuola Superiore Sant'Anna, Pisa, Italy

Paul D. Banick, MD, PhD, MBA, FACP, FCCP. Clinical Adjunct Professor, DeBusk College of Osteopathic Medicine, Lincoln Memorial University, Harrogate, Tennessee

John D. Banja, PhD. Professor, Department of Rehabilitation Medicine, Medical Ethicist, Center for Ethics, Emory University, Atlanta, Georgia

Jennifer S. Bard, JD, MPH. Professor, Alvin R. Allison Professor of Law and Director, Health Law Program, Texas Tech University School of Law, Lubbock, Texas

Donald A. Barr, PhD. Associate Professor (Teaching), Department of Pediatrics, Stanford University School of Medicine, Stanford, California

Jay M. Baruch, MD. Assistant Professor, Department of Emergency Medicine, Warren Alpert School of Medicine at Brown University, Providence, Rhode Island

Catherine Belling, PhD. Assistant Professor, Medical Humanities and Bioethics Program, Feinberg School of Medicine, Northwestern University, Chicago, Illinois

Nancy Berlinger, PhD. Deputy Director and Research Associate, The Hastings Center, Garrison, New York

Marina Boykova, MSc, RN. University of Oklahoma, College of Nursing, Oklahoma City, Oklahoma

Sherry L. Braheny, MD. Neurologist, Past Member of the California Medical Association, Council on Ethical Affairs, Grossmont Hospital, La Mesa, California

Alister Browne, PhD. Clinical Professor and Ethics Theme Director, Faculty of Medicine, University of British Columbia, Vancouver, Canada

Alexander M. Capron, LLD. University Professor, Scott H. Bice Chair in Healthcare Law, Policy and Ethics, Professor of Law and Medicine, Co-Director, Pacific Center for Health Policy and Ethics, University of Southern California, Los Angeles, California

Gretchen A. Case, PhD. Lecturing Fellow, Thompson Writing Program, Duke University, Durham, North Carolina, Adjunct Lecturer, Medical Humanities & Bioethics Program, Feinberg School of Medicine, Northwestern University, Chicago, Illinois

Lynette Cederquist, MD. Clinical Professor of, Internal Medicine, University of California, San Diego, California

René Claxton, MD. Clinical Instructor, University of Pittsburgh School of Medicine, Pittsburgh, Pennsylvania

Diana Cohen Agrest, PhD. Associate Professor of Modern Philosophy, School of Philosophy, University of Buenos Aires, Buenos Aires, Argentina

Felicia Cohn, PhD. Director of Medical Ethics, Department of Medicine, University of California Irvine, Orange, California

Henri G. Colt, MD. Professor of Medicine, Division of Pulmonary and Critical Care Medicine, University of California Irvine, Orange, California

Stephen Crawford, MD. Medical Senior Director, Cigna Health Care

Michael D. Dahnke, PhD. Assistant Teaching Professor, Health Sciences and Health Administration Department, College of Nursing & Health Professions, Drexel University, Philadelphia, Pennsylvania

Peter E. Dans, MD. Associate Professor of Medicine, Johns Hopkins University, School of Medicine, Baltimore, Maryland

Mohsen Davoudi, MD. Assistant Professor, Division of Pulmonary and Critical Care Medicine, University of California Irvine, Orange, California

Richard A. Demme, MD. Associate Professor of Medicine and Medical Humanities, Center for Ethics, Humanities, and Palliative Care, University of Rochester Medical Center, Rochester, New York

Arthur R. Derse, MD, JD. Director for Medical and Legal Affairs, Center for the Study of Bioethics, Director, Medical Humanities Program, Professor of Bioethics and Emergency Medicine, Medical College of Wisconsin, Milwaukee, Wisconsin

Douglas S. Diekema, MD, MPH. Professor, Department of Pediatrics, Department of Bioethics and Humanities, University of Washington School of Medicine, Seattle, Washington

Patricia Digilio, PhD. Professor of Philosophy, University of Buenos Aires, Argentina

Annette Dula, EdD. Advisory Board Member and Consultant, Tuskegee University National Center for Bioethics in Research and Health Care And Senior Associate, Womens Studies, University of Colorado, Boulder

Michael Farrell, MD. Assistant Professor of Internal Medicine, Pediatrics, and Population Health-Bioethics, Medical College of Wisconsin, Milwaukee, Wisconsin

Andrew Fenton, PhD. Project Manager, Situating Science Knowledge Cluster University of King's College and Member of the NTE Research Team, Novel Tech Ethics, Dalhousie University, Halifax, Nova Scotia, Canada

Marcia Santana Fernandes, PhD. Professor in Law, Faculty of Medicine–Federal University–UFRGS and Research Fellow, Laboratory of Bioethics and Science Research, Hospital de Clinicas, Porto Alegre, Brazil

David H. Flood, PhD. Professor, Medical Humanities, Medical Ethics, English Literature, Drexel University College of Nursing and Health Professions, Philadelphia, Pennsylvania

Cory Franklin, MD. Director Emeritus, Cook County Hospital, Chicago, Illinois

Lester D. Friedman, PhD. Chair and Professor, Media and Society Program, Hobart and William Smith Colleges, North Bethesda, Maryland

Thomas H. Gallagher, MD. Associate Professor, Departments of Medicine and Medical History and Ethics, University of Washington, Seattle, Washington

Christine Grady, RN, PhD, FAAN. Tenured Investigator, Department of Bioethics, National Institutes of Health Clinical Center, Bethesda, Maryland

Maren Grainger-Monsen, MD. Director, Program in Bioethics and Film, Stanford University Center for Biomedical Ethics, Palo Alto, California

James W. Green, PhD. Emeritus & Retired Faculty, Department of Anthropology, University of Washington, Seattle, Washington

Michael J. Green, MD, MS, FACP. Professor, Department of Humanities and Medicine, Penn State College of Medicine, Hershey, Pennsylvania

Joshua Hauser, MD. Assistant Professor, Buehler Center on Aging, Health and Society, Department of Medicine, Feinberg School of Medicine, Northwestern University, Chicago, Illinois

Jennifer Hawkins, PhD. Trent Scholar in Bioethics and Associate Research Professor in Philosophy, Duke University, Durham, North Carolina

April M. Herndon, PhD. Assistant Professor, English and Women's and Gender Studies, Winona State University, Winona, Minnesota

Edmund G. Howe, MD, JD. Professor of Psychiatry, Director, Programs in Ethics at Uniformed Services, University of the Health Sciences, Bethesda, Maryland

Jay A. Jacobson, MD, MACP. Emeritus, Professor of Internal Medicine, Infectious Disease and Medical Ethics, University of Utah School of Medicine, Salt Lake City, Utah

Bruce Jennings, MA. Director, Center for Humans and Nature, New York, New York

Anne H. Jones, PhD. Harris L. Kempner Chair in the Humanities in Medicine, Professor and Graduate Program Director, Institute for the Medical Humanities, The University of Texas Medical Branch, Galveston, Texas

Therese Jones, PhD. Director, Arts and Humanities in Healthcare Program, Center for Bioethics and Humanities, University of Colorado, Denver, Colorado

Albert R. Jonsen, PhD. Professor Emeritus, Department of Medical History and Ethics, School of Medicine, University of Washington, Seattle, Washington, Senior Ethics Scholar in Residence, California Pacific Medical Center, San Francisco, California

Timothy Krahn, BA (Hons). Research Associate, Novel Tech Ethics, Department of Bioethics, Faculty of Medicine, Dalhousie University, Halifax, Nova Scotia, Canada

Nicholas M. Lampros, BA. Creative Writing, University of California, Los Angeles, California

Stephen R. Latham, PhD, JD. Senior Lecturer in Political Science, Deputy Director, Bioethics Center, Yale University, New Haven, Connecticut

Solomon Liao, MD. Associate Professor, Department of Medicine, University of California Irvine, Orange, California

Sarah R. Lieber, BA. Pre-Doctoral Fellow, Department of Bioethics, National Institutes of Health, Bethesda, Maryland

David J. Loren, MD. Assistant Professor, Department of Pediatrics, University of Washington, Seattle, Washington

Carl Lundstrom, MD. Consultant, Division of General Internal Medicine, Department of Medicine, Mayo Clinic, Rochester, Minnesota

Robert C. Macauley, MD. Clinical Associate Professor, Department of Pediatrics, University of Vermont College of Medicine, Burlington, Vermont

Ignacio Maglio, PhD. Attorney at Law, University of Buenos Aires, Director, Legal Medical Risk Section, Hospital Fco. Javier Muñiz, Buenos Aires, Argentina

Irene Martinez, MD. Clinical Medical Ethics Fellow at MacLean Center at University of Chicago, Attending Physician, Internal Medicine, Primary Care, John Stroger Jr. Cook County Hospital, Chicago, Illinois

Marianne Matzo, PhD, GNP-BC, FAAN. Professor and Frances E. and A. Earl Ziegler Chair in Palliative Care Nursing, Sooner Palliative Care Institute, University of Oklahoma College of Nursing, Adjunct Professor, Department of Geriatric Medicine, Oklahoma City, Oklahoma

Thomas Wm. Mayo, JD. Director, Cary M. Maguire Center for Ethics and Public Responsibility & Associate Professor, Dedman School of Law, Southern Methodist University, Dallas, Texas

Keith G. Meador, MD, ThM, MPH. Professor of Psychiatry and Behavioral ciences, Center for Spirituality, Theology and Health, Duke University Medical Center, Durham, North Carolina

Lawrence Mohr, MD. Professor of Medicine, Environmental Biosciences Program, Medical University of South Carolina, Charleston, South Carolina

Letícia Ludwig Möller, LLM. Researcher at Bioethics Research Laboratory, Hospital de Clínicas de Porto Alegre, Brazil

Kristen R. Monroe, PhD. Professor of Political Science and Philosophy, Director of the UCI Interdisciplinary Center for the Scientific Study of Ethics and Morality University of California, Irvine, Orange, California

Stephen Murphy-Shigematsu, EdD. Center for Comparative Studies in Race and Ethnicity, Stanford University, Stanford, California

Deirdre Neilen, PhD. Associate Professor of Bioethics and Humanities, Center for Bioethics and Humanities, SUNY/Upstate Medical University, Syracuse, New York

Lawrence J. Nelson, PhD, JD. Senior Lecturer, Department of Philosophy, Santa Clara University, Santa Clara, California

Lois L. Nixon, PhD, MPH. Professor, Division of Ethics and Medical Humanities, Internal Medicine, College of Medicine, University of South Florida, Tampa, Florida

Bradley Olson, PhD. Assistant Research Professor, Foley Center for the Study of Lives, Human Development and Social Policy, Northwestern University, Evanston, Illinois

Kirsten Ostherr, PhD. Associate Professor of English, English Department, Rice University, Houston, Texas

Kayhan P. Parsi, JD, PhD. Associate Professor, Neiswanger Institute for Bioethics and Health Policy, Loyola University Chicago Stritch School of Medicine, Maywood, Illinois

Maria Luisa Pfeiffer, PhD. Doctor of Philosophy, Lecturer at the Faculty of Medicine of the University of Buenos Aires, Researcher, National Research Council (CONICET) of Argentina

Mark S. Pian, MD. Clinical Professor, Department of Pediatrics, University of California / Rady Children's Hospital, San Diego, California

Silvia Quadrelli, MD, PhD, MEd. Assistant Professor in Internal Medicine, University of Buenos Aires, Buenos Aires, Argentina

Elizabeth Reis, PhD. Associate Professor, Women's and Gender Studies Department, University of Oregon, Eugene, Oregon

Annette Rid, MD. Post-doctoral Fellow, Department of Bioethics, NIH Clinical Center, Bethesda, Maryland, Assistant Professor, Institute of Biomedical Ethics, University of Zurich, Switzerland

Jeffrey M. Ring, PhD. Director of Behavioral Sciences, Family Medicine Residency Program, White Memorial Medical Center, Los Angeles, California

David I. Rosenthal, MD. Medical Program Manager, Brigham & Women's Hospital, Harvard Medical School, Boston, Massachusetts

Alan Roth, MS, MBA, FAARC, FAAMA. Director, Respiratory Care and Rehabilitation Services, Memorial Medical Center, Modesto, California

Sadath A. Sayeed, MD, JD. Instructor, Division of Medical Ethics, Department of Global Health and Social Medicine, Harvard Medical School, Boston, Massachusetts

Carol Schilling, PhD. Visiting Scholar, Center for Bioethics, University of Pennsylvania, Philadelphia, Pennsylvania

Toby L. Schonfeld, PhD. Director, Center for Humanities, Ethics and Society, Associate Professor and Vice-Chair, Health Promotion, Social and Behavioral Health, College of Public Health, University of Nebraska Medical Center, Omaha, Nebraska

Judith Kennedy Schwarz, PhD, RN. Clinical Coordinator, Compassion & Choices of New York, New York, New York

Seema K. Shah, JD. Bioethicist, Clinical Center Department of Bioethics & Division of AIDS, National Institutes of Health, Bethesda, Maryland

Johanna Shapiro, PhD. Professor, Department of Family Medicine, Director, Program in Medical Humanities and Arts, University of California, School of Medicine, Irvine, Orange, California

Jerome Singh, PhD. Adjunct Professor, Program on Ethics and Commercialization, McLaughlin-Rotman Centre for Global Health, University of Toronto, Ontario, Canada

Rhonda L. Soricelli, MBBS (Sydney). Adjunct Assistant Professor, Department of Family, Community and Preventive Medicine, Drexel University College of Medicine, Philadelphia, Pennsylvania

Karma Lekshe Tsomo, PhD. Associate Professor, Department of Theology & Religious Studies, University of San Diego, California

Joseph Turow, PhD. Robert Lewis Shayon Professor of Communication, Annenberg School for Communication, University of Pennsylvania, Philadelphia, Pennsylvania

Delese Wear, PhD. Professor of Behavioral and Community Health Sciences, Northeastern Ohio Universities College of Medicine, Rootstown, Ohio

Alan Wertheimer, PhD. Professor Emeritus of Political Science, University of Vermont, Senior Research Scholar, Department of Bioethics, Clinical Center, National Institutes of Health, Bethesda, Maryland

September Williams, MD. Senior Physician Specialist (Geriatrics, Palliative Care, Bioethics), Laguna, Honda Hospital, San Francisco Department of Public Health, San Francisco, California, Writer-Director Ninth Month Productions, Mill Valley, California

Rebecca E. Wolitz, BA. Bioethics Fellow, National Institutes of Health, Department of Bioethics, Bethesda, Maryland

Nazanin Z. Rohani, MD. Research Associate, Department of Pulmonary and Critical Care, University of California Irvine, Orange, California

part one

personal reflections about film and ethics

frankenstein and the birth
of medical ethics

albert r. jonsen

BIOETHICS BEGAN AT THE MOVIES. To be less dogmatic, a movie inspired one of my first bioethics classes for medical students. I joined the faculty of the Medical School, University of California, San Francisco in 1972, as professor of bioethics, one of only a few such professors in American medical schools. Until that time, I had been teaching philosophy to college students and had no experience in medical education. I quickly learned that the airy abstractions of philosophical ethics floated far over the heads of medical students concerned with bodies and diseases, not theories and conjectures. I had to find a new mode of communication.

To learn a bit more about medicine and its culture, I sat in classes with students. These classes were filled with data; the professors were devoted to summarizing it and, on rare occasions, pointing it toward some future encounter with sick persons. Above all, the classrooms were darkened, illuminated only by slides that, one after another, showed charts or cells. Aha, I thought, if I could only put bioethics on slides it might appear to be a viable topic for medical education.

Bioethics then had no data, no numbers, and no charts. I recoiled from merely marking up slides with the words I was uttering. Then, a happy coincidence solved my problem. I saw director James Whale's classic 1931 film, *Frankenstein,* on television and, a few days later, found a paperback book that contained still photos of the entire film. Starring Boris Karloff as the monster and Colin Clive as the mad doctor, *Frankenstein* is a treasure trove of bioethical images. I bought the book and had slides made of most of its episodes—the oddest slides ever produced in the medical school's Classroom Aids department. Thereafter, the Creature, Dr. Frankenstein, and his assistant Fritz introduced my medical students to the problems of medical ethics.

Informed consent, the determination of death, life support, the ethics of research, and transplantation—usual topics of those early bioethics courses—were dramatized by the creature appearing at Dr. Frankenstein's clinic with a pleading look and begging for help, by Dr. Frankenstein lopping off and sewing together pieces of the cadavers he had filched from the local cemetery, by Fritz stealing from a research lab a pickled brain marked "Dysfunctional," and, best of all, by the triumphant moment when Dr. Frankenstein focuses lightning onto his stitched creature and bringing it to life. Much to my delight, I realized that there was hardly a bioethics issue that could not be illustrated by some scene from that wonderful film. In fact, Mary Shelley's novel of Dr. Victor Frankenstein (written in 1816) was an astute commentary on the collision between the human and the scientific world and, as such, provided an accessible pathway to understand why bioethics was coming into being as a field of study.

In the late 1960s, a few insightful persons who understood that the scientific and medical advances that marked the first half of the 20th century also contained moral dilemmas created the bioethics field. Those medical innovations and scientific advances that revolutionized the treatment of disease tapped into "secrets" of physiology and psychology that showed how to "remake" humans. They opened the mysteries of reproduction and heredity, and made it possible to "make babies" outside of the body and according to design. These possibilities bestowed creative powers on scientists and, with them, the capacity to do both good and evil. Such power recalls the tale of Frankenstein, the genius scientist who imparted existence to a lifeless bundle of parts collected from cadavers. Because Frankenstein did not know how to deal with his marvelous creature, it became a monster, dangerous to all humans and to itself.

Indeed, the name itself became an easily recognizable phrase for the dangers of medical research delving into realms beyond its control. Popular writers from the 1960s onward often referred to scientific accomplishments as "Frankensteinian." In the early days of organ transplantation, commentators sometimes compared surgeons to the mad scientist and patients to the poor patched creature. In the early days of molecular genetics, Frankenstein lurked in the laboratories. A politician opposed Harvard's plan to build a genetics laboratory with the alarm, "Frankenstein's monsters will crawl out of the sewers of Cambridge." Opponents of genetically engineered crops call them "Frankenfoods," and genetically engineered organisms are named "Frankenbugs."

This literary reference is extravagant but pointed. The Frankenstein story is a fable about modern scientific power. Dr. Frankenstein imparts life to a body he has pieced together from parts snipped from cadavers. He has discovered the "secret of life," and he makes dead matter alive. He also gives that living being a physical form (he intended it to be beautiful, but his hasty surgery created something ugly) and a psychological character (he intended it to be benign but, by his own mistreatment of it, it turned malign). He created it with the best of intentions—to solve the mystery of disease and death—but his good intentions went lethally wrong. Many commentators have found this riveting novel to be emblematic of modern science: it too has powers to create life, to sustain it, to shape its qualities. At the same time, it has not conquered death, and its mastery of nature is fallible. And it can go horribly bad. The bioethical questions acknowledge these powers and their limits and, above all, interrogate the responsibility of decisions that accompany the power of creation. At the root of bioethical probing lies an even more fundamental question: What is it to be alive or more particularly, to be alive as a human being, a person? What are the moral duties and constraints that confront us as we enhance the powers over who lives, who dies?

Mary Shelley wrote the Frankenstein narrative in an era when science was on the verge of the world that makes bioethics necessary. In the early 18th century, brilliant minds examined the mysterious workings of the human body with new interest and ingenuity. Chemistry, which for a century had dissolved minerals and fluids, began to turn to the composition of the human organism. Oxygen became a topic of avid study. In the early 19th century, the subject of "animal chemistry" encouraged scientists to study the processes of digestion and describe components even as we still do, into "oleaginous foods" (fats), "saccharinous foods" (carbohydrates), and "albuminous foods" (proteins). The field of physiological chemistry was born and, for the rest of the 19th century, unraveled the ways life originated and is sustained by respiration, nutrition, and elimination. The cellular theory and the germ theory revolutionized the understanding of disease. The structure of tissues and the hitherto hidden marvels of reproduction were observed through the microscope.

Also at the end of the 18th century, physics, which had lived in the glory of Newton's laws of motion and theory of gravity, began to investigate the physics of life. Electricity seemed to link nonliving and living matter. In 1792, Italian anatomist Luigi Galvani (or rather his wife) noted that the muscles of severed frog legs contracted and twitched when stimulated with an electric shock. "Galvanism" was coined to describe the power of electromagnetic force (imagined as a sort of fluid) to animate organic matter. In the same year, Alessandro Volta had published studies on the electrical stimulation of muscles, and several years later invented the battery to generate electrical power.

While chemists and physicists worked in their laboratories, a literary party vacationed at a lake near Geneva, Switzerland. Two of England's most famous poets, George Gordon Lord Byron and Percy Bysshe Shelley, rented adjoining villas. With Shelley was his lover and later wife, Mary, the 19-year-old daughter of philosopher William Godwin and feminist writer Mary Wollstonecraft (who died giving birth to her). Together, these literary neighbors passed balmy days sailing and stormy evenings telling ghost stories. On the evening of June 15, 1816, Byron, Shelley, and another guest, Dr. John Polidori (who later, in 1819 wrote the first vampire story in English) discussed "the principle of life." In the language of the time, "principle" meant origin, source, first cause. For example, John Hunter, a great English physician of the time, considered blood the "life-principle," distinguishing living from nonliving. Shelley and Polidori were both interested in scientific investigation and were familiar with the work of the esteemed scientist and physician, Dr. Erasmus Darwin (Charles Darwin's grandfather) who had investigated galvanism. During that evening conversation, the poets speculated that, "perhaps a corpse would be reanimated; galvanism had given token of such things; perhaps the component parts of a creature might be manufactured, brought together, and endued with vital warmth." Mary, "a devout but nearly silent listener" to that fascinating conversation, recorded those words. She could not sleep that night but saw "with acute mental vision" the shaping of a story. During that sleepless night, her imagination gave birth to her novel *Frankenstein*, the first text for bioethics.[1]

The story is well known. While still at university, Victor Frankenstein, a brilliant student of chemistry and physiology, becomes entranced by the idea of creating a living creature by means of galvanism. His motives are noble: "wealth was an inferior object; but what glory would attend the discovery if I could banish disease from the human frame and render man invulnerable to any but a violent death." His intense studies finally shed on his mind "a light so brilliant and wondrous... the astonishing secret... the cause of generation and life, nay more, I became myself capable of bestowing animation upon lifeless matter." He decides to compose a creature "like himself... and give life to an animal as complex and wonderful as man." He collects, gathers, and composes all the needed parts from cadavers, then jolts the stitched amalgam with an electric shock from a "powerful machine." The composite cadaver comes to life. Frankenstein, however, is horrified by his creation's hideousness and cruelly repudiates it. The "Monster" or "Wretch," as Frankenstein calls it, desperately seeks to understand how he came into being and to express his feelings in language. He yearns for acceptance by humans. He masters language but wanders alone, an outcast never welcomed into the human community. Rejection turns his originally compassionate nature to bitterness and then to violence. He tells Frankenstein, "I was benevolent and good; misery made me a fiend. Make me happy and I shall again be virtuous." His creator cannot make him happy and, in the end, the Monster, now called the Fiend, kills its creator—and everyone he loves. The 1931 film vividly, though rather inaccurately, visualized the novel and remains a staple of late-night movies.

Mary Shelley's novel was more than a chilling ghost story. It was a moralizing tale subtitled "The Modern Prometheus." Her readers, familiar with classic legend and literature, would have immediately understood this classical allusion: Prometheus was a rebel Titan who stole fire from the gods and brought it to mankind, a theft for which he was grievously punished by being bound to a rock while great eagles feasted daily on his liver only to have it grow back the next day to be eaten again. However, the classically trained reader would also recall Prometheus Plasticator, Prometheus the Maker, who shaped the human form from clay, readying it to receive heavenly fire, as the cause of its life and thought. Ancient literature portrays this artist as less than competent and relates the many human ills that result from his imperfect construction.

Victor Frankenstein, a modern Prometheus, hoped to create a beautiful being of great power and ingenuity but failed not in his vision but his execution of it. The Monster blames his creator for his unhappiness and for his crimes. Mary Shelley wrote a warning for those who would carry their science into the mysteries of the creation of life. To affirm that this fantastic story was not mere imagination, her husband, Percy, opened the preface that he composed for the first edition with the words, "The event on which this fiction is founded, has been supposed, by Dr. Darwin, and some of the physiological writers of German, as not of impossible occurrence." This was a moral tale about science and its future achievements.

I said that *Frankenstein* could be considered the first text of bioethics. That rather melodramatic claim needs some clarification. First, I do not mean that modern medicine and biological science is a horror story, telling how scientists create, willy-nilly, monsters rather than miracles. Bioethics is not a rounding condemnation of medical science (though some would make it so). It is not even a detective story, trying to find evil machinations behind each miracle. For, while science can go wrong, and medicine can harm instead of heal, the general direction has been toward human benefit. Only a kind of moralistic paranoia wants to suspect evil in every good.

Still, the story of Victor Frankenstein contains some of the essential elements of modern bioethics. First, it is a story about life, making alive and reviving life. The "bio" in bioethics means "life." The word "life" is itself ambiguous. It can mean the course of a person's history from birth to death. Its major moments can be listed in a "bio," or picturesquely or poignantly described in a biography. It can also mean the processes that sustain organic life, the complex activities of cells, programmed by genes, in interaction with a nourishing environment. All of the "bio" sciences; biology, biochemistry, and biophysics, study facets of these processes.

The fictional Victor Frankenstein immersed himself in these studies (in their very immature forms) and burns to bring them from theory to practice. By creating life in a cadaver, he has found "the principle of life." He wants to "banish disease from the human frame." His scientific quest has a healing goal; it is meant to provide ultimate success to the medical task that is, in Hippocrates' words, "to alleviate pain and lessen the violence of disease" (*The Art, iii*). Medicine deals with life in the biological sense and equally with life in the biographical sense. Physicians manipulate biological process, so that the life-course of an individual can progress without pain or disability. They must know the biography of their patients, as well as the biology. In dealing with the patient as a person, physicians must observe standards of behavior that we call "ethics," the other half of the word bioethics. Even more, the power of science must be ethically employed as it is brought into contact with human life. So, the Frankenstein story, in which a scientist revives a living being and then must decide how to behave in relation to it, is an anticipation of bioethics.

The practitioners of modern bioscience have yet to restore life after death has truly taken place. However, they can initiate life, imitating sexual reproduction in a laboratory dish, and can sustain life as a merely organic process long after personal life has disappeared. They cannot yet compose a complete human being out of exhumed organs and impart life to it. However, they can lift organs from a cadaver and implant them in a person whose own organs have failed. These men and women of medicine can substitute mechanical devices for organic parts and functions. Whenever they perform one of these actions, they encounter the standards of behavior we call ethics because the action is performed, not in a chemical preparation or physical device, but with a human person. The work of bioethics is to examine the points at which the biosciences touch human life, in individuals and in societies. The purpose of the examination is to discern how the science and its products can bring benefits with as little harm as possible. Bioethics seeks to form a picture of human persons and human society that can guide the vision and intentions of scientists.

Bioethics, however, is much more than a picture or a vision of an ideal world in which scientific discoveries and human dignity are in harmony. It is a field of practical ethics concerned with particular problems and cases of moral perplexity. *Frankenstein*, the film, contains many such moments of moral perplexity about how humans should treat the creature. The film does not linger on these perplexities, but sweeps to its dramatic ending. In real life, where scientific medicine meets the needs of particular patients, moral perplexities do—or should—bring a pause for reflection. The real moral case is a convergence of elements: the unique medical situation and possible medical responses; the desires, preferences, and choices of a particular patient; the judgments made about the worth and dignity of life, and particular life conditions and styles; the context of financial costs, laws, institutional constraints, and public welfare. All these converge into a case.

Bioethics has evolved as a form of moral philosophy that attempts to analyze these cases of moral perplexity and to render advice about how best to proceed, in the light of our understanding of moral principles. This form of bioethics is sometimes called *clinical ethics* to distinguish it from the broader vision of a humane medicine. Clinical ethics draws, consciously or unconsciously, on an ancient form of moral analysis called *casuistry*. Casuistry sorts out different kinds of moral dilemmas, governed by distinct moral values and principles.[2] It then attempts to fill out these general forms of moral dilemmas with the circumstances of the real case under consideration. It compares this case with other similar cases and with proposed solutions. This process has as its goal a decision about how to manage the medical case in a way that best meets standards of moral rightness, and also respects the very unique circumstances of real life.

Mary Shelley bestowed on Victor Frankenstein the title "The Modern Prometheus" because he sought to do what the legendary Titan did, namely, make a human being. The modern biosciences all conspire toward the same goal. The modern making of humans consists in the correction of the physical and mental faults and failures that bring disease and death. Making is an activity in which the mind forms an image of something that will come into being as the hands manipulate material to meet that image. Human purposes and motives guide the making and decide what is to be done with the product. Human purposes, however, are not only overarching goals filling a wide vision, but also many particular choices made at various juncture of human experience. These particular choices are the common, daily matter of our moral lives; the broad vision may be present, but it is often vague and unarticulated. Bioethics needs both. It must attempt to articulate the meaning, value, and dignity of human life, and it must respond to questions such as "under what conditions should this human life be saved?" The first task is a grand philosophical question; the latter task is casuistry. The Frankenstein story and the movies made from it point in both directions. It can be rightly honored as a beginning for bioethics.

REFERENCES

1. Shelley, M.W. *Frankenstein*, pp. 8, 39–40, 51, 97, 11, 40. London: Penguin Books, 1992.
2. Jonsen, A., and Toulmin, S. *The abuse of casuistry. A history of moral reasoning.* Berkeley and Los Angeles: University of California Press, 1987.

a personal journey using film to teach medical ethics

peter e. dans[i]

ROWING UP IN A COLD-WATER flat on Manhattan's Lower East Side, movies were a ticket out of the neighborhood and into other worlds.[1,2] As such, I was happy to find a way to incorporate them into my professional life. I first ventured into using films for teaching at the University of Colorado, during the 1970s, in the dark days before video recorders. Later, I used film while directing the required first year ethics and medical care course at Johns Hopkins University School of Medicine. A significant consideration in teaching medical ethics in a secular environment is that the students come from heterogeneous backgrounds and have diverse beliefs about both secular and spiritual issues. When they enter the classroom, they are strangers to one another and to their teachers. We were able to conduct a detailed, anonymous survey of incoming students at each yearly orientation from 1984 to 1990, however, in order to learn about their experiences in medical care, their understanding of ethics, their attitudes toward ethical issues, and the norms they used in making moral judgments.[3,4] We thus learned about their varying beliefs regarding contentious issues: whether life began at conception, birth, or somewhere in between; if they had cheated in college, high school, and elementary school; and when, if ever, was lying permissible.

The survey also served to help students understand that this course would not simply be a series of bull sessions or a rest-and-recreation period from "real" courses like anatomy and biochemistry. Rather, it was intended to foster their understanding that the discipline they were about to study, normative ethics, was as important to their personal and professional lives as the so-called "hard" sciences.

Normative ethics is that branch of moral philosophy that systematically and formally examines the rightness and wrongness of actions using general principles (e.g., autonomy and beneficence), theories (e.g., utilitarianism and deontology), standards (e.g., codes, virtues, and religious precepts), and nonstandardized approaches (e.g., cultural relativism, intuition, and secular humanism). Collating student responses allowed faculty members an infusion of insights, so that we could preview potential areas of discordance and concordance before students wrestled with contentious subjects in small discussion groups. We could also gauge the differing sophistication of class members depending on their background in philosophy and medicine, as well as their pluralism with regard to the norms used to resolve dilemmas.

The course was taught in three-hour sessions twice a week for nine weeks. Like many courses in moral judgment, topics consisted of what might be called mega-ethics, featuring true dilemmas in which opposing views cannot be easily reconciled, and in which the use of differing norms to resolve dilemmas often leads to disparate outcomes. For example, we studied abortion, a topic that had been excluded from the curriculum by the previous course director because it was considered to be too emotionally charged to be discussed with equanimity, especially in such a pluralistic setting. The session began by debating issues such as a woman's right to privacy over her body, where a fetus becomes a person on the continuum from conception to birth, whether it has rights and, if it does, when and to what degree they are commensurate with those of the mother. We insisted that all students participate in the lectures and discussion groups because, as caregivers, they would not be able to opt out of contentious issues when facing their patients.

The students' beliefs about personhood and attitudes toward abortion were thus displayed.[3] The concept of negative and positive rights, especially with regard to payment for abortion, was addressed.[5] Students were then shown the Public Broadcasting System film *Abortion Clinic*,[6] from the Emmy award–winning *Frontline* television program hosted by Jessica Savitch (initially aired on April 18, 1983). To prepare for this remarkably well-balanced program, Savitch had interviewed numerous women at the Reproductive Health and Counseling Center in Chester, Pennsylvania, and focused on two who chose abortion and two who did not. She interviewed doctors and nurses who worked in the clinic, as well as those protesting outside, including a pro-life physician. Students were thus able to put human faces on the women, the protestors, and the clinic personnel.

Heated arguments were avoided by encouraging students to use the technique of "active listening,"[7] which I had found particularly helpful while conducting pediatric oncology rounds, where nurses, social workers, and doctors held strong and sometimes-conflicting opinions about treatment choices. The technique consists of asking speakers, before they voice a forceful and contrary opinion, to restate what the previous speaker said, thus forcing him or her to listen and not simply rehearse their opinion while awaiting their turn to speak. Furthermore, rather than injecting their opinions, faculty moderated these sessions, thus allowing the discussion to flow among the students. The response to the sessions was very positive, with students gaining a better understanding of the arguments on both sides of the issue, while not necessarily changing their own opinions.

In the case of euthanasia, we prefaced the viewing of the film *Dax's Case*[8] by first discussing the distinction between active and passive euthanasia, as well as by discussing related issues of autonomy, competence, beneficence, and sanctity of life. This was followed by the half-hour film *Please Let Me Die*,[9] originally produced for a bioethics seminar at Southern Methodist University by Dr. Robert B. White, a psychiatrist at the University of Texas Medical Branch at Galveston, who had been one of the consulting physicians in Dax's case.

The film recounts how Donald "Dax" Cowart, a handsome Air Force Reserve pilot, was severely burned when his car's ignition set off a raging fire of propane gas that had leaked onto property he and his father were inspecting. He was massively disfigured, left blind and in considerable pain. Students were asked to focus on the various participants in the case and the various decision points. First, there was a farmer who had rescued Dax and had refused to give him a gun to shoot himself. Instead of walking away, which would have assured Dax's death, the farmer called 911, thus engaging the medical care system, beginning with emergency response of an ambulance and medics. Dax's father died in the ambulance, and Dax refused treatment en route; however, once he arrived at the emergency department of the rural hospital, physicians decided to stabilize him and then to refer him to the tertiary care center at Parkland Hospital in Dallas, all the while providing treatment against his wishes.

His mother had just lost her husband and did not want to lose her only son. She and her lawyer insisted that he be treated, even though it involved considerable pain, and they ignored his pleas to be allowed to die. Much of the debate centered on whether and when Dax was considered competent to make decisions about his care. Students discussed other factors affecting the reluctance of the staff to accede to his wish to be allowed to die: his favorable prognosis, the fact that he was not imminently and irreversibly dying, and that complying with his wishes would have meant essentially walking away from him and withholding food, water, and medicines unless direct active euthanasia was performed.

Believing that it was important for students to commit themselves before hearing the rest of the story, we asked them to vote on whether Dax should have been allowed to die, as they would have had to do if they had been in charge of the case. They were then shown a follow-up documentary produced by Keith Burton entitled *Dax's Case,*[10] which consists of interviews with the surviving participants. The students learned that Dax was discharged and, at one point was so adamant about dying that he escaped from his mother's house and made an unsuccessful attempt to reach a nearby road to get run over. Resigned to his fate, he married and pursued a law career devoted to championing patient autonomy.[ii] The students then discussed how what they learned about his subsequent life affected their beliefs as to whether he should have been allowed to die, and when and how that would have been accomplished had they acquiesced.

I also use film to teach "doctoring" from a historical perspective. We don't often have the luxury today of canvassing lecture attendees beforehand and feeding back their attitudes, nor is time allotted to show a complete film. So, except for rare occasions, I use scenes that focus on the portrayal of doctors in films dating from 1931 to the present, ranging from positive in early films to decidedly negative beginning in the 1980s.[2] By focusing on doctors collectively or as particular subsets (e.g., women doctors, medical students, specialists, etc.), these presentations aim at showing what patients value, or by contrast, are concerned about with regard to medical care, as well as medical ethics. It's important, therefore, to know the film well, in order to select the most instructive scenes. By viewing the film on multiple occasions, I am able to see things missed on first viewing and sometimes, even reevaluate a film once liked (*M*A*S*H**) or disliked (*The Interns*). What you get out of a film often depends upon what you bring to it, such as your stage in life, attitudes, and the cultural climate at the time you viewed it.

In large part, films provide snapshots of the conventional wisdom of the day. Filtered through the studio, screenwriter, and director, they illustrate the evolution of societal perceptions of a topic over time. In this way, films represent an intersection of medical ethics and history. For example, I began a presentation on abortion in film[11]—as part of a University of Michigan Medical School elective entitled "Contemporary Issues in Women's Health" (November 2007)—with a scene from *Men in White* (1934), in which a student nurse becomes pregnant, obtains an abortion, and dies of a pulmonary embolus. Tracing the trend line from there, the portrayal of abortion follows the evolution of its societal acceptance: from once being illegal and unethical according to the Hippocratic Oath and the American Medical Association (AMA) Code of Ethics, and considered generally immoral except when the life of the mother was at stake, to the present, where it is both legal and generally considered ethical except in Catholic hospitals, while remaining a highly contentious issue with respect to its morality.

Other films that show this progression include *The Interns* (1962), which also wrestles with the issue of euthanasia, in which an intern (Cliff Robertson) who tries to steal Pitocin to give to his pregnant girl friend (Suzy Parker) in order to induce an abortion is dismissed from the hospital; *Love with a Proper Stranger* (1964), in which the woman (Natalie Wood) walks out on the abortionist and ultimately marries the father (Steve McQueen) of her child; and the original *Alfie* (1966), in which a notorious womanizer (Michael Caine) arranges an abortion for the married woman involved in a one-night stand. In all three films, those performing abortions or wishing to do so are portrayed unsympathetically.

In several later films, however, those performing abortions were portrayed sympathetically and, as in *Cider House Rules* (1999) or *Vera Drake* (2004), in a laudatory manner. In turn, these portrayals have given way to movies in which abortion is rejected. This includes the remake of *Alfie* (2004), in which the woman (Nia Long), instead of having an abortion as in the original, leaves the abortion clinic and decides to have the baby. In *Waitress* (2007), a mother (Keri Russell), who despises her abusive husband, decides to go through with her pregnancy saying, "the child has a right to thrive." In *Knocked Up* (2007), a female television anchor (Katherine Heigl) decides to keep a child resulting from a one-night stand, and improbably marries the creepy father (Seth Rogen). In *Juno* (2007), an unwed adolescent mother (Ellen Page) leaves the abortion clinic and decides to put her child up for adoption. In *Bella* (2006), essentially the same thing occurs.

The reason for this attitude change in Hollywood films may relate to the ubiquity of ultrasound beginning early in pregnancy. In *Knocked Up*, this connection is fairly explicit when the parents see the beating heart at eight weeks and, during subsequent ultrasounds, recognize how early the fetus has a human appearance. From a historical perspective, issues such as personhood, rights of the unborn, whether the wishes of the father play a role in the decision to abort the pregnancy, and what, if any, lasting medical and psychological aftermaths occur after an abortion have come even more to the fore than when we were discussing this issue years ago.

Studying feature films from a historical perspective has also shown the virtual disappearance of references to codes of medical ethics that had been enshrined for over two millennia. If one asks physicians and even patients what comes to mind when they hear the term *medical ethics*, most would respond the Hippocratic Oath (although many might not be able to say what's in it, and its wording often differs from version to version[12]). Other codes, like that of Maimonides and later of Percival,[13] augmented rather than superseded the Oath.[iii] Scenes that feature the Hippocratic Oath are useful in discussing how it came to represent medicine and then how it was modified, beginning with the elimination of the proscription of both abortion and the administration of a deadly draught to the dying, into the many different versions in use today.[iv]

Exploring film from a historical perspective also provides insight into the evolution of the ethics of medical research. A number of older films treat this subject quite seriously. In *Arrowsmith* (1931), two scenes are particularly on point. The first is that showing Arrowsmith recite a researcher's prayer when he is given a laboratory in the McGurk Institute (representing the Rockefeller Institute in New York). The second is when Arrowsmith is shown testing plague vaccine in a randomized trial on a Caribbean island. The importance of a randomized trial in the development of an anthrax vaccine in sheep is shown in *The Story of Louis Pasteur* (1936), and in *Dr. Ehrlich's Magic Bullet* (1940), testing the efficacy of Salvarsan for the treatment of syphilis in humans. When one considers these films, along with the impassioned plea for research shown in *Madame Curie* (1943) and *The Citadel* (1938), one is impressed with how, unlike today, filmmakers did not feel the need to talk down to their audience or dumb down scientific concepts.

Having proposed the advantages of using film to study an ethics issue from a historical perspective, I should also describe some hazards. First, you need to know the composition of your audience. Setting the scene is important in all cases, but becomes most critical when there are marked disparities in a class's knowledge, attitudes, backgrounds, and experience. The second relates to how much time you have and whether you can break students into small groups for discussion and, if not, the possibility of meaningful interaction in the large group setting. While scene selection is easier because of DVDs, Internet sources, books, and screen-plays devoted to particular films, one should probably retain only enough frames to trigger discussion or make a point. By and large, the scenes should probably not exceed five minutes, sequenced on DVDs using menus that allow stopping and starting, as well as skipping around or truncating a presentation, if necessary.

A third consideration, especially if the subject is controversial and highly charged, is to wrap up the session by providing a substantive conclusion that encourages the attendees to continue rational discussions (since the intent is to continue to wrestle with it) rather than heated argumentation. In this respect, one should use caution when showing politically motivated or manipulative films, as well as those filled with falsehoods, unless that's the subject of the lesson. While films by Michael Moore and Oliver Stone represent the extreme in this regard, many films conflate or distort history to sway the audience.[v] In short, in selecting a film, the watchword should be caveat emptor.

I often ask students and residents about ethical dilemmas they encounter in daily practice. The vignettes they describe are rarely true dilemmas in that, after ascertaining more facts and the patient's preferences, the choice is usually clear. However, while not being examples of dilemma ethics, they are what might be called *everyday ethics* because caregivers, who are taught to practice beneficence (to do well by the patient), make many decisions daily, often without all available data and with limited time. Beneficence is manifested when these decisions are accompanied by a kind word, smile, or the simplest of actions to help patients cope with even the most mundane condition. That is why the doctor's character is a patient's most important safeguard.[vi] In *The Fugitive* (1993), one of my all-time favorite films, Harrison Ford plays a doctor who has been falsely convicted of killing his wife. He sets about trying to find the real killer, and although on the run from the law, can't help being a doctor. While posing as a janitor, for example, he is asked by a triage nurse to wheel a young boy with a fractured sternum to the observation area. Realizing the seriousness of the condition, he enters a note in the chart, and delivers the boy to the operating room. A nurse is scolded by a detective for not detaining Ford after realizing what he had done. Tired and wanting to go home after a long night, she can only answer that "He saved the boy's life." That's what the best of beneficence is all about; self-abnegation, denying one's needs and giving priority to another's. Health care professionals do that daily and, yes, they are practicing ethics while doing so.

NOTES

i. Dr. Dans authored the "Physician at the Movies" section of the Alpha Omega Alpha Honor Medical Society's quarterly journal Pharos, and a book on Hollywood's portrayal of doctors in film from Arrowsmith (1931) to Patch Adams (1998).[2]

ii. Despite his apparent successes, Dax still maintains that he should have been allowed to die and that medical professionals violated his rights.

iii. Percival's Code of the Gentleman served as the basis for the AMA Code of Ethics until the 1970s.

iv. Films in which the Oath is prominently featured include *Mary Stevens M.D.* (1933); *Men in White* (1934); *The Girl in White* (1952), the story of real-life physician Emily Dunning Barringer; *The Interns* (1962); and, for the Oath of Maimonides, *The Symphony of Six Million* (1932).

v. One example of such distortion and manipulation is the 1960 film *Inherit the Wind*, which is used in many high schools but whose portrayal of the Scopes Trial and its principals was totally debunked in Edward Larson's Pulitzer Prize winning 1997 book *Summer for the Gods*.[14] To a much lesser degree, the same holds for the 1992 film

Lorenzo's Oil, which painted a distorted picture of the researcher vis a vis the parents with regard to the development and use of an experimental treatment in a child fated to die from adrenoleukodystrophy.[2]

vi. To illustrate this, I have found the following films to be most useful: The Kildare films, including the first one wonderfully titled *Interns Can't Take Money* (1937); *Meet Doctor Christian* (1939); *People Will Talk* (1951); *The Last Angry Man* (1959); and *Awakenings* (1990).

REFERENCES

1. Dans, P.E. 2000. Doctors in the movies: Boil the water and just say aah! Bloomington, IL: Medi-Ed Press.
2. Dans, P.E., Lepkoff, R., and Wasserman, S. 2006. Life on the Lower East Side: Photographs by Rebecca Lepkoff, 1937–1950. New York: Princeton Archival Press.
3. Dans, P.E. 1992. Medical students and abortion: reconciling personal beliefs and professional roles at one medical school. *Academic Medicine* 67: 207–211.
4. Dans, P.E. 1996. Self-reported cheating by students at one medical school. *Academic Medicine* 71(Suppl): S71–72.
5. Segers, M.C. 1980. Political discourse and public policy on funding abortion: an analysis. In J.T. Burchaell (Ed.), *Abortion parley*, pp. 265–297. Kansas City, MO: Andrews and McMeel.
6. "Abortion Clinic." April 18, 1983. Produced by Mark Obenhaus. *Frontline*. WBGH Educational Foundation. This should not to be confused with the 2005 *Frontline* program "The Last Abortion Clinic."
7. Wikipedia.
8. Burton, K. 1989. A chronicle: Dax's case as it happened. In L.D. Kliever (Ed.), *Dax's case: Essays in medical ethics and human meaning*. Dallas: Southern Methodist University Press.
9. *Please Let Me Die*. 1974. Videotape produced by Robert White (see *Dax's Case*).
10. *Dax's Case*. 1985. Videotape produced by Unicorn Media Inc. for Concern for Dying.
11. Dans, P.E. 2008. Abortion in the movies. *Pharos* Spring: 32–34.
12. Crawshaw, R., and Link, C. 1996. Evolution of form and circumstance in medical oaths. *Western Journal of Medicine* 164: 452–456.
13. Pellegrino, E.D. 1986. Percival's medical ethics: The moral philosophy of an 18th-century English gentleman. *Archives of Internal Medicine* 146: 2265–2269.
14. Larson, E.J. 1997. *Summer for the gods*. New York: Basic Books.

movies help us explore relational ethics in health care

johanna shapiro

MANY MEDICAL SCHOLARS HAVE NOTED the potential of movies to address broad philosophical and ethical questions pertinent to the practice of medicine. For example, Baños argues that movies are a better way to teach about the patient–clinician relationship than are didactic presentations.[1] Yamada, Maskarinec, and Greene note that movies provide a forum for helping learners understand that illness has a moral trajectory as well as a medical course; and to help students in medicine, nursing, and related health professions to see themselves as moral actors.[2] Saab et al. point out that a good movie causes learners to ask reflective, introspective, self-critical questions about ethics in the context of relationships and emotion,[3] while Quadrelli, Colt, and Semeniuk demonstrate how it can teach students to resist social injustice.[4] Indeed, movies clearly are a valuable tool to encourage us to puzzle through questions about doing what is right, avoiding cynicism and disillusionment, and maintaining kind and compassionate hearts.[5] Movies facilitate reflection on such philosophical questions as the nature of medicine, sickness and health, life, death, and suffering.[6] Although movies can promulgate important truths about the human condition, they rarely offer entirely accurate factual scenarios. As such, they may persuade students to ponder the possibility that factual information is not the only source of learning[7]; therefore, questions about ethics and meaning, for example, may be more effectively examined through artistic media such as film than through didactic presentations.

Film is especially well positioned to help learners interested in the health professions recognize that caring for patients necessarily embodies principles of relational ethics and intrinsically contains both inherent moral value and incurs inevitable moral responsibility.[8] The theories and practices of relational ethics in health care have been developed primarily in nursing. Since one essay cannot do justice to the entirety of relational ethics as a moral philosophy, I will focus on only a few key themes often addressed in movies featuring serious illness and the patient–clinician relationship: empathetically understanding and respecting the experience and perspective of the suffering other; reflecting on the full range of personal emotions and judgments that emerge in response to the patient's situation; exploring the "proper" professional connection between clinician and patient; and considering how to translate these dimensions into meaningful relationships in "real" clinical situations. These foci reflect the essential elements of relational ethics,[9,10] that interactions with others are the location for ethical action[11] and a source of moral knowing[12]; that emotional engagement is as important as cognitive understanding in developing empathy for the other; and that mutual respect, including acceptance of difference, must anchor all relationships.

Within this essay, I will reference easily accessible American narrative films[i] that quickly capture a viewer's attention and engage him or her emotionally.[13] Such hallmarks focus learners on essential aspects of patients' illness experiences (a submersion in the phenomenological world of the suffering other) and on the core aspects of the patient–clinician encounter. These sanitized, and at times unabashedly romantic conceptualizations can sensitize learners to practicing relational ethics.[15] Specifically, engaging narrative illness movies may ultimately help learners refocus on the supremacy of relational ethics in promoting compassionate and effective health care.

awareness of and empathy for the other: the phenomenology of illness

A deep understanding of the other is fundamental to a relational ethics, especially the suffering (and therefore potentially threatening and disturbing) other.[16] Alexander et al.[17] coined the term *cinemeducation* to encompass the use of movie clips or whole movies as a method of helping educate learners about bio-psycho-social-spiritual aspects of health care. Essentially, cinemeducation assumes that movies provide insight about the phenomenology of illness—what happens to people when they become sick.[18] Movies tend to focus on how illness affects a person's life and relationships, not on the medical details that often become the primary concern of health profession students, thus encouraging an important rebalancing for these learners. This shift in focus helps students learn to situate patients both within their subjective experience of illness and within the relationships affected by this illness.

Movies are not neutral occurrences. Quite the opposite, they present definite points of view (or multiple points of view), according to the filmmaker's agenda. In a way that most other art forms do not, mainstream cinema often insists on a seamless binding together of the character's and spectator's points of view. Watching a film, the audience literally sees through the eyes of the onscreen character.[19] *The Diving Bell and the Butterfly* (2007) provides a striking example of this phenomenon. The protagonist Jean-Dominique Bauby (Mathieu Amalric), who suffered from locked-in syndrome after a massive stroke, is almost inaccessible to most viewers on a physical plane. But because director Julian Schnabel decided to tell parts of his story literally from the inside, through the juxtaposition of what he sees through his one still-functioning eye and in his vivid memories, the viewer experiences him empathetically and three-dimensionally. As in *The Diving Bell and the Butterfly*, illness films almost invariably lead the audience to sympathize with the plight of the patient.[20] In fact, medical educators report such connections when they use films with medical residents.[21,22,ii] Students participating in discussions of films used in medical education routinely pay great attention to the perspectives and viewpoints of others.[6]

Although contemporary films and television dramas often go to great lengths to achieve accuracy, medical content is always in the service of core story lines that are emotional and relational in nature.[23] Even when incorporating a diagnostic curiosity (e.g., *Mask* [1995] and Proteus syndrome; *Lorenzo's Oil* [1992] and adreno-leukodystrophy [ALD]), illness movies are primarily concerned with the relational implications that result from a specific medical condition. In the films *Stepmom* (1998) and *Terms of Endearment* (1983), for example, the central question revolves around how a mother dying of cancer can bear to part with her children, as well as prepare them to grow up without her and under the guidance of another woman with whom the protagonist has had a troubled relationship. For all the melodrama and tear jerking, the exploration and working through of this question is closer to how "ordinary people" experience their illnesses than how doctors experience their patients' illnesses.[24] Movies like *My Left Foot* (1989) or *Children of a Lesser God* (1986) are primarily about persons with physical difference (in the first case, severe cerebral palsy; in the other case, deafness) navigating in a majority nondisabled world and evolving a meaningful identity in relation to others that both incorporates and honors their physical circumstances.[iii]

Such films give learners invaluable opportunities to see medicine through the eyes of people (rather than patients). In the dark and quiet of the movie theater,[iv] viewers have a two-hour opportunity to reorient themselves, to adopt a different perspective on the meaning of illness that more closely parallels the agenda of the filmmaker rather than that of a clinician. Thus, movies offer an essential complement to the prevailing educational emphasis on the disease model and enable learners immersed in this perspective to see the patient and family situated in their lived lives.[25] A movie helps learners see wider relational dimensions and implications of illness than can be seen in a clinic visit.[26]

awareness of self: emotional education

Since relational ethics is predicated on the ability to forge an emotional connection, clinicians should be familiar with their own emotional responses, both positive and negative, toward their patients and be comfortable working with them in a way that promotes a conscious, intentional relationship that benefits the patient. Unfortunately, their education in general does a poor job of emotionally preparing students for clinical practice. Little effort is exerted to develop emotional honesty[v] in medical students or residents, for example,[27] either in terms of their own affective responses, or in terms of their awareness of others' emotions. Prosocial professional attributes of altruism, respect, compassion, and empathy are paid lip service, but are often not demonstrated by physician role models,[28] and students consequently spend little time learning how to cultivate such attitudes.[3] Conversely, while students often see displays of and personally experience negative emotions of fear, frustration, irritation, anger, and contempt toward patients, they only know that these feelings are "unprofessional" and should be stifled. Finding emotions so confusing, unsafe, and difficult, learners sometimes decide to adopt a position of emotional detachment and distance.[29]

Successful movies about illness, on the other hand, must be emotionally evocative and, as such, engage the learners' emotions.[30,vi] In terms of health professions education, film is a highly effective method for allowing learners to explore the affective domain by stimulating reflection.[14] Although some have argued that emotions evoked by movies are unimportant because they are not in response to "real" events, these emotions have depth and resonance because they are inexorably attached to the personal narratives of our own lives.[31] Thus, narrative films can provide valuable access to viewers' affective lives by "lighting up" disruptive or disturbing parts of the self that might otherwise be ignored or neglected. Movies allow learners to explore difficult emotions in nonthreatening ways,[21] in privacy, without judgment, and without the expectation of action or alleviating suffering. Because the characters portrayed in movies are not "real" (not even those based on "real" people), learners can be more honest about their reactions than if they were discussing actual patients. This emotional honesty becomes a starting point for exploring other emotional responses.

In the movie *Motorcycle Diaries* (2004), for instance, the medical student Che Guevara spends time in a leper colony, and through his modeling of caring attitudes, viewers' initial responses of revulsion have the potential to transform into caring and concern. In most illness movies, evolution in emotion occurs primarily as a result of the sympathetic portrayal of the characters. For example, films such as *The Elephant Man* (1980) or *Dying Young* (1991) intentionally evoke strong feelings of horror or aversion (in the first case to extreme physical anomaly, in the second to the visceral aftermath of chemotherapy), only to develop empathy for and identification with the initially grotesque protagonists. In this way, movies promote an ethics of relational engagement with the suffering other, rather than an ethics based on the detached, intellectual mastery of moral principles and theories.[32]

cinematic depictions of the patient–clinician relationship

Movies also provide both concrete positive and negative role models of relational ethics in the patient–clinician relationship. Films such as *The Elephant Man, Patch Adams* (1998), or scenes in *My Life Without Me* (2003) help guide emerging health professionals on a path that incorporates emotional self-awareness, commitment to and engagement with the patient, and respect and sensitivity to the subjective experiences of the patient. The relationship that develops between John Merrick, who suffered from a highly disfiguring medical condition, and his physician Sir Frederick Treves, in *The Elephant Man* shows an evolution from patient-as-exploited (scientific) object into one of mutual caring and respect. *Patch Adams* presents an idealistic medical student who defies his training to provide to patients health care that acknowledges their emotional needs and quality of life. In *My Life Without Me*, a young woman has advanced ovarian cancer. In the filmic depiction of breaking this bad news, the doctor clearly suffers along with his patient and mingles his helplessness and vulnerability with that of his patient.[20]

Contemporary television medical dramas also tend to represent physicians in a positive light. These doctors are not so much heroic as human, sensitive, vulnerable, fallible to be sure, but ultimately caring and committed.[23,34] While their tone is often soap-operish, the contextual seriousness (life and death are the stakes) often (although not always) retrieves these shows from pure silliness. Further, despite patently absurd situations (doctors falling in love with patients, violating all sorts of medical ethics codes to help them), they contain compelling depictions of physician–patient relationships, precisely because of these physicians' willingness to become emotionally involved with their patients.[35] Doctors who worry about and struggle with the suffering of their patients, even when they transgress appropriate professional boundaries to do so, provide fertile ground for viewers to examine the complex parameters of relational ethics.

Other portrayals of doctors in movies as greedy, egotistical, uncaring, unethical, materialistic, or caring more about science than patients create negative role models.[36,37] *Wit* (2001), for example, is replete with critical views of physicians as impersonal, emotionally distant, jargon-spouting, and insensitive.[38] In *Ikiru* (1952), the paternalistic physician lies about the patient's terminal diagnosis of stomach cancer, which protects himself, but not the patient.[20] The physician Jack McKee in *The Doctor* (1991) initially demonstrates a glib, insensitive, and indifferent attitude toward his patients.[19] Using examples from such films with learners to help build patient–doctor relational ethics entails an analysis of "anti-role modeling"; that is, encouraging learners to reflect on who they want to be as clinicians by contrasting it with what they witness on the screen.

translational applications: putting relational ethics into practice

The ultimate goal of cinemeducation is to facilitate students' ability to make links between movies they see and how they might feel and behave in actual clinical situations. Consequently, education using film must not stop with the evocation of learners' emotions—whether awareness of one's own emotions or empathy for the emotions of the suffering other—but further guide learners through discussions with peers and role models.[14] Such a group process is designed to assist learners in carrying forward their "movie learning" into their daily lives, by addressing the question of how to bridge the gap between the illusion of the movies and the reality of patient care.[4,15] Through various written and imaginative exercises, learners can practice putting themselves in the position of a particular patient's doctor and explore different ways to establish connection and caring; they can repeatedly imagine, rehearse, and play variations on their interaction.[20] Because the film's audience is expected to respond emotionally and cognitively, but not necessarily to act, it may help learners to think about their relationships with patients in more creative ways.[31] Finally, these discussions can assist learners to develop a healthy skepticism toward the excessive simplification and idealization that characterize many narrative illness movies, while maintaining awareness that such movies attempt to reach past the difficult complexities of the real world toward the essential humanity and connection that should bind together clinician and patient.

The nature of the medium itself is particularly powerful in this regard. Film, the audiovisual version of storytelling, emphasizes emotions and images. Movies are sometimes about language,[vii] but they are indelibly about powerful visual images,[39] usually supported by a musical score that intensifies the emotions evoked by the screen images.[40] A younger generation of learners that has come of age in the milieu of powerful visual and musical cues enjoys and benefits from learning about how cinematographic techniques strengthen the message of the film.[4] For example, the movie *Wit* raises many ethical issues about doctors' treatment of patients, the nature of clinical trials, and the coming to terms with one's own death with some dignity.[37] Yet, medical students who have viewed the film most often mention the visual impact of a single scene that transpires not between the physician and the patient (a John Donne scholar, Vivian Bearing played by Emma Thompson), but between the patient and her old teacher (Eileen Atkins). In this scene, Bearing is in great pain and dying. The professor has come to visit, but quickly realizes the extent of her former student's illness. She climbs into the hospital bed and begins reading a children's story. This scene becomes fixed in learners' minds as a metaphoric touchstone, an iconic representation for how they wish to care for terminally ill patients.

Integrating movies into medical education provides a powerful way to address relational ethics by presenting learners with moving scenarios rooted in relationship dilemmas and evolution. Watching a movie enables students to understand and emotionally resonate to the life experiences of a protagonist-patient; to explore problematic, shameful emotions while reflecting on how to transform them into more positive responses through their identification with the film's protagonist; and to observe in an emotionally engaged way various options for embodying or rejecting relational ethics in the patient–clinician relationship. Finally, through facilitated discussion, medical learners can rehearse different possibilities for uniting insights and attitudes toward self and other into an ethical, respectful, and caring clinical relationship.

NOTES

i. In the tactful words of a Brazilian family physician and medical educator who regularly incorporates film in his teaching, "American movies are particularly useful, since they tend to tell stories in a straightforward and uncomplicated manner."[14]

ii. Occasionally, this cinematic foundation collapses, as is evidenced in an article reporting that when family medicine residents viewed excerpts from the movie *Million Dollar Baby*, they resisted the director's agenda to elicit sympathy for the act of euthanasia performed by the character played by Clint Eastwood, and indicated that they would both desire a different outcome for themselves if they were in the same situation as the patient (a female boxer who, as a result of a fight injury, was paraplegic and an amputee), and would adopt a different position as the treating physician.[22]

iii. While I have heard anecdotal reports of medical student parties organized around the popular television drama *House* (and beer), with the goal of guessing the diagnosis of a new medical zebra before the brilliant Dr. Gregory House and his medical team identify it, the allure of this show is not primarily the revelatory diagnostic denouement but the playing out of witty, complex, and ultimately moving relationships among the emotionally damaged eponymous protagonist, his patients, his medical team, and the hospital administration.

iv. Increasingly younger generations choose to view films through a range of Internet-based modalities.

v. Directed inward, emotional honesty means admitting one's feelings and thinking about their implications (self-reflection). Directed outward, it means expressing one's feelings and acknowledging those of others (teaching and clinical care that appreciates the emotional, as well as technical/intellectual, development of physicians).

vi. In fact, movies are so good at creating emotional connection that one physiology professor uses still film clips to keep his students emotionally engaged during lectures![33]

vii. Witness the way the phrase "Make my day" has entered our modern lexicon.

REFERENCES

1. Baños, J.-E. 2007. How literature and popular movies can help in medical education: Applications for teaching the doctor–patient relationship. *Medical Education* 41: 918.
2. Yamada, S., Maskarinec, G., and Greene, G. 2003. Cross-cultural ethics and the moral development of physicians: Lessons from Kurosawa's *Ikiru*. *Family Medicine* 35: 167–169.
3. Saab, B.-R., Sidani, N., Merheb, M., Mahmassani, D., Ghaddar, F., and Hamadeh, G. 2009. Zooming in to health ethics: An action to promote ethics. *Family Medicine* 41: 17–21.
4. Quadrelli, S., Colt, H.G., and Semeniuk, G. 2009. Appreciation of the aesthetic: A new dimension for a medicine and movies program. *Family Medicine* 41: 316–318.
5. Winter, R.O. 2006. The wizard in you. *Family Medicine* 38: 241–243.
6. Blasco, P.B. 2001. Literature and movies for medical students. *Family Medicine* 33: 426–428.
7. DasGupta, S. 2006. Being John Doe Malkovich: Truth, imagination, and story in medicine. *Literature and Medicine* 25: 439–462.
8. Dobie, S. 2007. Reflections on a well-traveled path: Self-awareness, mindful practice, and relationship-centered care as foundations for medical education. *Academic Medicine* 82: 422–427.

9. MacDonald, H. 2007. Relational ethics and advocacy in nursing: Literature review. *Journal of Advanced Nursing* 57: 119–126.

10. Bergum, V., and Dossetor, J.B. 2005. *Relational ethics: The full meaning of respect.* Hagerstown, MD: University Publishing Group.

11. Katz, A.M., and Alegria, M. 2009. The clinical encounter as local moral world: Shifts of assumptions and transformation in relational context. *Social Science and Medicine* 68: 1238–1246.

12. Pauly, B., and James, S. 2005. Living relational ethics in healthcare. In C. Johns and D. Freshwater (Eds.), *Transforming nursing through reflective practice*. New York: Wiley, 27–37.

13. Alexander, M., Hall, M.N., and Pettice, Y.J. 1994. Cinemeducation: An innovative approach to teaching psychosocial medical care. *Family Medicine* 26: 430–433.

14. Blasco, P.G., Moreto, G., Roncoletta, A.F.T., Levites, M.R., and Janaudis, M.A. 2006. Using movie clips to foster learners' reflection: Improving education in the affective domain. *Family Medicine* 38: 94–96.

15. Shapiro, J., and Rucker, L. 2004. The Don Quixote effect: Why going to the movies can help develop empathy and altruism in medical students and residents. *Families, Systems, & Health* 22: 445–452.

16. Freedberg, S. 2007. Re-examining empathy: A relational-feminist point of view. *Social Work* 52: 251–259.

17. Alexander, M., Lenahan, P., and Pavlov, A., (Eds.). 2005. *Cinemeducation: A comprehensive guide to using film in medical education* Oxford: Radcliffe Publishing.

18. Alexander, M., Pavlov, A., and Lenahan, P. 2007. Lights, camera, action: Using film to teach the ACGME competencies. *Family Medicine* 30: 20–23.

19. Fischer, L. 2004. Big boys do cry: Empathy in *The Doctor*. In D. Friedman (Ed.), *Cultural sutures: Medicine and media*. Durham NC: Duke University Press, 149–165.

20. Belling, C. 2006. The 'Bad News Scene' as clinical drama Part 2: Viewing scenes. *Family Medicine* 38: 474–475.

21. Winter, R.O., and Birnberg, B.A. 2005. Family systems at the movies. *Family Medicine* 37: 96–98.

22. Winter, R.O., and Birnberg, B.A. 2009. Million dollar baby: Murder or mercy. *Family Medicine* 41: 164–166.

23. Makoul, G., and Peer, L. 2004. Dissecting the doctor shows: A content analysis of *ER* and *Chicago Hope*. In L.D. Friedman (Ed.), *Cultural sutures: Medicine and media*. Durham NC: Duke University Press, 244–260.

24. Toombs, S.K. 2007. *The meaning of illness: A phenomenological account of the different perspectives of physician and patient*. New York: Springer.

25. Elder, N.C., and Schwarzer, A. 2002. Using the cinema to understand the family of the alcoholic. *Family Medicine* 34: 426–427.

26. Weber, C.M., and Silk, H. 2007. Movies and medicine: An elective using film to reflect on the patient, family, and illness. *Family Medicine* 39: 317–319.

27. Poirier, S. 2009. *Doctors in the making: Memoirs and medical education*. Iowa City, IA: University of Iowa, 155–156.

28. Coulehan, J. 2005. Viewpoint: Today's professionalism: Engaging the mind but not the heart. *Academic Medicine* 80: 892–898.

29. Shapiro, J. 2008. Walking a mile in their patients' shoes: Empathy and othering in medical students' education. *Philosophy, ethics, and humanities in medicine* 3: 10.

30. Campbell, T.L. 2005. Foreword. In M. Alexander, P. Lenahan, and A. Pavlov (Eds.), *Cinemeducation: A comprehensive guide to using film in medical education*, pp. x–xii. Oxford: Radcliffe Publishing.

31. Heiserman, A., and Spiegel, M. 2006. Narrative permeability: Crossing the dissociative barrier in and out of films. *Literature and Medicine* 25: 463–474.

32. Milligan, E. and Woodley, E. 2009. Creative expressive encounters in health ethics education: Teaching ethics as relational engagement. *Teaching and Learning in Medicine* 21: 131–139.

33. Zagvazdin, Y. 2007. Movies and emotional engagement: Laughing matters in lecturing. *Family Medicine* 39: 245–247.

34. Vandekieft, G. 2004. From *City Hospital* to *ER*: The evolution of the television physician. In L.D. Friedman (Ed.), *Cultural sutures: Medicine and media*. Durham, NC: Duke University Press, 215–233.

35. Cohen, M.R., and Shafer, A. 2004. Images and healers: A visual history of scientific medicine. In L.D. Friedman (Ed.), *Cultural sutures: Medicine and media*. Durham, NC: Duke University Press, 197–214.

36. Flores, G. 2002. Mad scientists, compassionate healers, and greedy egotists: The portrayal of physicians in the movies. *Journal of the National Medical Association* 94: 635–658.

37. Flores, G. 2004. Doctors at the movies. *Archives of Disease in Childhood* 89: 1084–1088.

38. Lewis, P.R. 2005. The wisdom of *Wit* in the teaching of medical students and residents. *Family Medicine* 37: 396–398.

39. Friedman, L.D. 2004. Through the looking glass: Medical culture and the media. In L.D. Friedman (Ed.), *Cultural sutures: Medicine and media*. Durham, NC: Duke University Press, 1–11.

40. Winter, R.O., and Birnberg, B.A. 2003. Teaching the realities of child abuse. *Family Medicine* 35: 322–323.

4

visions of reality, sometimes larger than life

stephen crawford and henri colt

THROUGH FICTION AND TRUE-LIFE STORIES, medical movies depict larger-than-life characters and situations that entertain, educate, infuriate, and illuminate us about the human condition. Movies cause us to laugh and to cry, to lament about a poor production or to be enthralled by an astounding cinematographic experience. Whether illustrating ethical issues or humanistic perspectives, the best movies incite both our intelligence and imaginations; they provide us with a vision of reality, sometimes larger than life, that strikes the core of our emotional selves and often causes us to think beyond our standard responses to consider alternative ideas. As renowned Spanish painter, draughtsman and sculptor Pablo Picasso (1881–1973) so eloquently put it,[i] "Art is the lie that makes us realize truth."[1] Film records reality but sees it differently from ordinary human experiences.[2] With unequaled ability, film calls for our attention. Camera movements and angles, special framing of shots, and the power of sound to enhance the visual image[3] entices viewers to become more than passive observers of the images on a screen, but instead to participate, intellectually, emotionally, psychologically, and even physically in the story being told. "Cinema is form," said Alfred Hitchcock (1899–1980), "the screen ought to speak its own language, freshly coined, and it can't do that unless it treats an acted scene as a piece of raw material which must be broken up, taken to bits, before it can be woven into an expressive visual pattern."[4] Emotions are produced not only by the actor's performance but also by the associations brought about by the juxtapositions of scenes created by the filmmaker.[5] A gentle touch, the mournful lowering of an eyelid, the prolonged gaze of the onlooker: Emotions are portrayed in ways that seem to us fresh and original, made larger than life through kinetic symbolism: The isolation of a stairwell in *City of Angels*, the cutaways to fantasy in *Pan's Labyrinth*, the nuanced facial expressions seen in close-ups of Meryl Streep holding flowers in *The Hours*.

As a learning tool, film promotes enthusiasm, reflection, and discussion. We may associate with protagonists or feel like outsiders, eavesdropping on an intimate moment between partners. Even if we reject a film's context or are horrified by a storyline, the film's images, dialogue, movement, ideology, and symbolism can serve as starting points to initiate discussion and even debate. Famous Swedish director, writer, and film producer Ingmar Bergman (1918–2007) wrote "Film as dream, film as music. No art passes our conscience in the way film does, and goes directly to our feelings, deep down into the dark rooms of our souls."[ii] Bergman was a master dealing with the existential questions of mortality, love, and religious faith.

Using film to teach medical ethics allows us to go beyond the illustration of theories and principles, so that we might develop not only a range of rational and analytic skills, but also a range of emotional and interpretative ones, including those habits of the heart.[6] Film thus provides a matrix for a discussion of ethics topics that may also be ambiguous and filled with paradox. Like good literature, using film in the ethics classroom often stands in direct opposition to the standard models of ethical decision making so commonly taught in medical school classrooms: those step-by-step approaches necessarily seek answers, perhaps even one answer, to a particular dilemma, whereas a film strives to fling open doors to multiple questions and may never fully resolve an issue. Discussions among and with students and colleagues, independent of their level of knowledge and experience, are thought-provoking and can be intensely personal,[7] transforming ethics education into a pendulous experience that oscillates from scientific debate to an exciting and often uneasy voyage of moral inquiry.

All journeys are important for what we learn about the world, about ourselves, and about others, but none is more unsettling than exploring "the dark rooms of our souls." This fraught passage is transformative, personal, and fearfully awe inspiring. It is not readily begun without insight and reason, without some initiating event that turns our existing world upside down and forces us to reflect on who we are, who we have become, and who we long to be. In this sense, film, as art, can affect the root of our being.

Following an incident in which one of our colleagues lost a patient on the operating table, coldly announced the news to an anxious family, and subsequently retired from surgical practice one year later, we reflected on why so many physicians have difficulty showing compassion, and are yet deeply affected personally by the consequences of their professional lives. Concurrently, we discovered in film a larger-than-life story that helped elucidate the potential causes for such behaviors. In director Brad Silberling's *City of Angels* (1998), using a plot inspired by the 1987 classic *Wings of Desire* (screenplay written by Wim Wenders and Peter Handke), Berlin is moved to Los Angeles. Through the eyes of a brooding angel, Seth (Nicolas Cage), we see a multitude of heavenly hosts watch over their earthly souls. After he becomes involved with Dr. Maggie Rice (Meg Ryan), the heart surgeon of one of his charges, Seth chooses to abandon his celestial duties in order to become human and experience earthly love.

In an early scene,[iii] we discover Maggie, an archetypal tough, competent, self-sufficient, and confident cardiac surgeon. We watch as her patient dies suddenly and unexpectedly on her operating table, his heart in her hands. Shaken by her failure to save her patient from this unforeseen disaster, she leaves the operating room to deliver the bad news to her patient's waiting family. Tentatively, but stoically, she approaches the trusting and unsuspecting wife and teenage children. Haltingly, her hands welded in the pockets of a starched white lab coat, she introduces herself while standing in the center of the waiting room.

"Mrs. Balford?" She says.

"Where's the doctor?"

"I'm the doctor."

"I'm sorry," exclaims the wife, with some embarrassment.

"I operated on your husband."

"How is he?" the wife and children huddle together uneasily.

With a demeanor as stiff as her coat, Maggie informs them that he "did not survive" the open heart surgery. She goes on to recite a bewildering technical explanation for the physiological events after coming off coronary bypass. Her eyes furtively dart away from the shocked confusion of the family. She seems frozen in her own unease as the mother and children collapse together in a torrent of tears. "Excuse me," she mumbles to no one in particular, "I'm sorry."

Leaving the distressed family, Maggie flees to the solitude of a stairwell. Confusion and doubt wash over her like a rapid flood of thoughts in her anguish.

On the table – on my table, I'm sorry. I'm sorry. I'm sorry–
what happened, what happened? A graft occlusion? What?
It was textbook – it was textbook. It was textbook. I'm so sorry!
The room got so big – I was so small. How did I get so small?
I should have gone back on, I should have massaged longer,
I should have gone back on, I should have massaged longer.
I lost it… I lost it.

The scene ends with a concerned but unseen Seth tenderly watching the tears course down her cheeks.

Most of us will never witness a physician delivering bad news unless we ourselves are health care providers, or we are on the receiving end of the news itself. The scene from this film forces us simultaneously to feel the pain from both sides. As we look at this story, however, we likely sympathize with the grieving family. We are struck by Maggie's distance and lack of warmth. We expect physicians to help loved ones deal with death and loss. We expect compassion. Almost one hundred years ago, Sir William Osler[8] told medical students about the importance of understanding the individual, "It is more important to know what patient has a disease, than what disease the patient has." We are, therefore, disappointed in this surgeon, who seems to lack compassion and who obviously has not connected with her patient or his family.

The root of the word compassion reveals the true implications of its meaning. From the Latin roots, com- "together" and pati- "to suffer," compassion literally means to suffer together.[9] In City of Angels, everyone in the waiting room is suffering, yet each is in his or her own agony. Each is grieving. Maggie is not suffering together with the family. Instead, she seems to be suffering her own loss, and tortured by guilt, she remains aloof. Maggie's lament in the stairwell exposes her sense of failure and shame, but only to herself and, unbeknownst to her, an angel (and of course the audience as well). She did not merely fail to save her patient, she was a failure—she was too small. She *lost* control. *She* was the problem. She *"lost it."* While she mourns the loss of her patient, perhaps she mourns it less than she grieves for her own loss of self-confidence and power over life and death.

In the opening lines of *A Grief Observed* (1961), C.S. Lewis writes, "No one ever told me that grief felt so like fear. I am not afraid, but the sensation is like being afraid. The same fluttering in the stomach, the same restlessness, the yawning. I keep on swallowing."[10] Grief and fear seem closely linked: fear of the unknown, fear of life without *whom* or without *what* was lost. Maggie feared a future without her self-confidence—without her sense of absolute control within her operating room—control of her "world." She "lost it." This perception of "loss" can perpetuate the fear of being forever lost. Fear then paralyzes action. Fear places Maggie, hands in her pockets, in the center of the waiting room announcing the death of her patient.

On any given day, a health care provider, like Maggie, might experience the loss of a patient. This loss might be unavoidable, the natural result of disease, or the outcome of some misfortune, negligence, or harmful medical error. In these instances, in addition to feeling grief, one's sense of guilt may become overwhelming. Whether real or imagined, guilt in one form or another remains omnipresent in medical practice. It is not easily appreciated, however, because it is usually a hidden feeling, perhaps even repressed within the psyche of the health care provider. Guilt represents feelings of responsibility or remorse for some offense, crime, or wrongdoing, and reflects feelings of responsibility and accountability for our actions. Wrongdoing, whether defined as moral transgressions, a violation of some internal standard, or a betrayal of trust can be real or perceived, and the perception of wrongdoing can elicit guilt just as surely as if harm had actually occurred, and regardless of whether one has truly transgressed. Watching Maggie's behaviors helps illustrate how some health care providers might feel and behave in similar circumstances.

Guilt is a fundamental emotion essential to the development of our affective-cognitive structures of conscience and the affective-cognitive-action patterns of moral behavior.[11] It may come as readily and as frequently from omission as from commission—from failure to feel, think, or act in a certain way at a certain time, as well as from actual feelings, thoughts, or acts that violate moral codes or beliefs.[12] While there are some uniformities across cultures in the acquisition of guilt and guilt-related behaviors,[13] wide variability exists from individual to individual and culture to culture, often reflecting differing norms of moral, ethical, and religious standards or beliefs. Not necessarily explicit, these may be accepted intuitively, as individuals from childbirth onward incorporate or adopt an ethical framework that guides interpersonal relationships. Residual feelings of guilt become almost necessary in order to incite maintained vigilance against repeating those actions that cause pain to ourselves or to others. Guilt, unresolved, however, can have substantial adverse effects on human behavior, affecting private lives, professional decision making, social conduct, and an individual's concept of their "real, social, and ideal selves."[14] Of course, most would agree that the loss of a husband and father is far more important than the loss of self-confidence and the generation of feelings of guilt in a surgeon. Maggie, however, in addition to guilt, experienced profound grief. In fact, her behaviors suggest that in addition to losing her patient, she has lost her ability to fulfill her professional and moral responsibilities: "to cure sometimes, to relieve often, to comfort always."[15] Her duty, after losing her patient, was to extend her care and her caring to his grieving relatives. From within the grief of her loss should have emerged compassion.

For this, however, Maggie needed to be able to reappraise her values and standards. She needed to care for "the other"[iv] as much as, if not more than she might have cared for herself.[16] She needed to be able to quickly make amends, to forgive herself, and to recognize and accept her sense of guilt, so that she could empathize and express compassion for her patient's surviving family. Putting ourselves in Maggie's place, we too may feel that we could have "lost it." We may find that we are no more capable of pardoning ourselves than we are of standing on our own shoulders or looking ourselves in our own eye, and like others, we may find that it is more difficult to pardon[v] ourselves than it is to pardon others for the injury they do to us.

This film provides an example of how learning ethics, whether based on principles, values, moral and religious standards, codes, or behaviors, mobilizes all of our emotional resources. There is nothing better than art, in all its forms, to galvanize these emotions, and, as John Dewey points out, to communicate a moral purpose and convey messages that stimulate reflection on purposeful lives.[17] Man's imperfection is a reflection of his Human-ness. Like the lost sheep to the shepherd, the prodigal son to his father—perhaps what matters most, however, is not how often we stray from what we know is right, but only that we return. We cannot always repair what is broken by our actions any more than we can mend the cracked pot, shattered mirror, or broken covenant. On the other hand, a healthy sense of guilt allows us, perhaps, to start over—cast a new pot, buy a new mirror, or recraft a new covenant. While unable to forget the action or forgive ourselves for harm caused, we can ask to be forgiven. Thus humbled, we can learn to feel and manifest kindness "to notice the distress of a little boy wandering around lost, and to help him and his father or mother; or to volunteer to pick up the brother of a friend at the airport because the friend is not feeling up to it."[18] In the final analysis of the scene from City of Angels, however, it is only the angel, Seth, who shows compassion. He touched and was touched by Maggie's tears. He shared her anguish as though the loss were his. The picture is worth a thousand words.

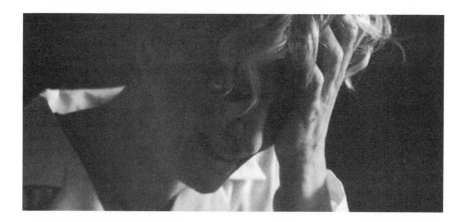

"On my table, I'm so sorry. What happened? A graft occlusion, It was text book. I am so sorry. The room got so big. I was so small. How did I get so small?"
Dr. Maggie Rice in *City of Angels (1998)*.

NOTES

i. From an interview with Marius de Zayas: Comments on Cubism "Picasso speaks" originally published in *The Arts*, pp. 315–326, New York, 1923. Translation approved by Picasso.

ii. Quoted by John Berger in "Every Time We Say Goodbye," in *Sight and Sound BFI*, June, 1991.

iii. Chapter 5, scene 00:13:16–00:15:44

iv. My responsibility for the other is the *for* of the relationship."

v. To pardon: ("to release a person from liability for an offense").[5]

REFERENCES

1. Harrison, C., and Wood, P. 2003. *Art in theory 1900–2000: An anthology of changing ideas*, pp. 39–40. Malden, MA: Blackwell Publishing.
2. Arnheim, R. 1957. *Film as art*. Berkeley, CA: University of California Press.
3. Carroll, N. 1985. The power of movies. *Daedalus* 114: 79–103.
4. Hitchcock, A. 1995. *Hitchcock on Hitchcock*, p. 256. S. Gottlieb (Ed.). Berkeley and Los Angeles: University of California Press.
5. Giannetti, L. 2008. *Understanding Movies*. 11th ed., p. 116. Upper Saddle River, NJ: Pearson, Prentice Hall.
6. Reich, W.T. 1995. History of the notion of care. In *Encyclopedia of bioethics*, vol.1. New York: Simon & Schuster/Macmillan.
7. Quadrelli, S., Colt, H.G., and Semeniuk, G. 2009. Appreciation of the aesthetic: A new dimension for a medicine and movies program. *Family Medicine* 41(5): 316–318.

8. Osler, W. 1919. *A way of life. An address delivered to Yale students on the evening, April 20th, 1913*. Springfield, IL: C.C. Thomas.

9. Dictionary.com. Online Etymology Dictionary. "Compassion." Douglas Harper, Historian. Retrieved October 4, 2009 from http://dictionary.reference.com/browse/compassion

10. Lewis C.S. 1961. *A grief observed*, p. 1. New York: Harper Collins.

11. Izard, C.E. 1991. *The psychology of emotions*, p. 355. New York: Plenum Press.

12. Izard, C.E. 1991. *The psychology of emotions*, p. 363. New York: Plenum Press.

13. Ausubel, D.P. 1955. Relationships between shame and guilt in the socializing process. *Psychological Review* 62: 378–390.

14. Katz, P.K., and Ziegler, P.K. 1967. Self-image disparity: A developmental approach. *Journal of Personality and Social Psychology* 5:186–195.

15. Anonymous. 1968. *Familiar medical quotations*, p. 410. M.B. Strauss (Ed.). Boston, MA: Little, Brown and Co.

16. Levinas, E. 2008. *Otherwise than being, or beyond essence*, p. 100. Pittsburgh, PA: Dusquesne University Press.

17. Dewey, J. 1934. *Art as experience*. New York: Perigee Books (Penguin Group).

18. Blum, L.A. 1980. *Friendship, altruism & morality*, p. 167. London: Routledge & Kegan.

part two

autonomy, justice, and informed consent

making autonomous decisions:
million dollar baby

jennifer hawkins

Million Dollar Baby (2004). Clint Eastwood, Hilary Swank, Morgan Freeman, Jay Baruchel, Mike Colter. Directed by Clint Eastwood. Duration: 137 minutes.

DVD chapter 31 scene 1:43:26 to 1:47:55

MILLION DOLLAR BABY tells the story of Maggie (Hilary Swank), a 31-year-old woman who becomes a boxer with the help of her trainer Frankie (Clint Eastwood). Despite Frankie's original concerns about a girl getting hurt, Maggie moves successfully into the world of female boxing, becoming a superstar at her level. Undefeated, she wants to move up. Reluctantly, Frankie arranges a fight with the middle-weight championship title holder. Maggie is holding her own in the match when her opponent, who has a reputation as a dirty fighter, hits her between rounds when her guard is down. Maggie falls backward and breaks her neck, becoming paralyzed from the neck down. Maggie thinks she can't bear a paralyzed life. She tries to kill herself, and when this fails, she asks Frankie to kill her. Frankie, although greatly distressed by her request, eventually agrees. He goes to her room, turns off her breathing machine, and injects her with something that allows her to die quickly.

Million Dollar Baby raises a number of ethical issues, but the most interesting of these are *not* obvious. Maggie's disabled life is agonizing, and death is clearly presented as the right option. The film leads the viewer to assume that Maggie has made the right decision, but cannot carry it out because of her condition. Her doctors (for reasons that are never explored) will not let her end her life. We thus seem to be presented with a simple case of autonomy thwarted by paternalism. Frankie's agonizing choice would not have to be made if only Maggie were allowed to request that her breathing machine be turned off. Today, however, that decision is a right that would likely be honored, assuming she was deemed mentally competent. The film aims to show us that death is sometimes the best choice, and that individuals should be allowed to make that choice—tragic though it may be—when they want. Frankie is a hero because he is the only one who respects her choice to die.

That paternalism is bad is an important message, although somewhat outdated, in this film. In the 1970s, right-to-die cases were a big issue because the law was in flux and the right of individuals to refuse treatment (and to have treatments stopped once they had been started) was hotly debated. Although the issues first arose when families petitioned to stop treatment for loved ones in persistent vegetative states (e.g., Quinlan, Cruzan),[1] the debate quickly spread to include questions about the right of disabled people. The case of Elizabeth Bouvia, a woman with cerebral palsy and degenerative arthritis who in 1986 won the right to refuse food and hydration, is illustrative.[2,3] But today, most patients in Maggie's situation could request that life support be stopped.

The more interesting question raised by this film is about what constitutes an autonomous decision. While the film presents us with a dramatic and heart-wrenching choice, it also gives a very misleading impression of what comprises an autonomous decision. Autonomy means "self-governing." Focusing on the "self" part, we tend to assume that any forcefully expressed decision coming from a competent individual—from a self—is autonomous. But we need to focus more on the "governing" aspect, which emphasizes *controlling, directing, influencing.* When the self's choice is reflective and so is *directed* or *controlled* by (a) adequate information, (b) a clear perspective on her values, and (3) an appreciation of her options, the choice is autonomous. Of course, in this model, autonomous choice is a degree concept (i.e., a choice can be more or less autonomous),[4] but some choices lack any significant degree of autonomy.

We focus on autonomous choices in medical ethics *both* because people typically want to make choices for themselves *and* because autonomous choices are more likely to be *right.* Of course, I mean "right for the particular individual." I don't assume the same decision is right for all people. But individuals sometimes make decisions that are good for them—that reflect their own values and help them to lead the kinds of lives they most want to have—and sometimes they also make decisions that are bad. It might seem obvious that Maggie's life has little left to offer her. But whether that is true depends on many things that the film never addresses, such as the material resources available, the kinds of emotional support she will have, and the deep facts about her personality that neither she nor we are likely to know in the first instance.

It can sometimes help to compare real-life stories. In the 1950s, two very different women contracted polio and were left paralyzed from the neck down, living first in iron lungs and then with respirators. One woman, Regina Woods, became paralyzed as a young girl and went on to live a meaningful life, including writing a memoir about her experiences.[5] There, she remarks on the fact that many people expect her to be angry and bitter about her life, although she is not. The other woman, Virginia Black, I know of only from the memoir of her daughter.[6] She developed polio as a young mother and never really adjusted to her disability. After two sad years, she died. Her daughter's description suggests that she was profoundly depressed, and that she did not have the kind of emotional support she needed. In particular, her marriage was rocky before polio, and after her illness, her husband could not accept the change. We could speculate at length on the differences between these two stories. Regina's success might be the result of greater emotional support. It might also have been easier to become paralyzed as an adolescent than as a young adult. In addition, Virginia probably suffered from depression that might be better treated today. Ultimately, however, the difference might just depend on deeper facts about their personalities. We will never know. But their stories remind us that not all stories of tragic disability are the same.

There is a strong temptation—one that *Million Dollar Baby* capitalizes on—to think we can judge from a person's past whether or not there is hope in their future. Thus, it is often said that so-and-so was a deeply independent person and would hate a life of dependency. Maggie has been a fighter both literally and meta-phorically all her life, and so the thought is that if she cannot box, her life will be pointless. But this may well not be true. Simply because Maggie has valued boxing up to now does not mean she can't adopt new values. It all depends. Being a boxer (literally) and a fighter (figuratively) might predict that an individual would only find a life of boxing worthwhile, but it could just as easily predict that a person would find meaning in new types of challenges and fight to overcome those.

The important point is that we can't tell what is going to be possible for a person in the immediate aftermath of a traumatic change. And neither can that person. Many aspects of the film seem designed to underscore the bleakness of Maggie's future. But these same aspects lead me to think that she may not be making a sufficiently autonomous decision. For example, in a pivotal scene Maggie's family pays her a visit. It becomes immediately clear that they do not care a shred for Maggie, but have come simply in the hopes that she will sign over her property to them. They are truly horrible people and leave Maggie with the sense that she is alone in the world. Sunk in feelings of isolation, it is not surprising that Maggie wants to die. But having no emotional distance on her situation, she is not able at that time to appreciate the fact that life might offer her other types of companionship in the future. A life of disability does not have to be a life of isolation and loneliness.

To make an autonomous decision, a person needs to really understand her options. She must know what her material existence will be like, but also realize the possibilities for human connection. It would probably help Maggie to meet individuals who have responded well to similar disabilities. Although it sounds paradoxical, *most people need the help of others to make truly autonomous decisions.* Minimally, they need information from others. They may also need someone to help them relate the information they have to what they care about. Finally, since most of us do not have a clear ranking of our priorities ready at hand for all situations, most of us need help figuring out what we care about *most* and how this relates to our current choice situation.[7]

Those who confront the disabled sometimes unintentionally undermine autonomous choice by simply failing to help with decision making. Able-bodied people who face those with disabilities often find it an extremely uncomfortable encounter, assuming that such lives are not worth living. They may communicate this view through body language, voice quality, and the like. Thus, rather than encourage a person to try to examine her options, they may unknowingly reinforce that individual's sense that she is "right" to want to die. In the extreme case, a physician might not even initiate a conversation about options with a severely disabled patient expressing a desire to die, because he or she may simply assume that because the patient is making the "right decision" no conversation is necessary.[8]

Many disability rights activists have criticized *Million Dollar Baby* for its portrayal of the disabled life as not worth living. They often insist that disabled people should *never* be allowed to choose death.[9,10] My point is more about the nature of decision making. I do not doubt that death is *sometimes* the best option, and when it is, an individual should be allowed to make that choice. But I do not think anyone can know which option is best in the immediate aftermath of a traumatic event. Moreover, even once the smoke has cleared, such choices must be made on the basis of reflection, with sufficient information, with proper emotional distance, and with support from others. Finally, I want to emphasize that one of the most common barriers to such support in the case of the severely disabled is the assumption on the part of the able-bodied that the choice is obvious.

REFERENCES

1. Pence, G. *Classic cases in medical ethics: Accounts of cases that have shaped medical ethics, with philosophical, legal, and historical backgrounds*, 3rd. edition, chapter 2. New York: McGraw Hill.
2. Annas, G. 1984. When suicide prevention becomes brutality: The case of Elizabeth Bouvia. *The Hastings Center Report* 14: 2: 20–21, 46.
3. Annas, G. 1986. Elizabeth Bouvia: Whose space is this anyway? *Hastings Center Report* 16: 2: 24–25.
4. Beauchamp, T., and Faden, R. 1986. *A history and theory of informed consent*, chapter 7. New York: Oxford University Press.
5. Woods, R. 1994. *Tales from inside the iron lung and How I got out of it*. Philadelphia: University of Pennsylvania Press.
6. Black, K. 1996. *In the shadow of polio: A personal and social history*. New York: Addison Wesley.
7. Emanuel, E., and Emanuel, L. 1992. Four models of the physician-patient relationship. *Journal of the American Medical Association* 267: 2221–2226.
8. Halpern, J. 2001. *From detached concern to empathy*, chapter 1. New York: Oxford University Press.
9. Longmore, P. 2003. *Why I burned my book and other essays on disability*, chapters 8 and 9. Philadelphia: Temple University Press.
10. Dolmage, J., and DeGenaro, W. (Eds.). 2005. Responding to *Million Dollar Baby*: A forum. *Disability Studies Quarterly* 25: 3. Retrieved from http://www.dsq-sds.org/article/view/590/767

2

informed consent: *extreme measures*

henri colt

Extreme Measures (1996). Hugh Grant, Gene Hackman, Sarah Jessica Parker.
Directed by Michael Apted. Duration: 120 minutes.

DVD chapter 34 scene 01:43:25 to 01:45:00

E XTREME MEASURES TELLS THE STORY OF Dr. Guy Luthan (Hugh Grant), an emergency room physician entering a neurology fellowship in a New York hospital. Luthan faces issues of conscience and professionalism after one of his patients, a homeless man with an identification wristband from a hospital Luthan has never heard of, dies and his body disappears. As the young doctor begins inquiries into the incident, he meets world-renowned neurosurgeon Dr. Lawrence Myrick (Gene Hackman), who performs experimental spinal surgeries on the homeless, without their consent, in an attempt to cure paralyzing spinal disorders.

In this scene, and throughout the movie, it appears that surgery has been performed without consent upon physically fit homeless individuals. The major protagonist of these actions, Dr. Myrick, declares that he is 68 years old and does not have time to follow the traditional protocol of first experimenting in rats and then in chimpanzees. He further justifies human experimentation in nonconsenting, uninformed individuals by saying that great advances in medical science can only occur when physicians do what they think is right, even if it involves breaking rules. "People die everyday," he says, "And for what? For nothing. What do we do? What do you do? You take care of the ones you think you can save. Good doctors do the correct thing, but great doctors have the guts to do the right thing."

I often use the plot lines of *Extreme Measures* as springboards for discussions about informed consent, and more recently, about the appropriateness of incorporating a "time out" prior to any surgical intervention, in order to help avoid performing inappropriate surgeries or operating on the wrong patient. With respect first to the surgery-without-consent issue, one needs to understand the legal notions of assault and battery. These were highlighted in the landmark case of *Schloendorff v. Society of New York* regarding a surgeon who performed a hysterectomy without consent. The law, which is based on the principle of self-determination,[1] states that a person has the right to remain free from aggression against one's person.

From a legal perspective, *assault* consists of a bodily threat and ability to do harm without a person's consent. Certainly, a surgeon has the ability to do harm either by operating inappropriately on a consenting patient, by performing procedures on a nonconsenting patient, and by performing the wrong procedure. Health care providers might also threaten to do harm by insisting on the performance of a procedure against a patient's wishes. *Battery*, on the other hand, consists of any intentional bodily contact that violates the personal physical security of another without that person's permission. The battered victim does not need to be aware that physical violation has occurred. Such a scenario would apply to a patient who has been sedated or rendered unconscious by anesthesia. Battery charges also do not require that actual damage be demonstrated.

From a historical perspective, the doctrine of informed consent derives from the 1947 Nuremberg Code. This required doctors to obtain voluntary informed consent prior to conducting medical experimentation and declared that all relevant information about a proposed procedure or treatment be provided prior to obtaining such consent. As a result of the Nuremberg trials, in which it was discovered that Nazi doctors had performed grotesque medical experiments on prisoners and work camp detainees, human subjects institutional review boards (IRBs) were created, in part to protect the rights of both patients and research subjects. With the World Medical Association's Declaration of Helsinki in 1964, an international code of ethics was also formulated to address concerns about the preservation of autonomy, beneficence, nonmaleficence, and justice for all human research subjects.[2]

Institutional review boards oversee research protocols, monitor drug and treatment trials, and help investigators maintain appropriate records in case of inquiry.[3] In the United States, the Code of Federal Regulations, Protection of Human Subjects (45CFR Part 46), directly results from various abuses of patient rights, such as those that occurred during the 30-year government-sponsored Tuskegee syphilis study: 300 black men were untreated for syphilis despite the recognized effectiveness of antibiotic treatment. Today, one of an IRB's major roles assures that medical researchers write informed consent documents in a way that all potential research subjects understand the risks and benefits of any proposed research.[4]

The American Medical Association has opinioned, however, that informed consent entails more than just informing patents about the risks and benefits of a proposed intervention or research project. It is a process of communication between a patient and a physician that results in the patient's authorization and agreement to undergo a specific medical intervention, ensuring that the patient has truly understood the elements of the procedure, as well as the consequences of undergoing or refusing to undergo the intervention.[5] It follows that physicians must disclose any and all conflicts of interest or compensation gained from any treatments or research being proposed. Similar recommendations have been issued by the British Medical Association, with emphasis on a patient-centered model of care whereby physicians take into consideration a patient's goals, values, and objectives, and provide information accordingly.[6,7]

While the Nuremberg Code insisted on consent from research subjects, subsequent arguments have been made that, in the case of therapeutic procedures on incompetent patients, and in research patients for whom there are no effective therapies, a strict requirement for informed consent may be viewed as contrary to the subject's best interests. Obviously, this argument cannot and should not be made in relation to this film, because the subjects of the experimental research in *Extreme Measures* are neither incompetent nor persons with diseases. The film thus prompts one to ask whether the research might have been justified if it were being performed on those individuals with neurological injuries, rather than on unwilling, disenfranchised, healthy, homeless subjects. Considering the ethical principles of autonomy, nonmaleficence, and a health care provider's duty to obtain informed consent, the answer to this question is a resounding no.

Regardless of place or type of medical practice, respect for individual autonomy mandates the informed consent process. Whether health care interventions occur from within a patient-focused or family-focused care model, informed consent represents shared decision making. Informed consent, as well as recently mandated surgical "time out" rules, helps ensure the satisfaction of legal and ethical obligations, and enhance the quality and safety of patient treatments and procedures.[8]

In addition, the health care provider's duties to do no harm reasonably trump any arguments that might be presented to justify assault and battery in the clinical setting. In cases in which there is a need for emergency intervention in incompetent patients, or in cases in which patients are without decision-making capacity and surrogate consent cannot be obtained, however, procedures might be performed on condition that patients could potentially benefit and that patient acceptance would be probable.

In *Extreme Measures*, however, justifications for performing surgery on individuals without their consent include the necessity to proceed with human experimentation because the results would benefit paralyzed patients. Another way to ponder some of the ethical dilemmas facing the health care providers in the film, as well as their administrative staff, therefore, is to reflect whether a common good (beneficence for society, or, in this case, specifically to the spinal-disorder patient community), might in fact, warrant the physical, emotional, and psychological harm done to the unknowing study subject. This is counter, of course, to the principles of respect for autonomy and the need to provide medical care while safeguarding a patient's best interests.

On the other hand, from a simple philosophical utilitarian perspective, one might argue that a greater good is accomplished for society as a whole, that the disenfranchised study subjects provide no benefit to society other than their availability as objects of experimentation. In *Extreme Measures*, Myrick tells Luthan that the homeless persons undergoing experimental surgical procedures without consent, are, in fact, heroes because losing one to save millions is worthy of their sacrifice. If society deems such an argument unacceptable, it is curious that similar perspectives are proposed to help justify the use and abuse of animals in research and procedural-based education, or the ready accessibility to patients, rather than to more costly low- and high-fidelity simulation in order to help health care providers improve their diagnostic and therapeutic procedural technical skills. Are these "extreme measures"?

REFERENCES

1. Bernat, J.L., and Peterson, L.M. 2006. Patient-centered informed consent in surgical practice. *Archives of Surgery* 141: 86–92.
2. Declaration of Helsinki. Accessed November 20, 2008 at http://www.wma.net/e/policy/b3.htm
3. Greenwald, Ryan, M.K., Mulvihill, J.E. 1982. *Human subjects research: A handbook for institutional review boards* New York: Plenum Press.
4. Colt, H.G., Mulnard, R.A. Writing for a human subjects institutional review board. *Chest* 130: 1605–1607.
5. Council on Ethical and Judicial Affairs. 2008. *American Medical Association Code of Ethics*, 1st ed. Chicago: American Medical Association.
6. Doyal, L., Tobias, J.S., Warnock, M., Power, L., and Goodare, H. 1998. Informed consent in medical research. *British Medical Journal*. 316: 1000–1005.
7. Bridson, J., Hammond, C., Leach, A., and Chester, M.R. 2003. Making consent patient centered. *British Medical Journal* 327: 1159–1161.
8. Berg, J.W., and Appelbaum, P.S. 2001. *Informed consent: Legal theory and clinical practice*, 2nd ed. New York: Oxford University Press Inc.

the ethics of self-determination: *the diving bell and the butterfly*

arthur r. derse

The Diving Bell and the Butterfly (2007). Mathieu Amalric, Emmanuelle Seigner, Marie-Josee Croze, Anne Consigny. Directed by Julian Schnabel. Duration: 112 minutes.

Scene: DVD chapter 7 scene 0:32:44 to 0:35:14

IN JULIAN SCHNABEL'S AWARD-WINNING FILM adaptation of Jean-Dominique Bauby's memoir,[1] we learn of Jean-Dominique's life of fast cars, good food, and beautiful women. He is 43, single, a father of two, and the editor-in-chief of *Elle*, a popular French fashion magazine. His personal drama begins on a country road, outside of Paris. Jean-Dominique is enjoying the day with his young son, driving in his sports car with the top down, when he has a stroke. He awakes in a hospital fully conscious but quadriplegic.

Initially, Jean-Dominique cannot communicate with his caregivers. They speak to him at times but are unsure if he is able to understand them. His right eye has been injured, and as a protective measure, the eyelids are sewn shut. The peripheral vision in his left eye is blurred. He has hearing loss in one ear. This former giant of the social world now lies paralyzed and silent, a Cyclops at the mercy of his therapists and far from family and friends. His treatment team and he discover that he can communicate—through eye movement and blinking. A more sophisticated communication develops between his therapist and him: he blinks his eye in response to the correct letter of the alphabet spoken out loud by his therapist. The letters are presented in order from the most frequently used to the least, and in this arduous way, words are spelled out. It is through this eyeblink communication that Bauby once again shares his thoughts and needs. He is no longer "locked in," and he can reflect on his past life and his new experience as a full-time patient. Through the medium of his therapist, Jean-Dominique writes a best-selling memoir of his struggle, which Julian Schnabel translated into film.

This scene from Schnabel's film illustrates the complexity of self-determination for the patient and medical staff. Jean-Dominique has already mastered the use of the eyeblink response to the alphabet presented by his speech therapist, Henriette. He spells out to her the words "I want." Henriette, who has been empathetic and patient with him, smiles and asks what he wants. It will be his first expression to her of his own wishes. With each blink of his eye, he spells out, letter-by-letter, "D-E-A-." As she vocalizes the next letter, "T," she realizes what he is spelling. In the process, her expression changes from empathy to confusion and hurt. She turns away from him, and when she turns back tells him, "How dare you! There are people who love you. To whom you matter. I hardly know you, and you matter to me already. You're alive! Don't say you want to die. It's disrespectful. Obscene!... . Let's hope you change your mind." She leaves the room abruptly. After several moments, she returns and apologizes. Jean-Dominique follows Henriette's movements and hears her apology but mentally asks, "For what?"

This scene exemplifies Jean-Dominique's assertion of his will to decide for himself what his choice will be, known as *self-determination*. Self-determination is also known by its synonym *autonomy*, from the Greek words for self-governance. Autonomy is a major principle—some would say the dominant principle—in the Western canon of bioethics.[2] The ability to determine for oneself one's choices about proposed medical treatment has been the cornerstone upon which the principles of informed consent and the ability to refuse medical treatment (including life-sustaining treatment) have been built. The principle of autonomy replaced centuries of traditional paternalism that characterized the doctor–patient relationship, in which patients were expected to submit unquestioningly to the superior knowledge and expertise of the physician.[3]

Over the past century, American law and medical ethics newly recognized that "[e]very human being of adult years and sound mind has a right to determine what shall be done with his [or her] own body,"[4] Not only must the patient give consent for medical treatment, but the patient must also be informed of the nature of the proposed procedure, as well as the benefits, risks, and alternatives.[5] Patients, who have the capacity to make decisions about proposed medical treatment (i.e., who have "decision-making capacity"), may refuse unwanted medical treatment, even life-sustaining medical treatment.[6] Self-determination has been recognized, for the most part, ethically and legally in a patient's right to refuse medical care rather than a right of the patient to demand certain medical care. The most dramatic examples of the right to self-determination have been for patients who refuse life-sustaining medical treatment, where their wishes may result in death.[7] If a patient is incapacitated, the right to refuse unwanted medical treatment may be asserted on the patient's behalf using a document known as an *advance directive* (e.g., directions about medical care in advance of incapacity, authorized by the aptly named Patient Self-Determination Act).[8]

This recognition of the centrality of self-determination in Western ethics and law is markedly different from other countries and cultures (e.g., Japan), in which respect for the medical profession and for family-focused care and decision-making are more highly regarded than patient self-determination and truth-telling. Nonetheless, the World Medical Association has incorporated the value of self-determination in its Code of Ethics stating, "A physician shall respect a competent patient's right to accept or refuse treatment."[9]

Jean-Dominique relies totally upon technological medical treatment for his survival and remains completely dependent upon his caregivers to be fed, to be moved, and to communicate. In this scene, he expresses his wish to die, although he cannot take any action to do so. As such, the scene aptly demonstrates that self-determination has its practical, ethical, and legal limits. Jean-Dominique's initial difficulty in communicating his wishes severely curtails his ability to assert self-determination. Bioethicists often cite communication as a major barrier to resolution of ethical dilemmas. The patient's treatment team, therefore, has an obligation to determine whether the patient can communicate with them and to use the best means available to allow the patient to assert his or her autonomous wishes.

In the *locked-in syndrome*, fully conscious patients are quadriplegic (i.e., cannot move arms or legs) and can only communicate through eye movements and blinking.[10] This syndrome occurs rarely and must be carefully distinguished from other neurological states in which patients are *not* conscious and do not have the potential ability to communicate, such as persistent vegetative state (PVS). Nonetheless, similar nightmarish scenarios to the locked-in syndrome do occur. Even as medical personnel shout questions at them repeatedly, patients who have various stroke syndromes attempt to speak, but are not understood, or attempt to move an arm or a leg but cannot. Ultimately, these patients may regain movement or improve their ability to communicate, and health care workers need to treat each patient as though they understand words and actions, despite their inability to express themselves. This film segment helps students understand this need for respect and patience.

Beyond practical limits to self-determination, there are also legal and ethical limits. Caregivers have no obligation to provide nonbeneficial treatments, even though patients or families may demand them (however, determining the likelihood and extent of medical benefit to the patient makes the ethical issue known as *medical futility* particularly vexing). In the United States, physicians may not intentionally administer medication to cause death (*euthanasia*, from the Greek words for "good death"), despite a request from a patient with decision-making capacity to do so. In the vast majority of jurisdictions, patients have the right to refuse medical treatment, but caregivers may not assist in suicide. Should the patient's wish to die result in a request for medication to do so, it would very likely not be fulfilled. In those jurisdictions that allow physician-assisted death, patients must have a terminal condition and have decision-making capacity. A person such as Jean-Dominique, diagnosed with locked-in syndrome, might not be considered to be terminal, and even if he or she were, the patient would be unable to fulfill another requirement—the ability to take the prescribed medication oneself.

Other limitations to self-determination include obstacles that exist within our health care system that prevent implementation of self-determination, such as family members who may be divided about what should be done for the patient, surrogate decision makers who do not accurately express the patient's known wishes or do not know the patient's wishes, physician and institutional bias toward (or against) treatment, and caregiver fear of litigation and practice of defensive medicine in refusing to allow the patient's wishes—often to forgo life-sustaining medical treatment.

When conflicts occur among patients, families, and caregivers concerning issues such as futility and requests to forgo life-sustaining treatment, or identified barriers to patient self-determination exist, ethics committees and ethics consultants may be helpful in facilitating communication and resolving these conflicts. Once the patient's autonomous wishes are known and are determined to be within acceptable ethical and legal limits, caregivers have an obligation to respect these wishes. In the scene described from *The Diving Bell and the Butterfly*, Henriette portrays the frustration and, at times, anger of a caregiver whose patient seems to be refusing beneficial and life-sustaining medical treatment. For her, it is not just a professional duty but also a personal investment in another person's life that he is rejecting. Although her feelings are understandable, she realizes quickly that she has stepped "out of line." Henriette knows she must ultimately respect her patient's wishes, even if she is disappointed by them.

Although the dialogue in the film is in French with subtitles, the bioethical issues need no translation. Self-determination, resistance from caregivers to patients who request to die, and communication barriers are well recognized across Western cultures. The technique of using Jean-Dominique's point of view for much of the film, and the depiction of the enormous effort it takes him to communicate his wishes is instructive of the central importance of self-determination for patients and caregivers alike. Ultimately, Jean-Dominique Bauby's ability to express himself and write his memoir becomes his temporary butterfly-like escape from his diving bell of locked-in syndrome. He died days after his book was published. That might have been thought a tragedy for his caregivers, but death is exactly what he told his therapist he really wanted.

REFERENCES

1. Bauby, J.-D. 1998. *The Diving Bell and the Butterfly*. New York: Random House Vintage International.
2. Beauchamp, T.L., and Childress, J.F. 2001. *Principles of Biomedical Ethics*. 5th ed. New York: Oxford University Press.
3. Junkerman, C., Derse, A.R., and Schiedermayer, D.L. 2008. *Practical Ethics for Students, Interns and Residents: A Short Reference Manual*, 3rd ed. Hagerstown, MD: University Publishing Group.
4. Schloendorff v. Society of New York Hosp. 211 N.Y. 125, 129–130, N.E. 92, 93 (1914).
5. Salgo v. Leland Stanford, Jr. University Board of Trustees, 152 Cal.App.2d 560, 317 P.2d 170 (1957).
6. Bartling v. Superior Court, 163 Cal.App.3d 186, 209 Cal. Rptr. 220 (1984). Bouvia v. Superior Court, 179 Cal.App.3d 1127, 225 Cal. Rptr. 297 (1986).
7. Meisel, A. 1993. The legal consensus about forgoing life-sustaining treatment: Its status and prospects. *Kennedy Institute of Ethics Journal* 2: 309–345.
8. The Patient Self-determination Act of 1990 (PSDA) (Sections 4206 and 4571 of the Omnibus Budget Reconciliation Act of 1990, PL 101–508). Effective December 1, 1991.

9. World Medical Association International Code of Medical Ethics. Adopted by the 3rd General Assembly of the World Medical Association, London, England, October 1949 and amended by the 22nd World Medical Assembly Sydney, Australia, August 1968 and the 35th World Medical Assembly Venice, Italy, October 1983 and the WMA General Assembly, Pilanesberg, South Africa, October 2006. Retrieved November 30, 2009 from http://www.wma.net/en/30publications/10policies/c8/index.html

10. Smith, E., and Delargy, M. 2005. Locked in Syndrome. *British Medical Journal* 330: 406–409.

paternalism and beneficence:
dark victory

marìa luisa pfeiffer and silvia quadrelli

Dark Victory (1939). Bette Davis, Brent Humphrey, Geraldine Fitzgerald, Ronald Reagan. Directed by Edmund Goulding. Duration: 104 minutes.

DVD Chapter 12 scene 00:33:00 to 00:34:37

DARK VICTORY TELLS THE STORY OF Judith (Bette Davis), a wealthy, vivacious young lady and her neurosurgeon, Doctor Steel (George Brent). Judith's recurrent headaches prompt consultation and surgery to remove a brain tumor, which turns out to be a malignant glioma. During the course of her treatment, neither Dr. Steel or Judith's family physician inform her of the diagnosis or that she will probably die within six months, stating instead, "I think I can promise a complete surgical recovery." In this scene, the doctors discuss her diagnosis with the pathologist in the physician's locker room and then proceed to the patient's bedside. They choose to hide the diagnosis, feign good cheer, and lie about the patient's status. Ultimately, Steel and Judith fall in love and wed. The surgeon retires from clinical practice, pursues his dream of becoming a researcher, moves to the countryside, and devotes his energies to assuring Judith's happiness. When she eventually learns the truth, the couple break up. But after Judith becomes conscious of the value of each instant of life, and learns to face her own impending death without fear, they renew their life together.

This scene, in addition to illustrating examples of deceit, suggests that physicians conferred upon themselves the power of a supreme father, responsible for life, death, and even the ways in which we live our lives.[1] In this regard, *Dark Victory* must be taken in the cultural context of the United States in the 1930s, a time when great advances were being projected in the medical sciences. The accepted practices of this period condoned the actions of Dr. Steele and his colleagues because the values portrayed were shared by much of society, including the expectation of a paternalistic relationship between doctors and their patients.

A scene like this would be almost impossible in a contemporaneous film because patients are accepted as moral agents who must be considered within the context of their culture and social environment. Yet, what appears as normative in many cultures may be aberrational in other societal settings. In China, for example, silence surrounds terminal illness, and disclosure of a diagnosis is often considered to be the family's responsibility,[2,3] while often, in Iran, only the patient's family is informed of a diagnosis such as cancer.[4]

In our daily lives, most people accept that a relationship founded on deceit can completely dominate another party's life. When members of a community cannot believe each other, the lack of truthfulness taints all evidence and makes viable judgments impossible. Consequently, we can say that truth is a fundamental value of ethics and coexistence. The question, however, is whether the doctor–patient relationship is in some substantial way different from other person-to-person relationships; in other words, are falsehoods admissible in the service of benevolent health care treatment?

At first, it appears obvious that the clinical encounter is based on a trust explicitly violated when physicians lie to (or withhold the truth from) patients. However, the degree of patient vulnerability that exists turns this relationship into a very unique interaction. Physicians frequently cite humanitarianism and compassion for another's suffering as justifications for hiding the truth. Proponents of this view invoke therapeutic privilege, especially if the physician believes the patient will harm himself if he learns the truth. Indeed, in many instances, the cost of telling the truth cannot be denied. Studies have shown that physicians favor providing frank and truthful survival estimates only 37% of the time to patients with terminal cancer being referred for hospice care and who might request such an estimate.[5]

Realism, optimism, and avoidance are common strategies physicians' use in discussing prognosis. None are completely satisfactory. Being realistic helps patients and physicians make more thoughtful medical decisions, but patients also report that such discussions can be blunt and sometimes brutal,[6] and when prognosis is not accompanied with effective empathy, behaviors can be perceived as uncaring. Data suggest that roughly 20% of patients, particularly those with advanced metastatic disease, do not want complete information about their prognosis,[7] whereas results from several studies report that while patients with cancer want their physicians to provide detailed prognoses, they also want to be given good news and shared optimism about their illnesses.[8]

Discussing prognosis means engaging the patient in a process of growing understanding about his or her situation, understanding the patient's evolving information needs, and providing information in a way that the patient can understand. Although truthtelling is a pillar of the respect for autonomy principle, allowing patients the ability to base decisions on accurate information, its value and impact must be weighed in the context of how autonomy was manifested during the patient's life. A person who has been dependant and with limited autonomy during his or her lifetime because of family circumstances, social position, illiteracy, chronic illness, or economic exclusion cannot be forced to assume full autonomy for the first time in what may be the most difficult moment of his or her existence.

Additionally, any medical whole truth is not a mathematical truth, objective and discernible to all parties, but assumes a margin of uncertainty. It is, therefore, closer to relative or probabilistic truth. Kaplowitz et al.'s study[9] of curable and incurable cancer patients found that a majority of patients want a qualitative prognosis, but that fewer than half want a quantitative estimate: those with poorer prognoses were less likely to request prognostic information altogether. Other investigators have shown that only half of patients want to be told how long they have to live when first diagnosed; many indicate that they want this information only if they ask for it directly.[10] It seems, therefore, that respect for autonomy also means allowing the patients' wishes, not the physician's preferences for disclosure, to dictate the flow and extent of information.

To prevent from succumbing to the temptation of paternalism, physicians can avoid aggravating patient vulnerability by actively listening and treating the patient as an equal, albeit devoid of substantial medical knowledge (although access to the Internet and other social media are rapidly changing this situation). Whereas the doctor possesses medical knowledge, the diseased person has more knowledge about himself, his familial and social surroundings, historical situation, and community engagement. When a patient explicitly requests not to be told, truth-telling can be forfeited, but in other instances, doctors, as virtuous professionals, cannot refuse their obligation of truth-telling in a way that can be found acceptable by that patient. Simple disclosure of data without carefully measuring its impact on the patient cannot be seen as fair behavior for a caregiver.

From a utilitarian perspective, hiding the truth may be acceptable in certain circumstances, such as when a physician is protecting his or her patient against potentially devastating consequences from learning, with no "practical" purpose, of a serious disease or poor prognosis. Principle-based ethics might argue that in these cases, beneficence trumps autonomy as it results in "the greater good" for the patient. The obvious weakness of this approach is that an external agent (the physician) is the one deciding unilaterally what is in the "best" interests of the patient. Sometimes, such decisions can be made in concert with family members or other caregivers. The eventual discovery of deception, however, can seriously damage a therapeutic relationship based on the premise that neither party has bad intentions. Deception also leads to mistrust and anger, often causing patients to become suspicious, litigious, socially isolated, and abandoned.[11]

From a Kantian perspective, lying is extremely difficult to justify. If we accept deceit as legitimate behavior, for example, we must accept it universally; that is, in any similar circumstance. Rationally (for Kant's approach is completely based on reason), as long The Lie is accepted, the concept of truth is denied, because it requires the existence of the lie as its counterpart to exist. Universalizing the acceptance of deceit, therefore, is against reason. When Kant denounced the paternalist state for benevolently restricting the subject's liberty, however, he was comparing it to a protector father who cares for an incompetent youngster, creating not a paternal behavior but a paternalistic one. Absolute custody, as in cases in which a father "owns" his sons, is thus applied to adults. Between doctors and patients, such behaviors can be viewed as a lack of recognition of equality, whereby the physician assumes power over the life, decision-making capacity, and future of the patient, before even receiving permission to do so. This Kantian approach presumes that highly developed universal moral agents make decisions, and that human beings have the consistent ability to make decisions exclusively on a rational basis. Ordinary life proves otherwise.[12]

In *Dark Victory*, we encounter Dr. Steele, the strongest of paternalists, who withholds information, intentionally lies, and falls in love with his patient, thereby finding justification for his behaviors. Dr. Steele never considers Judith's capacity for free will and autonomy. He makes all decisions on her behalf, and uses her illness and his need to care for her as his excuse to abandon his clinical career and become a researcher. He also deceives himself, as is often the case, by believing that he is acting in her behalf and in their "best interests." A more cynical viewer might argue that Dr. Steele has found a way to justify—to rationalize—his new career and someone with the funds to support his choice. A truly virtuous doctor, however, would characteristically respect a patient's' wishes, analyze the situation within the cultural context, reflect on what is right according to the patient's accounts, and act accordingly.

REFERENCES

1. Callahan, D. 1996. The goals of medicine: Setting new priorities. *The Hastings Center Report*.
2. Woo, K. 1999. Care of Chinese palliative patients. *Journal of Palliative Care* 15(4): 70–75.
3. Ross, M., Dunning, J., and Edwards, N. 2001. Palliative care in China: Facilitating the process of development. *Journal of Palliative Care* 17(4): 281–288.
4. Ghavamzadeh, A., and Bahar, B. 1997. Communication with the cancer patient in Iran: Information and truth. *Annals of the New York Academy of Science* 809: 261–265.
5. Lamont, E.B., and Christakis, N.A. 2001. Prognostic disclosure to patients with cancer near the end of life. *Annals of Internal Medicine* 134(12): 1096–1105.
6. Fried, T.R., Bradley, E.H., and O'Leary, J. 2003. Prognosis communication in serious illness: Perceptions of older patients, caregivers, and clinicians. *Journal of the American Geriatric Society* 51: 1398–1403.
7. Jenkins, V., Fallowfield, L., and Poole, K. 2001. Information needs of patients with cancer: Results from a large study in UK cancer centres. *British Journal of Cancer* 84: 322–331.
8. Weeks, J.C., Cook, E.F., O'Day, S.J., et al. 1998. Relationship between cancer patients' predictions of prognosis and their treatment preferences. *Journal of the American Medical Association* 279: 1709–1714.
9. Kaplowitz, S.A., Campo, S., and Chui, W.T. 2002. Cancer patients' desire for communication of prognosis information. *Health Communication* 14: 221–241.
10. Hagerty, R.G., Butow, P.N., and Ellis, P.A., et al. 2004. Cancer patient preferences for communication of prognosis in the metastatic setting. *Journal of Clinical Oncology* 22: 1721–1730.

11. Pfeiffer, M.L. 2000. Veracidad y consentimiento informado en la práctica médica. [Veracity and informed consent at medical practice]. *Jurisprudencia*. Argentina, Buenos Aires, N 6218.

12. Wolf, S. 1997. Moral saints. In: R. Crips, and M. Slote (Eds.), *Virtue Ethics*. New York: Oxford University Press.

5

consent, competence, and capacity: *a beautiful mind*

jay a. jacobson

A *Beautiful Mind* (2001). Russell Crowe, Jennifer Connelly, Christopher Plummer. Directed by Ron Howard. Duration: 136 minutes.

Scene: DVD chapter 16 Scene 01.39.05 to 01.42.3

A *BEAUTIFUL MIND*, INSPIRED BY A true story, explores the life, real and imagined, of John Nash Jr. (Russell Crowe), a brilliant, ultimately Nobel Prize–winning mathematician, who develops schizophrenia. His mind, still beautiful but now untrustworthy, is capable of solving even previously insoluble theoretical problems, but is not always capable of distinguishing reality from paranoid delusions and visual and auditory hallucinations. His medical treatment consisted of insulin shock treatments and an orally administered drug, both accompanied by significant adverse effects. The drug, however, was somewhat effective in controlling the symptoms of schizophrenia. Based on a delusional preoccupation with a conspiracy and his negative experience with treatment, Nash subsequently rejects treatment, leading to nearly catastrophic consequences. Ultimately forced, or at least coerced, into treatment, his heroic will and capacity to compartmentalize and separate reality from fantasy enable Professor Nash to pursue his passion for mathematics, manage his life and relationships, and do the complex work that eventually earns him international acclaim.

On a windy morning when John is responsible for bathing their baby, his wife, Alicia (Jennifer Connelly), steps outside to bring in clothes hanging on the line. The sound of a radio and a banging door draw her to a shed, where she is shocked by evidence of John's unabated schizophrenic delusions. Realizing that he is not taking his drug and fearful for the baby's safety, she rushes back inside the house, and finds and rescues the frightened, crying baby from a tub rapidly filling with water. Actively hallucinating, John imagines that his wife's call to his doctor constitutes a threat and knocks her down with their baby.

In the critical scene, Dr. Rosen has come to the Nash home. John admits that he stopped his medicine because of its side effects, and he acknowledges persistent visual hallucinations. Dr. Rosen warns him that, if untreated, schizophrenia will only worsen, and he recommends readmission to the hospital for more insulin shock and drug therapy. Reluctant to begin another traumatic hospitalization, John fears that it will never end. Dr. Rosen has commitment papers that Alicia can sign that mandate admission and treatment. John hopes that she won't sign, and wishes for more time to work this problem out. He affirms the doctor's judgment that, "I'm not safe anymore." When Alicia asks him if he would hurt her, he says, "I don't know."

This scene illustrates the problem posed by the multitiered concept of informed consent, especially in the context of mental illness, where decision-making capacity and competence are especially hard to isolate and evaluate. The policy and practice of voluntary informed consent arose in response to the forced, experimental, and even lethal treatment of prisoners in Nazi concentration camps. We now follow this principle in clinical settings as well. We grant patients with the mental capacity to make decisions a near absolute right to do so. We expect physicians to provide ample information and permit unforced consent or refusal. They should explain the indications for a treatment, its risks and benefits, and the comparative results of treatment, alternative treatment, and no treatment.

One prerequisite for voluntary informed consent is an environment free of a compelling force that will drive the decision in one direction and negate the patient's ability and freedom to choose. Another is the mental capacity to make a reasoned choice. One way to assess this capacity is to establish if the patient has a set of values and goals, if the patient can communicate and understand information, and can reason and deliberate about the choice.[1]

In this scene, we have a physician who makes an assessment and recommends the medically indicated treatment. He predicts what will happen without treatment. He doesn't address side effects, but also does not dispute the observations that John makes about the negative effects of drug treatment. John has prior personal experience with the risks and benefits of treatment. Thus, to some extent, the "informed" criteria for voluntary informed consent are met. What remains to be considered is whether John Nash, with his undeniable mental capacity for mathematical problem solving, has the mental capacity to make a reasonable and uncoerced personal treatment decision. If he lacks this capacity, others with his best interest in mind can and should make the choice for him. If he has the capacity and refuses the therapy that others think best for him, are there valid and ethical reasons to override that choice?

John, even in his unmedicated, self-acknowledged delusional state does seem to have sustained values and goals. His goal is to pursue his professional work, to solve problems. He values knowledge and his emotional attachment to his wife and child. He is able to communicate and to understand information from the doctor, although he reaches a different conclusion about treatment. Unfortunately, we've seen that he can't reliably discriminate between information coming from a real or an imagined source. He does, however, seem to reason about and give reasons for his choices. His belief about the result of another hospitalization demonstrates his ability to connect an intervention with an outcome, even if the outcome he foresees may not be the positive one for which the doctor and Alicia hope. It is a possible and plausible outcome.

A person's ability to make decisions is both ethically and legally important.[2] In law, it permits individuals to make choices, even choices judged unwise by others, and it makes individuals responsible for intentional actions that break laws or harm others. In medical ethics, it remains the basis for providing relevant information to patients prior to treatment or procedures and for respecting their decision to proceed or refuse. Legal cases about cognitive ability often arise in the context of financial matters, reproductive choices, or crimes. Medical ethics discussions of this ability usually pertain to decisions that affect the individual's health. The law presumes that individuals acquire sufficient decision-making ability when they become adults. The age of adulthood, rather than some demonstrated ability, becomes the standard and is set by statute. The law regards adults, absent evidence to the contrary, to be able and entitled to make their own decisions. The legal term for this is *competent*. Adults retain the right to make a full range of decisions for themselves unless a judge rules, based on evidence, that they are incompetent. Medical ethics is attentive to context and to individual differences in ability. In emergencies, for example, when medical decisions must be made quickly, if patients are temporarily mentally impaired or even unconscious, physicians generally proceed with treatment despite their patient's impaired or absent decision-making capacity, actions justified by the concept of implied consent.

When an adult patient's condition is not emergent and life-threatening, the law and medical ethics agree that consent for treatment is imperative. For patients who are obviously and permanently impaired and who don't refuse treatment, physicians turn to family members to make the decision they believe the patient would have made or, if that's unknown, the decision that would be best for the patient. When patients, who have been functioning independently and making their own decisions, refuse treatment for a dangerous and serious condition, doctors and concerned family members understandably question that patient's ability and right to make what seems to them to be an irrational and self-destructive decision. Before they can force an expressly unwanted medical intervention, physicians should attempt to understand the patient's reasons and capacity to make such decisions.[3]

This medical assessment could be as simple as asking the patient five questions: What is the medical problem? What treatment has been recommended? What will happen to you with and without the treatment? And, what is the reason for the decision? Patients with decision-making capacity demonstrate a correct understanding of the nature of the medical problem, its treatment and prognosis, and have a reason for their decision. When such patients offer a reason that seems irrational and unconnected with a personal, religious, or cultural set of beliefs and values, a more expert evaluation by a mental health professional is appropriate. The expert may conclude that the patient, even though mentally or emotionally ill, has the capacity to make medical decisions. If this expert decides the patient lacks decision-making capacity, the patient or someone on his behalf may still assert his legal competence and right to refuse treatment. If the patient appears to be a threat to himself or others, clinicians can temporarily take steps, such as hospitalization, to address that danger. However, to continue this beyond two or three days, or to begin treatment, will require that a legal determination of competence be made.[4]

Based on her questions to the patient, information from the family, and the opinion of experts, a judge decides whether a patient is competent. If so, the patient retains his right to refuse treatment. If not, the judge will appoint someone to be the guardian and decision maker for the patient. This could be a family member or someone specifically chosen for this task.

A Beautiful Mind doesn't include a legal determination of competence, and it is ambiguous about whether John Nash is ultimately persuaded or voluntarily chooses medical treatment. Fortunately for him and for the viewers, he somehow becomes able to manage the symptoms of his mental illness and resume a meaningful professional and family role. A patient's mental illness and impaired decision making often cause physicians and family members to feel frustration as they try to do what they believe is best for the patient, but encounter what they view as legal obstacles. The law, however, is there to safeguard competent patients' rights and protect their liberty to make even seemingly unwise decisions. The law does balance the rights of individuals to decide against the consequences of their decision for others. Interestingly, even competent patients may have their liberty curtailed if they refuse treatment for a readily communicated serious disease such as tuberculosis. Thus, imminent danger to others and self are reasons for hospitalization or institutionalization that doctors, families, and judges can all agree constitutes dangerous behavior.[5]

When diseases are dire and their treatments are safe, simple, well-tolerated, and inexpensive, highly effective, and life saving, doctors zealously advocate for them and most patients accept their recommendation. When we develop fully effective, better-tolerated treatments for mental illnesses such as schizophrenia, patients may be more willing to accept them and thus help us avoid the ethically, legally, and emotionally fraught decision to force treatment.

REFERENCES

1. Applebaum, P.S. 2007. Assessment of patients' competence to consent to treatment. *New England Journal of Medicine* 357: 1834–1840.
2. President's Commission for the Study of Ethical Problems in Medicine and Biomedical and Behavioral Research. 1982. *Making health care decisions: A report on the ethical and legal implications of informed consent in the patient practitioner relationship*, vol. 1. Washington, DC: Government Printing Office.
3. Brock, D.W., and Wartman, S.A. 1990. When competent patients make irrational choices. *New England Journal of Medicine* 323: 1353–1355.
4. Grisso, T., and Appelbaum, P.S. 1998. *Assessing competence to consent to treatment: A guide for physicians and other health professionals*. New York: Oxford University Press.
5. Kim, S.Y.H. 2006. When does decisional impairment become decisional incompetence? Ethical and methodological issues in capacity research in schizophrenia. *Schizophrenia Bulletin* 32: 92–97.

the challenge of personhood:
lorenzo's oil

michael d. dahnke

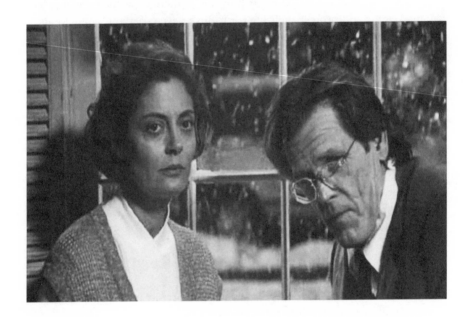

Lorenzo's Oil (1992). Nick Nolte, Susan Sarandon,
Peter Ustinov, Kathleen Wilhoite.
Directed by George Miller. Duration: 129 minutes.

DVD Chapter 13 Scene 01.40:58 to 01.42.37

L ORENZO'S OIL (GEORGE MILLER, 1992) tells the based-on-truth story of
Augusto (Nick Nolte) and Michaela (Susan Sarandon) Odone's efforts to
search for a cure for their young son's (Lorenzo) rare disease, adrenoleukodystrophy (ALD), a genetic disorder causing neurological debilitation and,
eventually, death. The parents research the disease and possible therapies, and
push the medical community for further research. Ultimately, the parents hit upon
a deceptively simple dietary therapy based on the oil of the rapeseed plant,
Lorenzo's Oil, which came to be a therapy for boys with ALD around the world.
By the end of the film, Lorenzo has improved, likely due to the oil. The real
Lorenzo lived to the age of 30, dying on May 30, 2008.[i]

In this scene, Lorenzo has debilitated to a state of immobility and unresponsive-
ness. Despite (or perhaps because of) her son's condition, Michaela constantly
speaks and reads to him. But even for Michaela, a human connection to this
unresponsive boy sometimes seems uncertain and tenuous. She asks her husband,
Augusto, "When you look at him what do you see?" He answers (in Italian), "It's
very difficult to know for sure what is left of our Lorenzo. If a person cannot
move, cannot see, cannot speak, how can we know what is in the soul? He is my
little boy. And my only wish is to have him back as he was before."[ii] Augusto clearly
and succinctly states the problem he and Michaela face: the defining of personhood.
It is unclear whether or to what degree Lorenzo is still a person. Contemplating
the state of Lorenzo at this point in the story provides an excellent opportunity to
investigate and study the concept and ethical challenges of "personhood."

the concept(s) of personhood

Person and *personhood* in philosophical and bioethical contexts are typically used
more conceptually than terms like *human* or *human being*, which are more biological in reference.[1] The concepts of person and personhood are thus much more

contentious matters of philosophical, legal, and even religious debate and negotiation.

Over 300 years ago, the French philosopher René Descartes (1596–1650) argued that our real self (person) is not our body but our mind: a singular, indivisible substance characterized by rationality, thought, and perception. This line of reasoning still deeply influences our conceptions of our selves. Although no consensus on the modern definition of personhood exists, qualities commonly associated with personhood include consciousness, reasoning, self-motivated activity, language use, and self-awareness.[iii] However, by focusing on these externally verifiable mental and psychological qualities, the personhood of infants, the vegetative, and the cognitively impaired becomes uncertain. At the same time, this concept of personhood might be inclusive of nonhumans. Aliens from outer space, higher mammals such as apes, and even computers[2] have all been put forward as potential candidates for personhood.[iv]

Legally, a person is understood as "a subject of legal rights and duties," which, like the philosophical concept of person, may not include all humans—e.g., infants and the incompetent.[v] The law also refers to natural and artificial persons. A natural person arises through natural means and would include all humans. The category of artificial (or unnatural) persons would include corporations and governmental entities, because they are persons as creations of the law, not nature. As legal, although artificial, persons, corporations and governmental entities have legal rights and duties. For example, they can own property and sue and be sued. However, this category is controversial since corporations and governmental entities are not singular coherent beings with their own intelligence and will, but legal fictions made up of persons.[vi]

The religious (Judeo-Christian) concept of personhood identifies the possession of a soul as the mark of personhood and the soul as responsible for the mental qualities of persons. However, even without these qualities manifest, a soul may still be present. Thus, religiously, personhood is often ascribed to fetuses and the vegetative, which are typically difficult and marginal cases in the philosophical and legal concepts. However, other difficulties may arise from basing personhood on an invisible, intangible, unverifiable soul. Essentially, personhood becomes a matter of faith.

Some critics of the concept of personhood have pointed out that this concept does not exist in the same manner in many non-Western cultures,[3] in which the individual is subsumed to the group, the community, or the whole.[vii] These cultures see "the contextual, relational nature of personhood" over the extreme sense of individual rationality and autonomy found in the Western conception of personhood.[viii] However, studying these non-Western concepts of personhood can "raise our own consciousness about some of the distinctive, singular, and even idiosyncratic features of the Western-American way in which we view personhood."[xi]

the ethics of personhood

Ethically, personhood operates as a mark of moral status, the condition of deserving moral treatment and moral consideration. Persons are distinguished from things or mere animals, to which we owe no moral consideration—although the point about animals is presently controversial. Most commonly, the question of personhood arises in the abortion debate. If one holds that a fetus is a person, then abortion is wrong. If a fetus is not a person, then abortion is permissible. Due to the difficulty and uncertainty of the concept of personhood, these arguments commonly reach a stand-still or attempt to bypass the concept of personhood.[x] And, of course, legal personhood is also an issue with abortion since the *Roe v. Wade* decision in 1973. Although the Court refused to make an explicit statement about the moral or philosophical personhood of fetuses, they attributed a minimal legal status to third-trimester fetuses by allowing states to outlaw abortion at that stage, with the exception of abortions to preserve the life or health of the mother. As a matter of faith, the religious concept of personhood contributes deeply to the controversy of abortion. Today, many Christians hold that conception marks ensoulment and the beginning of human life or personhood, thus making all abortions, other than those to save a mother's life, murder.

Recently, similar arguments have arisen regarding the issue of embryonic stem cell research, which could potentially lead to treatments for serious conditions like Parkinson's disease and Alzheimer's disease. However, such research necessitates the destruction of embryos in order to harvest stem cells. If embryos are persons, such research would be ethically troubling. Questions of personhood also arise in issues involving other "marginal" persons such as the comatose, the vegetative, the cognitively and mentally impaired, and even infants and children. In all these cases, questions arise as to what rights are owed these marginal persons, what it means to respect beings in these states. Also, viewing apes as marginal persons raises questions about medical research involving them.

is lorenzo a person?

Later in the film—and years later in the story—Michaela is rewarded for her steadfastness and hope. She is still reading Lorenzo the stories he enjoyed as a small boy. Finally responding to the treatment researched and devised by his parents, Lorenzo communicates that he wishes more age-appropriate material. Still unable to speak, he has developed minimal control over his body, enough to communicate simple desires. It is unclear whether Lorenzo was always a person temporarily trapped in an unresponsive body or if in some way he lost and regained his personhood. This partial recovery, however, does not provide any easy answers. His fortunate outcome cannot inform our reaction to any other specific case of marginal personhood. Such cases will forever remain uncertain in the clinical setting. But, in the words of palliative care physician Ira Byock,[4] "Our task as clinicians is not to provide ultimate answers. Our task is to manifest ultimate commitment… if we are to be of service in the face of persistent suffering, it seems we must allow ourselves to become a vehicle for a more profound and subtle knowledge."[xi] In the spirit of Dr. Byock's statement, the conceptual and practical difficulties and challenges of Lorenzo's personhood dramatized in this film can provide us with greater understanding of such cases and acknowledgment of the need for compassion both for such patients and their families.

NOTES

i. "Obituary: Lorenzo Odone" (2008). Available from NewScientist. Retrieved March 12, 2009 from http://www.newscientist.com/article/dn14060-obituary-lorenzo-odone.html.

ii. Lorenzo's Oil.

iii. These are the qualities identified by Mary Anne Warren in her landmark paper "On the Moral and Legal Status of Abortion." They are not a list of necessary and sufficient conditions but reflect the common types of qualities identified throughout the literature. Warren, M.A. 1973. On the moral and legal status of abortion. *The Monist* 57(1): 43–61.

iv. If an alien species exhibited the mental and social qualities of personhood, we might have to accept them as persons. Regarding computers, see Turing, A.M. October 1950. Computing machinery and intelligence. *Mind*, LIX (236): 433–460. Regarding apes, the Great Apes Project, founded by philosophers Peter Singer and Paola Cavalieri, advocates for the extension of human rights to apes. They have so far found success in New Zealand and Spain. See Glendinning, L. 2008. Spanish parliament approves 'human rights' for apes. Guardian.co.uk, June 26. Retrieved August 25, 2008 from http://www.guardian.co.uk/world/2008/jun/26/humanrights.animalwelfare?gusrc =rss&feed=networkfront.

v. Gray, J.C. The Nature and Sources of the Law. Quoted in *Legal theory lexicon 027: Personhood*. Retrieved August 25, 2008 from http://lsolum.typepad.com/legal_theory_lexicon/2004/03/legal_theory_le_2.html.

vi. *Legal theory lexicon 027: Personhood*. Retrieved August 25, 2008 from http://lsolum.typepad.com/legal_theory_lexicon/2004/03/legal_theory_le_2.html

vii. See De Craemer, W. Winter 1983. A cross-cultural perspective on personhood. The Milbank Memorial Fund Quarterly. *Health and Society* 61(1).

viii. De Craemer, W. Winter 1983. A cross-cultural perspective on personhood. The Milbank Memorial Fund Quarterly. *Health and Society* 61(1): 32.

ix. Ibid.

x. Pro-life "potentiality" arguments asserted that fetuses may not be persons but were at least "potential" persons and should be respected on that status. These arguments, however, ran into logical problems of attributing qualities to a being that belong to a still ontologically distinct being. Judith Jarvis Thomson's famous "violinist" thought experiment assumes the personhood of fetuses in arguing that abortion could still be justified in some cases with that assumption. Don Marquis's pro-life argument replaces personhood with what he calls a "future-like-ours" standard of moral status. See Jarvis Thompson, J. 1971. A defense of abortion. *Journal of Philosophy and Public Affairs* 1: 47–66; Marquis, D. April 1989. Why abortion is immoral. *Journal of Philosophy* 86(4): 183–202.

xi. Quoted in Bretscher, M.E. and Creagan, E.T. August 1997. Understanding suffering: What palliative medicine teaches us. *Mayo Clinic Proceedings* 72(8): 786. Retrieved August 21, 2008 from http://proquest.umi.com.ezproxy.library.drexel.edu/pqdlink?index=23&did=13655414&SrchMode=3&sid=1&Fmt=4&VInst=PROD&VType=PQD&RQT=309&VName=PQD&TS=1236960186&clientId=18133&aid=1.

REFERENCES

1. Macklin, R. 1983. Personhood in the bioethics literature. *The Milbank Memorial Fund Quarterly. Health and Society* 61(1): 35–57. http://www.jstor.org/stable/3349815 (accessed August 21, 2008).

2. Turing, A.M. 1950. Computing machinery and intelligence. *Mind*, LIX, no. 236,: 433–460.

3. De Craemer, W. 1983. A cross-cultural perspective on personhood," *The Milbank Memorial Fund Quarterly. Health and Society* 61(1): 19–34.

4. Bretscher, M. E. and Creagan, E.T. 1997. Understanding suffering: What palliative medicine teaches us. *Mayo Clinic Proceedings* 72(8): 785–787.

the clinician's role in addressing social ills: *vera drake*

felicia cohn

Vera Drake (2004). Imelda Staunton, Phil Davis, Peter Wight, Adrian Scarborough, Heather Craney, Daniel Mays, Alex Kelly, Eddie Marsan, Jim Broadbent. Directed by Mike Leigh. Duration: 117 minutes.

DVD chapter 13 Scene 00.57.46 to 00.59.34

VERA DRAKE (IMELDA STAUNTON) IS a typical working-class woman living in London in 1950. Like many women of her era and class, she spends her days cleaning houses for the upper class, caring for her sick neighbor and elderly mother, and doting on her family. Unknown to her family, however, she also secretly visits women to help them induce miscarriages for unwanted pregnancies, always without remuneration. Although abortion (a term Vera does not use) was illegal in 1950s England, Vera believes she is merely helping women in need, something she simply "has to do." She treats these women with respect, kindness, and compassion. Her portrayal is far from that of the greedy, dirty, and dangerous back-alley abortionist whom the law must stop. Vera has engaged in this practice for "a long time," probably a couple of decades, and the technique she uses is depicted as relatively safe and effective. Then, a woman, whose husband is serving in the military overseas, becomes pregnant as the result of an affair and suffers complications following Vera's assistance; ultimately, she must go to the hospital, and this causes the police to investigate the circumstances of her condition. The criminal proceedings devastate Vera and her family. The film's sympathetic depiction of a kindly abortion provider appears designed to challenge the legal prohibition of abortion. In addition, the movie presents consequential and deontological arguments about abortion and raises questions about the role of law enforcement and the ends of criminal justice. But my focus here is on a different ethical issue.

Nested in this tale of unwanted pregnancy and illegal abortion is a scene that highlights the physician's role in addressing social ills. After the woman described above comes to the hospital showing signs of infection, the physician caring for her questions the patient's mother about her daughter's condition. The mother admits to having called for help to bring about a miscarriage, but initially refuses to say anything more. The physician demands that she reveal who she called and that she contact the police stating, "If you don't call the police, I will." This scene is useful for providing context for discussing questions about the health care professional's responsibility for addressing social problems, mandatory reporting, and the use of coercion.

Privacy and confidentiality are fundamental values that generally refer to the maintenance of personally sensitive information. Functioning within traditional norms may also mean avoiding interference in "private" family matters. As a result, respect for privacy and confidentiality may mean two things for health care professionals: first, an obligation to protect the private information of their patients from others; and second, a focus on treating the presenting symptoms without attention to the personal or social context in which they arise. The duty of confidentiality described in the first sense has persisted since at least the Hippocratic Oath, which requires the physician to swear that, "What I may see or hear in the course of the treatment or even outside of the treatment in regard to the life of men, which on no account one must spread abroad, I will keep to myself holding such things shameful to be spoken about."[1] The American Medical Association's Code of Medical Ethics states that "[t]he information disclosed to the physician during the course of the relationship between the physician and patient is confidential to the greatest possible degree."[2] International codes, such as the World Medical Organization's Declaration of Geneva[3] and the International Code of Medical Ethics[4] also require confidentiality, even after a patient's death. Such codes, reinforced by law, went into effect under the U.S. Health Information Privacy and Accountability Act (HIPAA) in 2003, which protects all forms of individually identifiable personal health information and applies to all health care organizations, providers, and related services (e.g., billing, insurers, information systems).[5]

Although an essential ethical and legal responsibility, privacy creates a conundrum in the practice of medicine highlighted by the second sense of privacy. The goals of privacy and confidentiality are to protect the patient, prevent harm, and maintain trust within the intimate relationship between health care professional and patient. However, protecting a patient's information can be problematic in at least two ways. First, some providers may use privacy as an excuse not to intervene in matters deemed by society to be private, regarding the reasons for a patient's broken bones, knife wound, or miscarriage to be none of their business.[6] Second, protecting private information may become harmful itself, particularly when a victim of some form of violence or illegal activity is returned to that setting and that person or someone else may be harmed if the activity continues.[7]

These problems suggest why health care professionals may bear a responsibility for addressing the social context of a patient's illness, whether that means breaching confidentiality or not. Health care professionals have access to information about individuals not readily shared with others. Patients willingly reveal information about such issues as lifestyle, eating habits, and sexual practices, believing that disclosing such intimacies is necessary to receive the best care possible. Whether a health care professional asks or not, a patient may describe the conditions that resulted in the current illness, such as abuse endured at the hands of her spouse, home-made efforts to end a pregnancy, participation in a crime, or attempts at suicide. The patient may have no one else with whom to share his or her concerns, and nowhere else to turn for guidance and help. Intervening in these social and legal issues themselves may not fall within the scope of clinician practice, but addressing the patient's concerns certainly is the responsibility of the health care professional. Addressing the issue may involve anything from simply listening compassionately to the patient, to making referrals for further help, to enlisting law enforcement. This is the dilemma of the physician in *Vera Drake* and, as such, the scene provides the opportunity to discuss several important issues: whether the physician had an ethical obligation to intervene in this situation; to consider the health care professional's role in law enforcement; to weigh his obligation to patient privacy and confidentiality against his obligations to seek redress for harms to his patient and to protect the public health; and to speculate about his intentions and beliefs (about abortion) and their impact on his decision to notify the authorities.

It is these notions of patient protection and respect for the law that underlie mandatory reporting requirements. Health care professionals' perspectives are often only footnotes in abortion and other contentious societal debates, if mentioned at all. They are expected to obey the law, either refusing to provide illegal services or to provide services that are legal, even if they violate the practitioner's personal values. The law, however, often imposes a role on physicians and other health care professionals, encouraging or requiring them to report illnesses and injuries that arise in the context of activities deemed to be a threat to the public health. Health care professionals may be mandated reporters. Because in the ordinary course of their work they have regular contact with children, disabled persons, senior citizens, or other identified vulnerable populations, health care professionals are required to report physical, sexual, financial, or other types of abuse observed or suspected, including evidence of neglect, knowledge of an incident, or an imminent risk of serious harm. In the United States and other countries, health care professionals may be required to report gunshot and knife wounds, various forms of family violence, and various sexually transmitted diseases.

Mandatory reporting laws[8] may be created with the best intentions, but have become controversial. Consider, for example, mandatory reporting laws for intimate partner abuse and neglect. The goals of the laws may include improvement of the health care response to the underlying cause of illness, aid in victim referral, and assistance with perpetrator prosecution. Clinicians, however, express concern about the impact on the clinician–patient relationship, particularly a reduction in patient trust and concerns about confidentiality, a decrease in health care–seeking behavior, the potential for an escalation in violence if the report is discovered by the perpetrator, creating a false sense of security for the victim, a lack of referral services, inadequate response from law enforcement and assistance organizations, and personal threats to the clinician's safety. As a result, many health care professionals conscientiously object to existing reporting laws. In addition, the reporting laws may serve as a barrier to screening for family violence, as clinicians cannot be obligated to report what they do not know. Victims themselves are ambivalent about reporting requirements. Many believe these requirements can be helpful, but also that the decision to report should be the victim's, due to concerns about increased risk and loss of control. The controversy demonstrates how the important ethical principles—e.g., beneficence, nonmaleficence, patient safety, patient autonomy, justice, and respect for authority—on which medical practice is built may clash. It is unclear whether the physician in *Vera Drake* was subject to a mandatory reporting requirement, but given his knowledge of a crime, he appeared to believe that the authorities must be contacted. Therefore, this scene can serve to raise questions about whether various health care professionals should be mandatory reporters and allow students to consider the benefits and risks of reporting requirements.

Rather than reporting the illegal and botched abortion to the authorities himself, the physician in *Vera Drake* demanded that the patient's mother make the report. He left her little choice, stating that either she could contact the police or he would. Similarly, a physician might insist that a patient reveal a positive human immunodeficiency virus (HIV) test to a spouse or a sexually transmitted disease to sexual partners, that an abused person turn in the abuser, or that a colleague report a drug abuse problem to a supervisor. In some cases, the physician may be legally required to report the findings, as with some sexually transmitted diseases that must be reported to public health agencies, or child abuse that must be conveyed to child protective services. Even if an informing requirement exists, the clinician may attempt to compel the person to provide an account, reveal the information to another person, or seek help him- or herself, either in addition to or instead of the clinician's report. Some might describe such behavior as coercive or manipulative, tactics that are not generally believed to be ethically acceptable. *Coercion* refers to the intentional use of a credible and severe threat of harm or force to control another (e.g., physical or financial). *Manipulation* (informational) involves a deliberate act of managing information in a nonrational, forceful, or misleading manner that alters another's understanding of a situation and thereby motivates that person to do what the agent of influence wants. Examples include lying, withholding information, exaggerating, or using a strong tone. Respect for individual autonomy entails allowing another to make informed, voluntary decisions.[9] Both coercion and manipulation inhibit voluntariness and are contrary to the principle of respect for persons and thus not generally considered ethically appropriate in medical practice, although they may be acceptable in law enforcement. One may attempt to persuade another to believe something or to act. *Persuasion* occurs when one person advances reasons to convince another person to believe in something based on the merit of those reasons. Such discussion or argumentation is ethically acceptable, and sometimes may be considered ethically obligatory. This scene in *Vera Drake* is useful for considering the distinctions among coercion, manipulation, and persuasion; how far health care professionals should go in asserting their beliefs over patients; and clinician responsibility for convincing another person to do what the clinician believes to be right. It also provides context for differing perspectives. Some may argue that the physician was coercive, threatening to report the attempted abortion regardless of the patient's mother's refusal, whereas others may maintain that he effectively persuaded her to do so, based on consequential arguments that things would go better for her if she did. If deemed coercive, some might contend that the physician's behavior was justified by the legal prohibition against abortion, an obligation that all citizens report crimes, and a responsibility for physician's to use their special knowledge of a patient's case to intervene in such situations. Others might assert that the physician should have focused on the medical care of the patient, limiting his involvement in the social or legal issue only to making efforts to persuade the patient and her mother to contact the authorities themselves.

REFERENCES

1. Oath of Hippocrates. 1995. In W.T. Reich (Ed.), *Encyclopedia of bioethics,* vol. 5, p. 2632. New York: Macmillan.
2. Opinion 5.05. In *Code of medical ethics.* Chicago: American Medical Association.
3. World Medical Association Declaration of Geneva. In W.T. Reich (Ed.), *Encyclopedia of bioethics*, vol. 5, pp. 2646–2647. New York: Macmillan.
4. World Medical Association International Code of Ethics. Retrieved January 17, 2009 from http://www.wma.net/e/policy/c8.htm
5. Moskop, J.C., et al. 2005. From Hippocrates to HIPAA: Privacy and confidentiality in emergency medicine. Part I: Conceptual, moral, and legal foundations. *Annals of Emergency Medicine* 45(1): 53–59.
6. Cohn, F., and Rudman, W. 2004. Fix the broken bones and the broken home: Domestic violence and patient safety. *Joint Commission Journal on Quality and Safety* 30: 11 636–646.
7. Cohn, F. 2008. The veil of silence around family violence: Is protecting patient privacy bad for health? *Journal of Clinical Ethics* 19: 4 319–327.
8. For more information see, Cohn, F., Salmon, M.E., and Stobo, J.D. 2001. *Confronting chronic neglect: The education and training of health professionals on family violence.* Washington, DC: National Academy Press.
9. Beauchamp, T.L., and Childress, J.F. 2009. *Principles of biomedical ethics*, 6th ed. New York: Oxford University Press.

research and racism: *miss evers' boys*

annette dula

Miss Evers' Boys (1997). Alfe Woodard, Lawrence Fishburne, Joe Morton, Craig Sheffer. Directed by Joseph Sargent. Duration:118 minutes.

DVD chapter 10 Scene 00:53:42 to 00:55:36

MISS EVERS' BOYS, IS A fictionalized account of the Tuskegee Syphilis Study (formally known as "The Tuskegee Study of Syphilis in the Untreated Negro Male"), in which the government enlisted over 400 Macon County, Alabama, black men in a study that lasted from 1932 to 1972. The movie is largely an account of Nurse Evers' relationship with four of the men. It opens with the 1972 Senate committee hearing. The committee is determined to get at the truth of the Tuskegee Study. Alfe Woodard—acting the part of Nurse Eunice Evers—is testifying before the committee about her role in the study. The movie flashes back and forth between the 1972 hearing and the history of Miss Evers' participation in the study.

Nurse Evers and Dr. Brodus (Joe Morton), the black medical team caring for blacks in a Macon County hospital, find many health conditions that affect their patients. Among them is syphilis. A northern philanthropic organization has decided to use some of its resources to wipe out syphilis in the colored male in Macon County, Alabama. Enter Dr. Douglas (Craig Sheffer), a white physician who becomes the third member of the team treating Negroes for syphilis. All three are elated by the good they are about to bestow. Even before recruitment for treatment begins, the medical team decides—at the suggestion of Nurse Evers—that the men will not be told they have syphilis; rather, the team will label their condition as "bad blood."

The movie focuses on four men with whom Miss Evers develops strong caring relationships, including a romantic relationship with one of the men, Caleb (Lawrence Fishburne). The four comprise a music/dance troupe who desires to go to the Cotton Club in Harlem. In return for signing up for treatment, Miss Evers provides transportation for them as they compete in various area talent shows. In gratitude, they name themselves "Miss Evers' Boys."

When the philanthropic organization is affected by the 1929 economic crash, funds, treatment, and Miss Evers' job dry up. To salvage the situation, Drs. Douglas and Brodus go to Washington to see if they can receive help from the United States Public Health Service (USPHS). They do receive help, but at a cost: the team must study, rather than treat the men. Thus begins the sad saga that lasts for 40 years. The two doctors perceive the turn of events differently. For Dr. Douglas, it is a chance to be a scientist and to contribute to medical knowledge. After initial hesitation at nontreatment, Dr. Brodus brushes away his qualms and convinces himself that it is an opportunity to prove that syphilis is the same in the Negro male as in the white male: the experiment is for the greater good of the race.

Miss Evers' job is restored. The scene where Nurse Evers is informed that no treatment will be given is important; it sets the stage for the rest of the movie. Nurse Evers happily returns to her beloved work, presumably to continue treating the men. Dr. Brodus breaks the news to her: the men will be studied—not treated. Dr. Brodus convinces her that, within a year, the men will again receive treatment for syphilis. Her stunned and unbelieving response inevitably evolves (as the years go by) into sad resignation, acceptance, and ultimately her appearance before the Senate committee 40 years later.

The rest of the film reflects on Nurse Evers' inner conflicts: (1) her knowledge that the men think they are being treated, when they aren't; (2) her love of the men; and (3) her own romantic involvement with Caleb, the one recruit who knows about the deception. Near the end of the movie, for the first time, Nurse Evers finally shows her anger at a racist political system that turned a blind eye to the long study: Nurse Evers angrily retorts to the Chair of the Senate hearing, "the PHS would never have agreed to do the study and Congress would never have voted year after year to fund the study if the men had been white… but because they were black no one cared."

The Tuskegee Syphilis Study is well known across professional, academic, and research communities, including bioethics, public health, medicine, social anthropology. It has remained a particularly prickly thorn in researchers' efforts to enlist people of color in clinical trials. Thousands of articles and many books force us to remember this blatant violation performed on the nation's most vulnerable population. The ethics of the study has been debated, scrutinized, mulled over, and even justified ever since Peter Buxton, through Jean Heller, forced the experiment into the consciousness of the whole world in the *Washington Post* in 1972. James Jones points out that: "… Miss Evers' Boys…[and] the revelations of other kinds of Research that trampled on the rights of subjects… all help to introduce different understandings to broader and broader members of the public and research communities."[1] In that vein, the film actually opens a broader discussion regarding many ethical concerns and suggests several questions for consideration. These include the following:

- *Maintaining the line between care and research.* In the film, we see how easily the role of the provider shifts to that of researcher. In his paper "Experimentation with Human Beings," bioethicist Jay Katz warned that physician-investigators confront a dilemma. As physicians, they are dedicated to caring for their patients; as investigators, they are dedicated to caring for their research.[2] Nurse Evers as provider built up incredible trust. She took that trust with her as she became a researcher. Thus, she easily retained her patients as subjects for experimentation. Such role-shifting also raises several contemporary questions. What is the role of one's physician in patient recruitment? Should a physician caring for patients facilitate a researcher's access to patients? Should an emergency doctor/investigator on duty when a patient is brought to the emergency room be allowed to enroll the patient in her own research? Current restrictions prohibit, for the most part, enrolling research participants without their informed consent, largely a result of outrage over the TSS; but, there are exceptions: Institutional Review Boards can waive consent in planned emergency research if certain conditions are met. Is waiver of informed consent for physicians as researchers ever justifiable, and do physicians ever have a moral justification to enroll their patients in clinical trials without their consent?

- *Unequal power relations.* In addition to the inherent unequal power that the institution of racism maintains, more specific unequal power relations permeate the medical system. The relationship between the two doctors appears to be equal. Yet, the final arbiter of decisions, the white doctor, is merely a proxy for the powerful white institution—the USPHS. In fact, the medical team all become objects to achieve the USPHS's end. In what sense might one argue that providers stand on equal power footing with pharmaceutical and insurance companies? Can Dr. Douglas also be seen as a victim of unequal power?

- The power relations between physicians and nurses are also clearly marked. On a number of occasions, Dr. Brodus, in the presence of his patients, almost threateningly asserts and reasserts to the nurse that the doctor knows best and even demands agreement from her. Constant affirmation of one's skills to others can lead to physician arrogance. At first Nurse Evers gladly accepts that "the doctor knows best." She finally breaks that hold by seizing her own personal power, stealing penicillin, and giving it to one of her "boys." Regrettably, it is too late. After Nurse Evers seizes power, she does not hold on to it, but again accepts the nontreatment of her patients. What explanations might one offer about the way in which Nurse Evers thereby participates in her own oppression as a woman and as an African American?

- *Conflicts of interest.* Does the romantic relationship between Caleb and Nurse Evers present nurse–patient ethical issues? Are there conflicts of interest between Dr. Douglas and the USPHS? Between the two doctors? Nurse Evers uses the government car to take men to musical competitions. Can this be seen as bribery, coercion, or compensation?

- *Communication between black patients and white doctors.* In the movie, Dr. Douglas addresses the men using incomprehensible medical jargon. Nurse Evers translates, so that the men understand what he is saying. Facial expressions change as understanding sets in. Several studies have found that African American patients rate their visits with physicians as less participatory than whites; there is less information exchange between white physician and black patients, although African Americans would like to have more information from white physicians than they are given.[3] A 2008 study from Johns Hopkins found that black patients had shorter office visits, less exchange of biomedical and psychosocial information, and less rapport building with doctors than did their white counterparts.[4] Given that problems in communication often result from unequal power, what reforms are needed to improve communication and understanding, thereby improving health outcomes? Should it be important who treats African Americans (and other minority or underserved populations), given that they have such poor health?

- *Health disparities.* At the time of the Tuskegee study, black people faced numerous health problems and unnecessary deaths, including from tuberculosis (TB), malaria, excessive malnutrition, pellagra, syphilis, and lynchings. Today, health disparities persist between whites and the nation's minority populations and poor people. Almost 80 years after the start of TSS, African Americans still face excessive health disparities in cancers, heart disease, asthma, acquired immune deficiency syndrome (AIDS), infant mortality, and longevity (to name only a few),[5] and, in this second decade of the 21st century, unnecessary deaths still occur due to inequalities in health status, access, and quality of care. To what extent might racism still play a role in the poor health of African American and other racial/ethnic minorities? What kinds of reforms are needed to eliminate health disparities among U.S. populations? At the time of the Tuskegee study, end-of-life care meant access to a decent burial. What does end-of-life care mean to African Americans today?

Several years ago, when I was giving a talk on the TSS at a workshop for researchers, one of the workshop participants voiced anger at having to listen to "more stuff on Tuskegee." She was, she said, well aware of the study, and another presentation wasted her time and workshop money. But Tuskegee is only one example of such abuses of power. Others, occurring at the same time as the Tuskegee consciousness, began to appear in popular media in the 1980s and 1990s: the Holmesburg Prison's experimental research program lasted 23 years, from 1951 and 1974.[6] Between 1946 and 1974, the U.S. government sponsored radiation experiments on human subjects without their consent. What conditions in the United States allowed all three studies to last so long?[7]

In a recent book, Rebecca Skloot[8] narrates the development of a cell line from the cancer cells of Henrietta Lacks. Lacks, an African American, died of cervical cancer in 1951. Before her death, cells were removed—without her knowledge or consent—from her cervix. The first immortal cell line ever grown in culture was established from these cells. Both science and individuals have benefitted enormously. Her cells were used to develop polio vaccine, and they help advance in vitro fertilization, cloning, and gene mapping. The sad irony here is that this African American woman contributed much to the fight against cancer and many other diseases. Yet, the benefits of her contribution continue to be shared disproportionately with African Americans as health disparities continue decade after decade.[5]

So, to answer that sceptical workshop participant: Yes, providers, researchers, and the general population still need TSS narratives, movies like *Miss Evers' Boys*, books like Susan Reverby's *Tuskegee's Truths*,[9] and Jones' *Bad Blood*,[10] and other reminders of tragedies and harms caused by the injustices of both unequal care and research abuse—twin tragedies often heaped on our most vulnerable populations.

REFERENCES

1. Jones, J.H. 2000. Foreword. In S. Reverby (Ed.), *Tuskegee's truths*, pp. xi–xiii. Chapel Hill, NC:University of North Carolina Press.
2. Katz, J. 1993. Human experimentation and human rights. *St. Louis Law Journal* 38(1): 7–54.
3. Cooper-Patrick, L., et al.1999. Race, gender, and partnership in the patient-physician relationship. *Journal of the American Medical Association* 282: 583–589.
4. Cené, C.W., Roter, D., Carson, K.A., Miller, E.R., and Cooper, L.A. 2009. The effect of patient race and blood pressure control on patient-physician communication. *Journal of General Internal Medicine* 24(9): 1057–1064.
5. Orsi, J.M., Margellos-Anast, H., and Whitman, S. 2010. Black–white health disparities in the United States and Chicago: A 15-year progress analysis. *American Journal of Public Health* 100(21): 349–356.
6. Hornblum, A.M. 1998. *Acres of skin*, p. 297. New York: Routledge.
7. Faden, R., Lederer, S.E., and Moreno, J.D. 1996. US medical researchers, the Nuremberg doctors trial, and the Nuremberg Code: A review of findings of the Advisory Committee on Human Radiation Experiments. *Journal of the American Medical Association* 276: 1667–1671.
8. Skloot, R. 2010. *The immortal life of Henrietta Lacks*, p. 169. New York: Crown Publishers.
9. Reverby, S. 2009. *Examining Tuskegee: The infamous Syphilis Study and its legacy*, p. 384. Chapel Hill: University of North Carolina Press.
10. Jones, J.H. 1981. *Bad blood: The Tuskegee Syphilis Experiment*, p. 272. 1981. New York: Free Press.

9

justice, autonomy, and transhumanism: *yesterday*

september williams

Yesterday (2004). Leleti Khumalo, Kenneth Khambula, Harriet Lenabe, Lihle Mvelase, Camilla Walker. Directed by Darrell Roodt. Duration: 96 minutes.

DVD chapter 9 scene 01.09:55 to 01.10:58

YESTERDAY IS ABOUT A YOUNG black South African mother with human immunodeficiency virus/acquired immune deficiency (HIV/AIDS). Yesterday (Leleti Khumalo) lives with her daughter, Beauty (Lihle Mvelase), in her husband John's remote rural village in the Kwazuli Natal province of South Africa. In the economic tradition, not yet abolished by the end of apartheid, John (Kenneth Khambula) works as a migrant miner. Yesterday, an uneducated outsider in John's village, is attracted to the grace of the village's new teacher (Harriet Lenabe). While her daughter is not yet school age, Yesterday develops a persistent cough, a sign of AIDS. Her husband, who ultimately becomes terminally ill, batters her after she travels hundreds of miles to the mine and informs him of her infection. Supported by the Teacher, Yesterday combats inadequate health care, ignorance, fear, abuse, and alienation. Facing death, she establishes her own goals, completing universal tasks associated with the developmental stage of life's end. By exercising her autonomy, Yesterday brings meaning to a life assaulted by injustice.

Yesterday provides ample opportunities to facilitate consideration of: (1) medical triage justice issues in resource limited circumstances, (2) autonomy in cross-cultural geopolitical context, and (3) how the discipline of clinical medical ethics, and the clinically relevant 21st century philosophical movement, transhumanism, intersects the course of the HIV/AIDS pandemic.

The scene of primary interest is no longer than a sigh. Yesterday attempts to access hospital care for her husband. She walks into the hospital, which has become a hospice for people dying of AIDS. A close-up, foreground shot of a man similar to John reminds viewers that Yesterday's husband is but one of many. The camera pans, like Yesterday's eye, looking for a way to help her husband. The only empty bed on the ward is being cleansed of negative spirits by a traditional ceremony, in preparation for its next occupant, who will clearly not be John. A kind but realistic nursing sister offers to place John on a waiting list. The film's ever-present background music has stopped, leaving Yesterday disconnected from her inner self as she speaks with the nurse. A wide camera angle, with a deep focus, expands the volume of the sick, overwhelming the viewer with the hopelessness of Yesterday's quest. In an earlier scene, Yesterday herself was also denied access to a clinic. Her own cough had worsened, and she had walked a long twisted road to the clinic with her daughter Beauty. Because the two could not walk there early enough to make the cutoff in the queue, both were turned away without seeing a doctor.

In these two scenes, Yesterday and John are triaged by two separate models. They are triaged irrationally on both the *first-come, first-served* and *limited resource* models. Clinicians utilize the limited resource model during war, trauma, and disaster. Wartime triage says, "expend resources only on those likely to benefit."[1] This means that those most likely to die with or without medical attention are left to die. The first-come, first-served model is used for minor non–life threatening issues. It is the muddled rationale for their denial, in the face of medical knowledge, that leaves us uneasy. Clinical medical ethics helps dissect the discomforting events seen on the screen. Analyzing such discomforting "eyebrow-raising events" often exposes ethical conflicts.

In clinical medical ethics, the principle of beneficence obligates clinicians to apply known medical knowledge appropriately. In Yesterday's case of "cough," medical knowledge supports early serological diagnosis, antiretroviral intervention, pneumocystis (a sentinel pulmonary disease in AIDS) treatment or prophylaxis, interventions to block further HIV transmission, and tuberculosis evaluation. All of the above were eventually offered to Yesterday in the film, so they were available. South Africa is relatively wealthy in material resources, as opposed to other countries caught up in the sub-Saharan HIV/AIDS epidemic. John, although terminally ill, should have been offered inpatient-based hospice support to diminish his suffering. Based on the similarity between John and the other patients shown, the hospital is clearly only providing palliation.

Yesterday's care delay was not because South Africa has limited drug resources. Drugs are only one of the technologies impacting the HIV/AIDS pandemic. The rules of clinical triage required that the nurse managing the clinic's access ask Yesterday about her illness. After assessing her risks, her position in the line should have been determined. Her symptoms of persistent and worsening cough would have flagged an increase risk. Similarly, the nurse in the hospital was not portrayed as having asked risk stratifying questions about John and Yesterday's illnesses.

Triage is facilitated by communication. If the depicted nurses (likely representing a protocol established by a doctor) elicit answers to the appropriate questions, the outcome for triage is based on medical indications, or beneficence. Yesterday would bump the line based on increased need and risk. Gunshot victims access emergency services ahead of those with stubbed toes. Yesterday's risks of death *and* spreading AIDS could have been diminished by earlier appropriate triage. John's, Yesterday's, and Beauty's suffering would have been diminished by his admission to the hospital for palliative care. The benefit of intervention beyond the single individual is essential in triage during epidemic management.

Often, as in this case, a nagging eyebrow-raising event is not the true ethical issue. The apparent clinical ethical conflict in the scenes of interest is not primarily violations of justice, but violations of beneficence. They are examples of "bad medicine," because neither nurse in either scene asked the questions that appropriate triage science demands. The two scenes differ, therefore, in their role in the story. While the clinic scene foreshadows Yesterday's lack of information and assertiveness as a barrier to overcome, the hospital scene flags the end of her victimization and anticipates her radical increase in autonomy.

Clinical medical ethicists (1) clarify ethical conflicts, (2) facilitate paradigm shifts to promote clinical ethical decision making, and (3) recommend ethically acceptable courses of clinical action. Clinical medical ethics is an applied arm of bioethics and as such is predetermined to result in action. For better or worse, clinical medical ethics uses both casuistry and ethical principles–based analysis to explore clinical ethical conflicts. Casuistry uses case- or story-based narratives to enhance moral reasoning.[2] Tensions between competing "goods" or ethical principles are dissected from the case.

The most often taught clinical medical ethics decision-making paradigm explores tensions between ethical principles in ranked order: beneficence (medical indications), autonomy (respect for the rights of persons in the context of culture and family), and justice (equitable distribution of benefits and burdens in the context of geopolitical structures).[3] Ranking ethical concerns is a device for prioritizing considerations to facilitate clinical action. Anecdotally, reversing the order of clinical ethical analysis, say beginning with justice, rarely promotes timely clinical ethical response because geopolitical and other social contextual features often range beyond patient and clinician control. Instead, when clinical ethicist stay "close to the bedside," focused first on medical indications and the individuals involved, clinical evidence induces justice as a collateral benefit.

The field of clinical medical ethics and HIV/AIDS share the same historical timeline (both beginning in the 1970s). Clinical medical ethics emerged as a separate clinical field to operationalize the Belmont Commission Report on the Protection of Human Research Subjects.[4] The Belmont Commission was the U.S. federal government's response to research and clinical violations of the U.S. Public Health Service Syphilis Study at Tuskegee (1934–1974).[5]

Many clinical medical ethical decisions have influenced the HIV/AIDS pandemic course.[6] These influences include new technologies applied to (1) prevention and public health[7]; (2) delivery of health care and provision of care to individuals and unborn children[8]; (3) advancing relevant biomedical and behavioral research; (4) stringency of informed consent across race, class, and culture related to clinical practice and biomedical/behavioral research[9,10]; (5) assuring appropriate application of palliative care, and (6) geopolitical analysis of security by the United Nations Security Council in defining sub-Saharan HIV/AIDS as a threat equivalent to war.[11] "Technology" is used here specifically to mean the applied arm of all sciences, physical and social. Ranking beneficence concerns first in the analysis of ethical conflicts often exposes gaps in medical knowledge. The assumption that HIV/AIDS can be controlled and cured derives from a transhumanist approach.[12]

Transhumanism is a philosophical movement that assumes a moral imperative for human beings to live longer and better. The goals of transhumanism focus on developing science and technology practically aimed at expansion of the human lifespan. The expansion of lifespan by the systematic removal of barriers to longevity is a fundamental force in the advancement of medical knowledge and public health. Transhumanists believe that technology is the answer to maximizing human potential beyond its current constraints, including morbidity and mortality. Although transhumanism is operant in technologies from cryogenics use in organ death prevention to disease eradication by vaccines, most are familiar with the movement's agendas through its influence on futurist films. These films provide "compelling illustrations for independently worked philosophical ideas."[13] A chasm exists between the transhumanist agenda and the reality of the sub-Saharan African HIV/AIDS epidemics.

Sub-Saharan Africa remains the region most heavily affected by HIV worldwide, accounting for two-thirds of all people living with HIV, and for three-quarters of AIDS deaths in 2007. An estimated 1.9 million people were newly infected with HIV in sub-Saharan Africa in 2007, bringing to 22 million the number of people living with HIV in that region.[14]

The gap in understanding of this pandemic's drivers persists not only among the HIV affected on the ground in Africa and elsewhere, but also in academic ivory towers. Health care delivery systems will not expand their understanding while academic disciplines are slow to do so. Clinical medical ethics is a tool for the analysis of such gaps in understanding. One strength of *Yesterday* is its exploration of slow understanding in overwhelmed health care system providers, compared with role modeling rapid growth in understanding for our heroine. There is wide variation between how people understand. Bioethicists Beauchamp and Childress say, "An analysis sufficient for our purposes is that persons understand if they have acquired pertinent information and justified relevant beliefs about the nature and consequences of their actions."[15]

Yesterday portrays, with cross-generational aesthetic accessibility, a young black South African woman who learns to understand her HIV/AIDS. She acts in her own best self-interests as a consequence of her understanding. The AIDS community reports: "Sub-Saharan Africa's HIV/AIDS epidemics vary significantly from country to country. Those regions with improving burdens of HIV/AIDS have consistently used a multifactorial approach of education, barrier prevention, antiretroviral and most importantly, the enhancement of the autonomy of women."[14]

Practitioners of clinical medical ethics use both principle-based and narrative case analysis to enhance moral reasoning. A film such as *Yesterday* illustrates numerous clinical ethical concerns and exemplifies how film narrative can be used to enhance health understanding. In its portrayal of a young South African woman's burgeoning autonomy, *Yesterday* also earns a place in the futurist film genre. Its story, written in an ancient tribal language, is set against the stark minimalism of rural Kwazulu Natal, and provides a futurist view of the strength of a people to transcend HIV/AIDS. Resource-stressed triage issues become a minor theme in the face of Yesterday's transformation to autonomy-driven justice. Indeed, through the film's astounding nonviolent climax, Yesterday emerges as a super-heroine, building from the peri-apartheid neocolonial rubble a new place transcending the confines of her sick body and shortened lifespan.

REFERENCES

1. Jonsen, A., Winslade, W., and Siegler, M. 2002. *Clinical medical ethics,* 4th ed., p. 173. New York: McMillan.
2. Jonsen, A., and Toulman, S. 1988. *The abuse of casuistry: A history of moral reasoning.* Berkley: University of California Press.
3. Jonsen, A., Winslade, W., and Siegler, M. 2002. *Clinical medical ethics,* 4th ed. New York: McMillan.
4. The Belmont Commission Report Federal Registry 1974.
5. Clinton, W.J. 1997. *Remarks by the president in apology for the study done in Tuskegee.* Washington, DC: The White House, office of the Press Secretary.
6. Williams, S. 2000. The need for autonomy driven HIV prevention and treatment. In M. Secundy, A. Dula, and S. Williams (Eds.), *Bioethics research concerns and directions for African-Americans,* pp. 98–106. Tuskegee University National Center for Bioethics in Research and Health Care.
7. Editorial. *Washington Post* June 17, 1995: A 16.
8. Benatar, S.R. 2008. Global health ethics and cross-cultural considerations in bioethics. In P.A. Singer, and A.M. Viens (Eds.), *The Cambridge textbook of bioethics,* pp. 341–349. Cambridge: Cambridge University Press.
9. Dula, A., and Williams, S. 2005. When race matters. *Clinics in Geriatric Medicine* 21: 239–253.
10. Karim, Q.A., Karim, A.S, et al. 1998. Informed consent for HIV testing in a south African hospital: Is it truly informed and truly voluntary? *American Journal of Public Health* 88(4): 637–640.
11. Kofi Annan. *Report of the Secretary-General on the Work of the Organization.* General Assembly Official Records Fifty-fifth session Supplement No.1 (A/55/1). New York: United Nations, 2000, p.4. Retrieved December 10, 2010 from http://www.un.org/documents/sg/report00/a551e.pdf.
12. Retrieved December 4, 2010 from http://humanityplus.org/learn/transhumanist-declaration/
13. Shapshay, S. 2009. Introduction: Pedagogical function of film. In *Bioethics at the movies,* p. 5. Baltimore, MD: The Johns Hopkins University Press.
14. Retrieved December 4, 2010 from http://data.unaids.org/pub/globalreport/2008/20080715_fs_regions_en.pdf. Source:http://data.unaids.org/pub/GlobalReport/2008/jc1511_gr08_executivesummary_en.pdf.
15. Beauchamp, T., and Childress, J. 1994. *Principles of bioethics.* New York: Oxford University Press Inc. p. 88.

10

another kind of dnr: *titicut follies*[i]

therese jones

Titicut Follies (1967). Black-and-white documentary by Frederick Wiseman.
Duration: 84 minutes. Purchase or rental of VHS or DVD is available from
Zipporah Films, Inc.

DVD Chapter 5 (45:43 to 53:43)

ITICUT FOLLIES IS THE FIRST major, full-length documentary by Frederick
Wiseman, considered to be the most successful independent filmmaker in
the United States. Critics aptly describe Wiseman's films as both "artistic
experiences and social documents," revealing the complex politics of American
institutions and exploring difficult legal, social, educational, and scientific issues.[1]
Titicut Follies (the title is taken from an annual talent show produced by inmates
and staff) was filmed at the Massachusetts Correctional Institution, in Bridgewater,
a sprawling facility of four divisions, one of which was the state hospital for the
criminally insane. Of the 2,000 men warehoused there in the 1960s, only 15% had
ever been convicted of a crime. Yet, the institution was administered by the
Department of Corrections rather than the Department of Mental Health—units
representing very different and contradictory goals. Both the correctional and
medical staff were undertrained and underpaid, and physicians "marginal within
their own profession" often provided treatment. At the time of the filming, only
two psychiatrists and one trainee were caring for the 600 men in the hospital
section.[1]

Believing that public awareness of the terrible conditions at Bridgewater would
create an impetus for reform and a demand for improvement, Wiseman represented
to administration and staff the goal of his proposed film project as educational,
ultimately gaining unlimited access to the facility. Using relatively new technology
such as high-speed film that enabled shooting in natural light, telephoto lenses,
and a directional microphone that picked up usually inaudible sounds, the crew
freely and openly photographed naked inmates periodically hosed down, tor-
mented by guards, or confined to bare, unlit cells. The result was a bitterly critical,
shockingly brutal documentary account of the prison hospital, and despite initially
giving Wiseman permission to make the film, the Commonwealth of Massachusetts
quickly moved to ban its release upon completion. In September 1967, just days
before it was to be screened at the New York Film Festival, the attorney general
filed an injunction that would permanently forbid the documentarian from ever

showing the film to anyone. In 1969, the Massachusetts Supreme Court permitted
its use with doctors, lawyers, health care professionals, and students, and finally, in
1991, the courts allowed its release to the general public. *Titicut Follies* is the only
American film "whose use [has had] court-imposed restrictions for reasons other
than obscenity or national security."[1]

The scene featured in this chapter occurs in the middle of the documentary. It
begins with a physician quickly and casually checking on an inmate through the
small opening in the cell door. He subsequently reports to other medical personnel
that the inmate has not eaten in at least three days and orders that he be force-fed.
Accompanied by several large, uniformed guards, the naked and shrunken inmate
appears totally unresponsive, either unwilling or unable to comply with the
physician's request that he ingest the liquid feed by mouth. He remains silent and
docile as the guards tie his hands and feet to the corners of a gurney before the
physician carelessly proceeds to snake an ill-lubricated tube (he swipes it around an
empty jar of petroleum jelly several times) into the inmate's nostril.

In this scene, Wiseman chooses to use both close-up shots and didactic editing.
The camera moves slowly back and forth among the physician's frown of concentration, the patient's stoic countenance, and the guard's nonchalant expression.
Moreover, Wiseman consistently juxtaposes the callous force-feeding of the ema-
ciated with images of this same man after death. The physician is so unconcerned
about the patient's well-being and so disrespectful of his personhood, that the ash
from the doctor's cigarette, which has dangled from his mouth throughout the
procedure, falls into the funnel at the end of the tube. The director crosscuts these
images with the quiet, reverential preparation of the corpse by another staff
member who gently lathers the inmate's cheeks, carefully fills his eye sockets with
cotton, and finally dresses him in suit and tie. At the end of the scene, the doctor
dismisses the inmate with a compliment, "Very good patient... very nice," as he is
escorted down an empty and dismal prison corridor. That image is immediately
followed by the coroner closing the morgue drawer on which the casket is placed.

If we apply any of the criteria that Gregory Pence uses to specify what he calls
"classic cases in medical ethics," those cases that have shaped our laws, our
institutions and our consciousness,[2] then the complicated production and legal
history of *Titicut Follies* would qualify it as a landmark case in documentary ethics.
The film serves as a paradigm case in any examination of issues endemic to the
documentary enterprise, such as the balance of risks and benefits, the principle of
informed consent, the norms of privacy, and the question of voyeurism. Moreover,
when the subjects of a film are patients—in this instance, wards of the state in a
prison hospital—ensuring their decisional capacity and their individual preferences, as well as protecting their privacy, becomes highly problematic.

balancing risks and benefits

In his famous 1926 essay, "First Principles of Documentary," John Grierson
described documentary as the "creative treatment of actuality," and posited it as

an incredibly powerful tool for social reform and political communication. The defining and redefining of the medium has been an ongoing process "as each decade has brought social upheavals that cried for documentation" and produced technological innovations to meet the challenges."[3] However, one demand of documentarians has remained consistent albeit naïve—objectivity. Describing his own work as "reality fictions," Wiseman dismisses any claims of film truth: "the events are all real, except they have no meaning except insofar as you impose a form on them and that form is imposed in large measure, of course, in the editing."[1] In essence, documentarians make endless choices, and each choice is an expression of a point of view. Moreover, because the documentary tradition is driven by a desire for social justice yet relies on the impression of authenticity, there is often an inherent conflict between persuading and informing, advocating, and entertaining. As scholar Bill Nichols notes, "Of what risks should filmmakers inform their subjects? To what extent can filmmakers reveal their intentions?"[4]

While social activists promote protection in inverse relationship to power, documentary filmmakers work the other way around, and collateral damage of the powerless, the group in need of the most protection, can result. A 2009 report from the Center for Social Media at American University, "Honest Truths: Documentary Filmmakers on Ethical Challenges in Their Work," concludes that documentarians feel bound less by the need to be fair than by the desire for social justice, and they admit to manipulating institutions, individuals, and images to help viewers grasp the documentary's higher truth.[5] For instance, Eric Steel, director of the *The Bridge* (2006), which photographed jumpers from the Golden Gate Bridge over the course of one year, was sanctioned by authorities who felt they were misled when he obtained permission for the project. Although the documentary achieved its objectives—forcing the city to reconsider the issue of suicide barriers and calling attention to the plight of the mentally ill—the footage of individuals committing suicide can be rightly considered cruel and grotesque. When the Commonwealth of Massachusetts argued that *Titicut Follies* was a sensational, exploitative product of dubious educational value, Wiseman's defense countered with the public's right to know what transpires in a public-supported institution: "public scandal cannot be revealed without scandalous revelation."[1]

obtaining informed consent

The dominant mode of *Titicut Follies* is observational, also called "direct cinema," which was popularized by Wiseman. It stresses the nonintervention of the filmmaker, relies on editing to enhance the impression of real time, and is characterized by synchronous images and sounds at the moment of filming, affording viewers an opportunity to look in on and overhear the lived experience of others and creating an effect that what they see is what occurred spontaneously before the camera, with little or no intervention or modification. This film especially exposes the substantial but not uncommon gap between the ideal of informed consent and the practice of direct cinema. Similar to health care professionals, a wide consensus exists among documentary filmmakers that consent is not valid unless it is given under conditions free of coercion and deception and with knowledge of the procedures and anticipated effects by someone competent.[1] Thus, a documentary filmed at a state institution that functions as both a prison *and* a hospital strains such conditions of validity. When challenged by the state about specific shots, such as the verbal and physical abuse of a nude inmate, the intake interview between a psychiatrist and a child molester, and the force-feeding of the naked, catatonic patient, Wiseman's response was simple: He assumed that all subjects were competent unless the staff informed him otherwise, putting the moral burden and ethical responsibility squarely back on institutional personnel. Much like the conflicts of interest that arise when documentarians, determined to right social wrongs, must first get access and support to make a film and next, get people to see it, the issue of informed consent often highlights the inherent conflict between ethics aesthetics: "Without the informed consent of the subjects, the form lacks ethical integrity; without freedom for the filmmaker, it lacks artistic integrity."[1] Two recent documentaries, *Out of the Shadow* (2006) and *Thin* (2004) also represent the tension between photographing subjects who are extremely mentally ill in order to focus attention on the inadequacies of the systems designed to care for them. In *Out of the Shadow,* filmmaker Susan Smiley includes one troubling scene in which she and her sister lie in order to coerce their psychotic mother, Millie, to consent to treatment. The viewer can only assume (and hope) that Millie had an opportunity to consent to the inclusion of this scene after the fact. Although the mostly underage girls hospitalized for eating disorders speak coherently and act reasonably in *Thin*, the corporeal reality of their grave illness—their starving bodies—challenges that assumption. Yet, filmmaker Lauren Greenfield gains access to individual and group therapy sessions, morning weigh-ins, and private bathrooms where girls smoke or vomit secretly.

protecting privacy and questioning voyeurism

In fiction films, scenes are contrived so that a viewer oversees and overhears someone, an actor, who is playing a role. In documentary, a viewer witnesses the lived experience of actual persons. As Nichols points out, looking through the documentary "keyhole" can simultaneously exploit subject and viewer.[4] Not surprisingly, Wiseman was charged with violating the rights to privacy of both inmates and staff in *Titicut Follies*. At the time, the American Civil Liberties Union (ACLU) struggled with how to "rein in technology's power to surveil, record and disseminate the details of a person's life... yet [use] that power for positive purposes," and the Massachusetts Supreme Court issued a contradictory ruling: that while the film was a "collective indecent intrusion into the most private aspects of the lives of unfortunate persons," it was valuable as a social document and might indirectly benefit inmates by leading to improvements at Bridgewater.[1] Another significant case in medical ethics is the story of Dax Cowart, whose competent and consistent refusal of life-saving treatment is documented in *Please Let Me Die* (1974). Although Dax fully and freely participated in a taped interview with psychiatrist Robert White, the footage of his naked body during segments that begin and end the film are problematic when considering his inability to see the video camera because of his blindness or to cover his genitals because of his injured hands. Interestingly enough, Dax would not include these scenes in the follow-up documentary, *Dax's Case* (1985), and later would have an editor obscure his genitals in the educational materials that were eventually published with the original *Please Let Me Die*.

Questions about privacy and voyeurism in regard to making groundbreaking documentary films—How does Wiseman's disavowal of even the most basic conventions of respectfulness prevent his being influenced by the institutions he films? How does Dax's sightlessness and helplessness intensify the exposure of his body? How does witnessing suicides prevent suicides? How do adolescent girls behave differently in front of a camera?—are especially complicated in settings with patients who are vulnerable, dependent, and impaired. As viewers watch the actual death of Tom Joslin in the documentary, *Silverlake Life: The View From Here* (1993), there may be little distinction between their feeling of being permitted by the filmmaker to witness his end and their feeling of being forced to witness his end.

Unlike fiction films that picture a world that makes sense in terms of cause and effect, documentaries reveal a world filled with moral contradictions and ethical conundrums—much like the filmmakers themselves. Wiseman readily admits that all of his films, including *Titicut Follies*, are "manipulative... biased, condensed, compressed but fair" and that he has "an obligation to people who have consented to be in the film," regardless of how that consent was obtained.[6]

NOTE

i. "Do Not Record" is a play on the now-standard acronym for "Do Not Rescuscitate," found in medical records and hospital charts.

REFERENCES

1. Benson, T.W. and Anderson, C. 1989. *Reality fictions: The films of Frederick Wiseman*. Carbondale: Southern Illinois University Press.
2. Pence, G.E. 1990. *Classic cases in medical ethics*. New York: McGraw-Hill.
3. Barnouw, E. 1993. *Documentary: A history of the non-fiction film*. 2nd edition. New York: Oxford University Press.
4. Nichols, B. 2001. *Introduction to documentary*. Bloomington: Indiana University Press.
5. Cieply, M. September 14, 2009. At Toronto Film Festival, cautions on documentaries. *New York Times*.
6. Poppy, N. "Fredrick Wiseman." *Salon.com*. Retrieved December 12, 2010 from http://dir.salon.com/story/people/conv2002/01/30/wiseman/index.html

part three

professionalism

the bounds of physicians' authority:
dr. kildare's strange case

joseph turow

Dr. Kildare's Strange Case (1940). Lew Ayres, Lionel Barrymore, Laraine Day, Shepperd Strudwick. Directed by Harold S. Bucquet. Duration: 76 minutes.

DVD Chapter 3 scene 00:35:06 to 00:37:41

DOCTOR KILDARE'S STRANGE CASE, AN installment in the popular MGM *Dr. Kildare* movie series of the late 1930s and early 1940s, centers on intern Jimmy Kildare (Lew Ayres), who learns the medical ropes in Blair Memorial Hospital, guided by Dr. Leonard Gillespie (Lionel Barrymore). The "strange case" of this film's title begins when Gillespie assigns Kildare to work with Dr. Gregory Lane. Lane is a surgeon whose professional self-confidence has been crushed by a string of failed surgeries and resulting patient deaths. In this scene, he confronts a patient with a skull fracture who, Lane says, will die if he doesn't get an immediate operation. As Lane goes off to arrange it, the woozy patient insists to Kildare he does not want the operation. Kildare tells the patient— about whom he and Lane know nothing, not even his name—that he must go through with it to survive. In the meantime, Lane wavers about whether he should perform the surgery or wait. Kildare exhorts him to perform the procedure in view of his initial diagnosis. He quotes Dr. Gillespie's opinion that Lane has "the best hands in the hospital." He adds more Dr. Gillespieisms saying that "sometimes we have to act, with life in one hand and death in the other" and that "the true test of a doctor is his faith in his own judgment even though he knows someone is going to die if he's wrong." Hearing that, Lane exclaims, "We'll operate immediately." We next see him walking into the operating room as he says: "This patient has refused the operation, but I take full responsibility."

Whenever I play this clip, physicians, medical students, and even people not affiliated with the medical profession, erupt in laughter. They immediately recognize that the final line of the scene—about the patient refusing the operation but the physician going ahead anyway—would today be considered a clear case of malpractice. When the laugher dissipates, I suggest it is highly unlikely that audiences in 1940 would have reacted that way to what was clearly a serious scene in a melodrama. The audience agrees, and the moment opens a space to discuss my key point about how doctors are supposed to act toward patient: What a doctor's authority is and how he or she should express it—has changed over the decades. Comparing then and now can generate a useful discussion about the contemporary nature of a doctor's power in relation to his or her patients and the ethical boundaries of that power.

Dr. Kildare's Strange Case was produced at a time of growing optimism about the promise of American medicine to solve individual health problems. Just 60 years earlier, before the 20th century, medicine was a sometimes near-subsistence occupation whose practitioners used methods with severely ill patients (bloodletting, for example) that often did not heal and that scared people away from visiting doctors. One 19th century observer wryly observed that heroic medicine was "one of those great discoveries which are made from time to time for the depopulation of the earth."[1] The prognosis for American medicine began to change slowly in the late 19th century. A number of circumstances converged to greatly increase physicians' credibility. The most important occurred when leaders of the American Medical Association (AMA), state medical societies, major medical schools, and major hospitals hitched their profession's star to the rising success of science. The new technologies and medical discoveries that came in rapid succession, along with the sharp reduction in hospital deaths, did wonders to increase the legitimacy of regular medicine in the eyes of the rest of society, as well as to encourage people's dependence on physicians.[2] To be sure, many still hurled devastating criticism at the emerging private medical structure that focused less on general public health and more on the individual patient's well-being. But by 1940, the general public accepted a physician as a popular culture hero. Stung by attacks by the AMA against Hollywood for negative portrayals of physicians, the major studios hired physicians to advise them on films with doctors. Joe Cohen, who produced the Kildare series for MGM, recalled that he tried to make sure that the central characters contradicted medical evils of the day by portraying the possibilities, the ideals, of American medical practice.[3]

What characteristics distinguished an "ideal" physician of the day and their guided interactions with patients? As reflected in this scene, the doctor was likely to be white, male, and Anglo Saxon. Increasingly, too, he was a specialist who used the hospital and its expensive technology as his workplace. Beyond these institutional features, though, a widespread belief in certain values and their origin gave physicians special cultural authority. Popular culture presented Americans with the idea that an admirable doctor possessed membership in an elect group, a special person born to succeed in the profession and then shaped by the profession. (Dr. Gillespie's comment that Dr. Lane has "the best hands" in the hospital echoes this belief.) The elect status came with responsibilities to the patient that, the norm dictated, took precedence over personal comfort (for example, it emphasized the need to work long hours) and payment (the salaries of interns and residents were notoriously as low as their hours were long). But the elect status also brought with it a huge amount of authority as the young knight made it through the training gauntlet. The physician stood at the center of the medical profession. Not only did health workers (especially nurses) have to obey his orders, but patients did as well.

Linked to the idea of the physician as authoritative expert is his individualism. Note that all the decisions in the scene revolve around the individual physician. The radiology technicians hand the doctor the x-rays, note their conclusions, and leave. The surgeon stands alone in making the decision to operate—egged on by neophyte intern Kildare—in the absence of discussions with any other specialists, nurses, or admissions personnel. There may be poetic license in this movie, but it is clearly a value producers believed the audience and the medical establishment would accept. As Kildare notes, his profession (in the form of the great "diagnostician," Dr. Gillespie) accepted as ideal a doctor whose confidence in his abilities and judgment was so important that it would even override whether he was right or wrong—or successful or not—with respect to a particular patient. The key goal was to allow the physician's talent to emerge.

Compare the values reflected in the *Kildare* scene with those associated with physicians today—both in popular culture (think of the series *ER*, for example) and in the norms medical schools teach. The value of saving a person's life in an acute situation certainly remains with us—and at the core of television's presentation of medicine. So, too, physicians still stand as the captains of care (to the chagrin of some health care professionals). The medical establishment certainly agrees that today's physician population ought to be quite a bit more diverse than its Depression-era counterpart from the standpoint of gender, race, and ethnicity. Also dramatically different is the belief about the physician's authority and its origins. Neither the profession nor the larger society accepts the idea that doctors are members of an elect group blessed with powers that, if used correctly, give them the right to place their decisions above those of everyone else. The ideal of the physician as a determined individualist who has the right to make lone decisions dictating patient care has given way to a belief that doctors are part of a web of parties responsible for developing the approach to a patient's care—including (if possible) the patient and people related to him or her.

Steeped in this new belief, contemporary audiences immediately recognize that early 21st-century norms of physician behavior do not allow dismissing a patient's desire to forego an operation. Physicians and other health care practitioners readily accept the current regime that dictates doctors' relationships with patients and health care professionals as clearly more ethical, and smarter about physicians' purview, than that of the era in which *Dr. Kildare's Strange Case* was made. Yet comparing the mid-20th-century medical culture with that of the early 20th century underscores that what seems obvious regarding medical authority is really culturally rooted. It is interesting to consider which beliefs that the contemporary medical institution and larger society accept as clearly ethical will be considered less than ethical—in fact, wrong-headed—60 years from now.

REFERENCES

1. Ehrenreich B., and English, D. 1978. *For their own good: 150 years of expert advice to women*, p. 48. New York: Anchor.
2. Star, P. *The social transformation of American medicine*, pp. 1–200. New York: Basic Books.
3. Interview with Joe Cohen, Summer 1986.

medical narcissism: *malice*

john d. banja

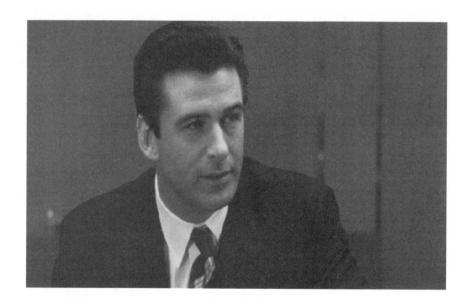

Malice (1993). Alec Baldwin, Nicole Kidman, Bill Pullman, Peter Gallagher, Bebe Neuwirth, Anne Bancroft. Directed by Harold Becker. Duration: 107 minutes.

DVD Chapter 16 Scene 00:49:31 to 54:24.

"I AM GOD!" SEETHES DR. JED Hill in *Malice*, one of Hollywood's most memorable portrayals of a pathologically narcissistic physician. Deliciously played by Alec Baldwin, Dr. Hill's narcissistic rant occurs at a deposition in which he is defending himself against the malpractice allegations of a former patient, Tracy Safian.

The events leading up to Dr. Hill's malpractice suit begin with his meeting an old high school chum, Andy Safian (Tracy's husband, played by Bill Pullman). Andy invites Dr. Hill—who has just moved to town—to rent the top floor of Andy and Tracy's home. The Safians are remodeling the house and are sorely in need of cash. Andy's lovely wife Tracy (Nicole Kidman) wants to become pregnant but is worried about severe and recurring abdominal pain. During an acute attack, she is rushed to the hospital and is seen by Dr. Hill. He discovers that she is pregnant and decides that both her ovaries are diseased. Refusing to heed the advice of another physician to wait for lab results, Hill removes Tracy's ovaries and the fetus aborts. When the pathology results come back indicating that at least one of Tracy's ovaries wasn't necrotic, she sues Dr. Hill. Typical of the narcissist who believes he can do no wrong, Dr. Hill decides to defend himself against the lawsuit.

Dr. Hill's self-deification is hardly surprising. Whether he is mesmerizing the operating room staff with his surgical virtuosity or sweeping women off their feet, Dr. Hill personifies a typical narcissistic mix of charm, brilliance, and grandiosity. During his deposition, he points out that his M.D. is from Harvard; that he is board certified in cardiothoracic medicine and trauma surgery; that he has been awarded citations from seven different medical boards; and that he is "never, ever sick at sea." Dr. Hill seems the perfect DSM-IV, advanced narcissist: pompous, arrogant, immensely accomplished, seductive, swashbuckling, and never, as he says, sick at sea.[1]

Had *Malice* continued this story line, it might well have become a very popular teaching film in medical schools and residency training programs. Would Dr. Hill be exonerated at or before trial? Did his behavior constitute an unreasonable departure from the standard of care? Would his narcissism be knocked down a peg or two by the experience? What effect would the lawsuit have on Tracy and Andy? Unfortunately, though, the film takes a decided Hollywood turn and becomes an improbable (and remarkably convoluted) story of betrayal, greed, and murder.

Nevertheless, Dr. Hill's brand of narcissism is worth consideration by any medical student or resident. Physicians daily confront temptation after temptation to develop an unhealthy narcissism. Because they work long and often excruciatingly hard hours, they must be convinced of the social worth and the preciousness of their skills. While they occasionally experience crushing disappointment, they will more often experience exhilarating gratification. Physicians routinely receive the adoration, indeed the genuflection, of patients and their families on a daily, sometimes hourly, basis. For narcissists like Dr. Hill *who have an exaggerated need to feel awesome*, the practice of medicine provides the perfect setting to accommodate, one might even say nurture, their narcissistic cravings.[2]

Nevertheless, while Alec Baldwin's Dr. Hill was a not uncommon medical personality some decades ago—recall that the film appeared in 1993—his over-the-top narcissism seems less common today, although the popular TV show *House* demonstrates its continuing presence in the contemporary medical world. Over the last century, the ethical sensibilities of medicine have steadily evolved patient-centered constructs, such as honoring informed consent, respecting privacy and confidentiality, and practicing empathy and compassion. In so doing, medicine is following the overarching sensibility of modern Western ethics, which is that principled moral behavior tends overwhelmingly to be *other-regarding*. As moral philosophy's greatest theorist Immanuel Kant argued 250 years ago, acts done purely out of self-interest or performed instinctively have no serious moral standing, save that their selfish character makes them morally vacuous. Utilitarians make the point even more starkly: The moral act is the one that does not satisfy or accommodate the interests of the actor, but the one that realizes the most happiness for the most people.[3]

The pathological egocentricity of narcissists like Dr. Hill represents the antithesis of the other-regarding stance. Narcissists like Dr. Hill tend to be ideologically and psychologically inflexible. The only beliefs, feelings, and ideas that count are theirs. If they are abundantly charming—which they frequently are—it is because they want something and will manipulate the other to deliver it. Almost by definition, they have poor listening skills. What they unconsciously hear in conversation is largely the provocation "How does this talk apply to me and my need to feel important?" It is extremely hard for them to admit error, and they often feel above rule following. They tend to be remarkably unempathic because they primarily focus their attentional (or libidinal) energy on themselves. Thus, Dr. Hill seems oblivious to the impact of his self-deifying rant on his listeners because he's not in the habit of considering what others think or feel. Indeed, to admit parity with others is to lose the very thing—a calcified "cut above the rest" conviction—that narcissists pathologically require to sustain a belief in their worth and lovability.[2,4,5]

Unfortunately, virtually no empirical literature explicitly examines the pitfalls of an unhealthy narcissism in medicine, although anecdotal observations abound. Martin Leichtman has movingly discussed the liabilities of having a narcissistic physician father or husband,[8] while any risk manager observing Dr. Hill's narcissistic outburst at deposition would doubtlessly recommend what Hill's attorney did: settle the case as soon as possible rather than allow this pompous boor to enrage a jury.

A study by Robert Murden and his colleagues suggests how narcissistic behaviors can present themselves as early as medical school. The team wondered whether various types of professional deficiencies observed in first-year medical students might predict poor performance two years later, when they commenced their clerkships.[9] Interestingly, the investigators found that first-year students who "exhibited paternalistic and controlling behavior during interviews, often focused the interview on self rather than patient, did not listen to, respond empathically to, or establish rapport with patients (p. S46)."[9] had significantly lower third-year grades in their clerkships. This cluster of traits proves extremely suggestive of an unhealthy narcissism. The study additionally implies that medical students often begin their professional training with a narcissistic self-formation intact.

Another study reported by Gerald Hickson and his colleagues found that a high number of obstetrical patients' complaints about their physicians strongly correlated with the physician's being in a high-frequency malpractice group (i.e., was sued relatively often).[10] The investigators reported that patients of these "high complaint" obstetricians were particularly critical of the latter's interpersonal skills. The physicians were reported to appear hurried, uninterested in patients, and unwilling to listen and answer questions—traits that are somewhat suggestive of a narcissistic formation. Importantly, the research team noted that there was no difference in the technical adequacy of the care that was delivered by the various physicians groups surveyed. The difference was largely manifested in the high malpractice frequency group's poorly developed relational and empathic skills.[10]

What is especially worrisome about a narcissistic formation in medicine is how it disenables the physician's ability to manage self-esteem threats that, unfortunately, occur all the time. Managing the patient whose therapeutic course is profoundly frustrating or disappointing, disclosing a medical error, treating a dying patient, caring for an irascible one, or delivering bad news like an upsetting diagnosis are daily experiences for many physicians. But the more unhealthy one's narcissism, the more difficult it will be to dispatch these tasks artfully and therapeutically because they all challenge the narcissist's extreme vulnerability to self-esteem loss.[2,6]

Psychiatrists would likely predict that a calcified narcissist like Jed Hill is beyond help.[6] (Hickson's group suggested that the interpersonal difficulties of high-frequency obstetricians are probably resistant to change.[10]) First of all, such persons resist therapy because they have a very difficult time admitting that they are in any way responsible for their relational failures. And even if they enter therapy, they tend to drop out as their defenses will not tolerate the therapist's exploration of their imperfections or weaknesses.[6] On the other hand, less-hardened narcissists need to recognize that the opportunities to develop an unhealthy narcissism abound in medicine.[7] Self-therapy for "softer" narcissists might consist in the purposeful and deliberate practice of non-narcissistic behaviors. Psychologist Albert Bernstein recommends that narcissists practice listening skills and empathy, ask for constructive criticism and resist defending against it, avoid talking about themselves, discuss mistakes and errors with colleagues, spend time with people who are different from them, practice developing a curiosity about them, do charity work, and, perhaps most difficult of all for the narcissist, "never miss an opportunity to do an anonymous good deed" (p. 177).[11]

Physicians need a healthy sense of self to survive the psychological rigors of their work and to maintain therapeutic relationships with patients, especially when things go poorly. Arguing that Jed Hill's narcissism is justified by his awesome technical skills is itself an idealizing, narcissistically based rationalization that only perpetuates that kind of pathological behavior. Narcissists like Jed Hill have no place in medicine (or in any profession), and allowing their behavior to go unaddressed redounds to no one's advantage.

REFERENCES

1. Millon, T., with Davis, R.D. 1996. *Disorders of personality DSM-IV and beyond*, 2nd ed., pp. 393–427. New York: John Wiley & Sons, Inc.
2. Banja, J. 2005. *Medical errors and medical narcissism*. Sudbury, MA: Jones & Bartlett Publishers.
3. Beauchamp, T., Childress, J. 2001. *Principles of biomedical ethics*, 5th ed., pp. 340–355. Oxford, UK: Oxford University Press.
4. Akhtar, S. 1989. Narcissistic personality disorder: Descriptive features and differential diagnosis. In Kernberg, O., ed., *Narcissistic personality disorder. Psychiatric Clinics of North America* 12: 505–529.
5. Otto Kernberg, "An ego psychology object relations theory of the structure and treatment of pathologic narcissism: An overview," In Otto Kernberg, ed., *Narcissistic Personality Disorder. Psychiatric Clinics of North America*, 12(1989): 723–729.
6. Masterson, J.F. 1988. *The search for the real self.* New York: The Free Press.
7. Novack, D., Suchman, A., Clark, W., Epstein, R., Najberg, E., and Kaplan, Craig. 1997. Calibrating the physician: Personal awareness and effective patient care. *Journal of the American Medical Association* 278: 502–509.
8. Leichtman, M. 1988. The occupational hazards of having a physician father. In G.O. Gabbard and R. Menninger (Eds.), *Medical marriages*, pp. 103–119. Washington, DC: American Psychiatric Press.
9. Murden, R.A., Way, D.P., Hudson, A., and Westman, J. 2004. Professionalism deficiencies in a first-quarter doctor-patient relationship course predict poor clinical performance in medical school. *Academic Medicine* 79: S46–S48.

10. Hickson, G., Wright Clayton, E., Entman, S., Miller, C., Githens, P., Whetten-Goldstein, K., and Sloan, F. 1994. Obstetricians' prior malpractice experience and patients' satisfaction with care. *Journal of the American Medical Association* 272: 1583–1587.

11. Bernstein, A. 2001. *Emotional vampires: Dealing with people who drain you dry.* New York: McGraw Hill.

3

disclosure of harmful medical errors: *the verdict*

david j. loren and thomas h. gallagher

The Verdict (1982). Paul Newman, Jack Warden, James Mason, Charlotte Rampling. Directed by Sidney Lumet, screenplay by David Mamet, based on the novel by Barry Reed. Duration: 122 minutes.

DVD Chapter 19; Scene 1:47:28 to 1:54:3

HE VERDICT, A STORY OF personal redemption, medical malfeasance, and deception, is also one of the few Hollywood portrayals of a harmful medical error. As the movie opens, lawyer Frank Galvin (Paul Newman) struggles with a lost professional reputation and a failing practice. A stroke of luck sends him a referral: the tragic case of Deborah Ann Kaye, a woman left in a coma after a Cesarean section delivery. The operation, at a fictional well-known Catholic hospital (St. Catherine's) in Boston, was complicated when the patient threw up into her anesthesia mask, aspirated, developed cardiac arrest, and was resuscitated but left in a persistent vegetative state. First motivated primarily by the financial reward of the case, Galvin later becomes invested in seeking justice and pursues the case to its dramatic courtroom revelations.

Exactly what happened in the operating room four years prior to the events depicted in the film remains incomplete until almost the end of the story. We first learn that something may have gone wrong when Galvin (the plaintiff's lawyer) interviews an anesthesiologist as an expert witness who purports that the comatose patient was mismanaged by two renowned physicians: "... those doctors murdered her, they gave her the wrong anesthetic." The film suspends the viewer between Galvin's pursuit of what happened in that operating room and the defense lawyer's zeal for keeping those facts hidden. We discover that the crucial question to be answered is exactly *when* did Deborah Ann last eat before she was administered general anesthesia. Were the two anesthesiologists in that operating room negligent in their care, or just unfortunate bystanders in a complication of appropriate care? In the final courtroom scene (time codes noted above), we learn not only that a serious error occurred in Deborah Ann's care, but also that her admission record was falsified to cover up the mistake.

This movie provides a dramatic depiction of one of the most vexing medicolegal intersections, disclosure of harmful medical errors. This final courtroom scene offers a potent departure point for the classroom discussion. I let the audience see the climax first, pose multiple questions to stimulate debate, and then look back to the preceding scenes to focus the discussion around each individual question. What is a medical error? What are the imperatives for disclosure? Is there a rationale for nondisclosure? When might disclosure of a medical error pose a genuine ethical dilemma? Who benefits from disclosure? How do we balance a patient's wishes for culpability and justice with the health care worker's desire for a blame-free medical environment?

Arguments supporting the disclosure of harmful medical errors are robust. Patients (or parent/family surrogate decision-makers) need to know and understand the current status of their health in order to make fully informed decisions regarding their care. If a patient has been injured during medical care, he or she can participate in informed consent for further care only if the details that led to that injury are fully comprehended. Furthermore, withholding information germane to a patient's health care can only be interpreted as dishonesty in the eyes of a patient. Such obfuscation undermines the physician's fiduciary relationship with a patient. During an early scene, as Galvin recruits an expert witness, we hear what may be a remarkably simple philosophical foundation for disclosure: "Why are ya doin' this?," "To do the right thing, isn't that why you're doing it?" However, such a deontological motive does not provide much guidance regarding the practical details of actually telling a patient that something "went wrong."[1]

The events of this film unfold in the early 1980s, in Boston. During this era, the American Medical Association (AMA) issued its first code of ethics related to communication of unanticipated outcomes.[2] Professionalism code E-8.12 (1981) framed disclosure of medical errors in the context of physician honesty and patient autonomy: patients need "... to be free of any mistaken beliefs concerning their conditions." Additionally, the AMA urged that "... concern regarding legal liability which might result following the truthful disclosure should not affect a physician's honesty in dealing with the patient."[2]

Discussions about medical errors can be challenging on many levels, beginning with the lack of consensus regarding a clear definition of medical error. The Institute of Medicine, in the groundbreaking 2000 publication *To Err Is Human: Building a Safer Health System,* framed medical error as the "failure of a planned action to be completed as intended or the use of a wrong plan to achieve an aim." An adverse event, "harm that is the result of the process of health care rather than the patient's underlying disease," is distinctly different from a medical error and refers to a specific outcome, rather than a breakdown in the process of care.[3] Employing these terms in our classroom discussion can engender strong emotions among the discussants. Errors by definition are not intentional and not the result of reckless behavior. In the process of causing harm to a patient, we may feel responsible for causing the error but reject a sense of fault and blameworthiness.

If your group could rewrite the story in this movie, how would they counsel the operating room team to communicate this medical error to Deborah Anne's family? Research over the past decade has demonstrated that virtually all patients want to be told about serious medical errors, and most even want to be told about minor errors.[4] When told about a medical error, patients want to hear an explicit statement that an error occurred, what happened, and why, as well as implications for their ongoing health care.[5] Patients seek solace in knowing that their suffering might prevent harm to someone else and thus want to know how the medical team will prevent a recurrence of the error. Last, the majority of patients wish to hear a sincere apology that recognizes the harm they have experienced.[6]

Heeding these simple directives has proven to be complicated in practice. Research into physician attitudes and experiences with medical error disclosure has demonstrated that physicians want to disclose medical errors. However, they report that they experience multiple barriers in the disclosure process, including lack of training in leading these emotionally charged conversations, fear of disciplinary actions or harm to their reputation, and skepticism that disclosure has benefits for the patient. Last, many physicians express a fear of being sued after disclosing a medical error. Consequently, a growing number of studies in the United States and Canada have demonstrated that physicians disclose medical errors at rates much below what is desired by patients and families. Furthermore, physicians appear to disclose medical errors less frequently when the patient is not aware that an error occurred.[7]

The interaction among medical error disclosure, apology, and litigation is complex. In an effort to propel medical error disclosure by reducing physicians' fear of litigation, a number of states have enacted legislation that excludes a health care worker's apology from an admission of liability. On the other hand, intentional obfuscation of the error (e.g., by deletion, tampering, or destruction of medical records), as depicted in this movie, may be employed as evidence of malpractice in a civil suit. Furthermore, such spoliation of evidence may also be considered a misdemeanor violation of state or federal statutes. Indeed, allegations of medical record alteration may lead an insurance carrier to refuse payment of a settlement or even cancel the implicated physician's malpractice coverage. While outright lying on the part of a physician may inspire a patient to file a lawsuit, exactly why some patients seek legal counsel against a physician is not well understood. Some authors contend that greater error disclosure could increase the rate of litigation surrounding medical errors as more patients learn about the errors that occur in their care.[8]

Physicians have described concerns that disclosure may be further injurious to a patient, viewing nondisclosure as patient-centered care.[9] In that light, who then are the beneficiaries of disclosure in general? On an interpersonal level, disclosure of a medical error begins to fulfill the patient's sense of being wronged. Disclosure also begins the process of self-reconciliation and forgiveness that appears to be strongly desired by physicians who have been involved in causing a medical error. Institutionally, disclosure of medical errors is one component of a culture of accountability, open communication, and transparency. Disclosure of medical errors clearly entails risks as well. Disclosure can be very alarming to a patient or family. After learning about a medical error, a patient may lose trust and confidence in an individual physician, care team, or health care institution, and as a result, the patient may refuse further beneficial treatment. Could knowledge of a medical error tip a severely depressed person to suicide? A consequentialist approach might argue that some errors should not be disclosed.

Exploring the conflicts of interest posed by the disclosure of a medical error provides insight into the challenges of navigating this ethical dilemma. Disclosing a medical error places a tension between a patient's desire for knowledge about what happened during his or her medical care and a physician's or hospital's interest for self-preservation and limited information sharing with a patient. Contemporary developments in the relationship between risk managers and physicians may serve as an effective illustration of the evolution in transparency within health care settings. Historically, risk managers have been perceived as protectors of a hospital's financial interests and have counseled physicians to refrain from disclosing errors. Recently, risk managers have assumed a more proactive role in protecting the hospital—and the patient—by encouraging adverse event reporting and the disclosure of medical errors. Indeed, present experience with medical error disclosure suggests that, contrary to the classical paradigm of "do no harm to the organization" (e.g., do not tell patients about any errors), open and honest communication about unanticipated outcomes actually leads to safer health care systems and greater patient trust in those organizations.[10]

The Verdict implicates the decisions of one physician in the serious error that led to Deborah Anne's coma; however, medical errors are more commonly the result of a complex interplay among personnel, clinical processes and practices, technology, and organizational factors. Potent interprofessional issues arise when errors are not due to the actions of one individual. How does a physician disclose an error when that physician may not have been the only, or most proximal cause of that error? How does a team decide who will lead an error disclosure, and how can team members ensure that they will not be implicated during a disclosure conversation? Answers to these questions are at present elusive and currently fuel research efforts into the efficacy and methodology of error disclosure.[11]

Whether framed in the context of justice, patient autonomy, or truth-telling, disclosure of harmful medical errors is increasingly gaining both public and academic scrutiny. Thirty years after the events of The Verdict took place, the current research agenda in error disclosure reflects health care's growing intimacy with how to admit when we violate our fundamental principle of *primum non nocere*, "first, do no harm."

REFERENCES

1. Wu, A.W., Cavanaugh, T.A., McPhee, S.J., Lo, B., and Micco, G.P. 1997. To tell the truth: Ethical and practical issues in disclosing medical mistakes to patients. *Journal of General Internal Medicine* 12(12): 770–775.

2. American Medical Association Council on Ethical and Judicial Affairs. 2004. *Code of medical ethics, annotated current opinions: Rules of the Council on Ethical and Judicial Affairs.* Southern Illinois University at Carbondale School of Law (Ed.). Chicago, IL: American Medical Association.

3. Gallagher, T.H. 2009. A 62-year-old woman with skin cancer who experienced wrong-site surgery: Review of medical error. *Journal of the American Medical Association* 302(6): 669–677.

4. Gallagher, T.H., and Lucas, M.H. 2005. Should we disclose harmful medical errors to patients? If so, how? *Journal of Clinical Outcomes Management* 12(5): 253–259.

5. Mazor, K.M., Simon, S.R., Yood, R.A., Martinson, B.C., Gunter, M.J., Reed, G.W., and Gurwitz, J.H. 2004. Health plan members' views about disclosure of medical errors. *Annals of Internal Medicine* 140(6): 409–418.

6. Lazare, A. 2006. Apology in medical practice: An emerging clinical skill. *Journal of the American Medical Association* 296(11): 1401–1404.

7. Loren, D.J., Klein, E.J., Garbutt, J., Krauss, M.J., Fraser, V., Dunagan, W.C., et al. 2008. Medical error disclosure among pediatricians: Choosing carefully what we might say to parents. *Archives of Pediatric Adolescent Medicine* 162(10): 922–927.

8. Studdert, D.M., Mello, M.M., Gawande, A.A., Brennan, T.A., and Wang, Y.C. 2007. Disclosure of medical injury to patients: an improbable risk management strategy. *Health Affairs (Millwood)* 26(1): 215–226.

9. Gallagher, T.H., Waterman, A.D., Ebers, A.G., Fraser, V.J., and Levinson, W. 2003. Patients' and physicians' attitudes regarding the disclosure of medical errors. *Journal of the American Medical Association* 289(8): 1001–1007.

10. Shapiro, E. 2008. Disclosing medical errors: Best practices from the "Leading Edge. In *Disclosure: What's morally right is organizationally right.* At the 18th Annual IHI National Forum on Quality Improvement in Health Care. Orlando, Florida.

11. Shannon, S.E., Foglia, M.B., Hardy, M., and Gallagher, T.H. 2009. Disclosing errors to patients: Perspectives of registered nurses. *Joint Commission Journal on Quality and Patient Safety* 35(1): 5–12.

abandonment: *mr. jones*

kayhan p. parsi

Mr. Jones (1993). Richard Gere, Lena Olin, Delroy Lindo, Anne Bancroft, Tom Irwin, Bruce Altman, Lauren Tom, Lisa Malkiewicz, Thomas Kopache. Directed by Mike Figgis. Duration: 114 minutes.

Scene: DVD chapter 23 Scene 01.28.52 to 01.30.56

MR. *JONES* CARRIES ON THE tradition of several dramatic films that highlight a specific psychiatric disorder (in this case, bipolar disorder) and the relationship that ensues between the patient (Richard Gere) suffering from the illness and his treating psychiatrist, Dr. Elizabeth Bowen (Lena Olin). The movie begins with a manic Richard Gere singing to himself (with James Brown's "I Feel Good" in the background) as he bounds down a sidewalk. He comes upon a building site and persuades a skeptical foreman (Bill Pullman) to let him work on a construction job. On the roof, he strikes up a conversation with a fellow worker (Delroy Lindo), who appears bemused with Mr. Jones' antics until he walks out onto a high beam looking at airplanes flying low above and shouting "I'm gonna fly!" Lindo's character (Howard) successfully rescues Mr. Jones, whereupon he is admitted to a psychiatric hospital. The remainder of the film explores Mr. Jones relationship with Dr. Bowen, culminating with an intimate encounter.

This film provides excellent opportunities to explore professional boundaries in the psychiatric field. There is widespread consensus that any sexual contact between a psychiatrist and patient (whether current or former) is unethical. Clearly, Dr. Bowen transgresses this professional boundary. I will not, however, focus on this primary issue. Rather, I will concentrate on a brief scene late in the film. After having sex with Mr. Jones, a clearly troubled Dr. Bowen informs one of her colleagues, Dr. Patrick Shaye (Tom Irwin), that she would like to take herself off the Jones case. She then informs him that she slept with Mr. Jones. Incredulous, Dr. Shaye tells Dr. Bowen: "For Christ's sake! What the fuck do you think you were doing? Twelve years of training as a psychiatrist, and you blow it off! First of all, you'll be fired. Then, if Mr. Jones, solid, stable citizen that he is… chooses to press charges, you could be prosecuted. You could go to jail." Dr. Shaye then tells Dr. Bowen that she cannot see Mr. Jones again and that he will be transferred to another hospital with no further explanation from her.

The central ethical issue here is whether Dr. Bowen's and/or Dr. Shaye's decision constituted patient abandonment. Edmund Pellegrino defines abandonment as "unilateral withdrawal by a physician from a patient's care without first formally transferring that care to another qualified physician who is acceptable to the patient… leaving the patient without care."[1] In this scene, Dr. Bowen attempted to unilaterally transfer Mr. Jones to Dr. Shaye, without first discussing this change in care with the patient. Her feelings of guilt prompted her to "turf" Mr. Jones to another professional. Dr. Shaye refused.

Moreover, professional guidelines govern the proper termination of a physician–patient relationship. For instance, the American Medical Association (AMA)'s Code of Medical Ethics contains the following statement: "Physicians have an obligation to support continuity of care for their patients. While physicians have the option of withdrawing from a case, they cannot do so without giving notice to the patient, the relatives, or responsible friends sufficiently long in advance of withdrawal to permit another medical attendant to be secured."[2] Again, in this case, Mr. Jones received no proper notice. Because of shame, guilt, and/or embarrassment. Dr. Bowen purposefully avoided confronting Mr. Jones and attempted to pass her patient on to her colleague. Moreover, by not directly addressing Mr. Jones, she compounds the emotional abandonment of this vulnerable patient.

Principle VII in the AMA's Code also speaks directly to this issue: "A physician shall, while caring for a patient, regard responsibility to the patient as paramount."[3] In caring for Mr. Jones, Dr. Bowen exhibited a great deal of care and compassion for her patient. Yet, her sexual feelings toward a seductive patient created great ambivalence for her. Scared and disappointed, Dr. Bowen did what many would probably do—she tried to distance herself from her patient after the fact. Dr. Shaye admonishes his colleague in this scene, telling her that she could never see him again, and that Mr. Jones would be transferred to another hospital. Dr. Shaye threatens her by saying that if she sees Mr. Jones again, he will report her to the authorities. This, of course, raises another ethical issue—did Dr. Shaye have an obligation to report his colleague, regardless of any agreement between him and Dr. Bowen?

Patients routinely leave their physicians. A patient may do so for a variety of reasons—dissatisfaction with the physician, a new job, relocation, etc. Physicians also routinely terminate their relationships with patients. Physicians close practices, move, or take on new positions. Terminating a physician–patient relationship, however, is different from abandonment. Termination suggests that the physician has taken the necessary steps of informing the patient, giving enough time, and ensuring the patient has a new physician. Abandonment, however, can give rise to a lawsuit. In a typical malpractice case, a plaintiff has to show that a physician had a duty toward the patient, there was a breach of duty (a deviation from the standard of care), an injury occurred that was caused by this breach, and there were some damages due to this injury. In some states, a claim of abandonment may not suffice as a legal cause of action. In others, however, this may be seen as a viable cause of action. For instance, in the case *Tierney v. University of Michigan Regents*, a physician terminated his relationship with his patient because the patient was suing him.[4]

He did not give reasonable notice. The patient sued him on the basis of abandonment. Although the physician won at the trial level, the appellate court stated that:

> The physician has a definite right to withdraw from the case provided he gives the patient reasonable notice so as to enable him to secure other medical attendance. Such a withdrawal does not constitute an abandonment. ... [A] physician who is generally engaged to attend a patient is liable for any damages caused by his abandoning the case without sufficient notice or adequate excuse, provided injury results from his action.

In this case, not only did Dr. Bowen risk discipline by her state board for sexual misconduct (and perhaps even criminal charges), she also exposes herself to liability for her abandonment of Mr. Jones.[5]

Some commentators have identified appropriate reasons for a physician to terminate a physician–patient relationship. These occur when a physician believes that the patient needs the services of someone more skilled or knowledgeable, when the physician believes that the patient acts inappropriately (e.g., sexually or in a violent manner), or when the physician believes that his or her cultural/religious values prohibit him or her from doing a certain procedure.[6] The relationship between Dr. Bowen and Mr. Jones already crossed certain boundaries even before it became sexualized. In several earlier scenes, they share time together outside of a formal clinical encounter in her office or hospital. In light of this, Dr. Bowen could have referred Mr. Jones to another physician. Despite these early warning signals, Dr. Bowen acted upon her attraction toward Mr. Jones.

This scene illustrates not only the danger of sexual misconduct between therapist and patient, but it also realistically portrays how such relationships end precipitously, abruptly, and often very badly. The therapist's behavior adds insult to injury in such a case: after first violating a patient's trust through sexual contact, therapists will often abandon the patient and not refer him or her to another clinician. As one commentator has mentioned: "This failure to provide for ongoing care not only brings about the very abandonment that many patients in therapy fear, but also is a brutal indicator of how little therapists who have sex with their patients really care about them as people with psychological needs."[7] One could argue that Dr. Bowen truly did care for Mr. Jones but that her care shifted from a compassionate concern in a clinical context to become highly personalized and even romanticized. This unprofessional journey from couch to bedroom ultimately leads to abandonment.

Having facilitated seminar discussions with psychiatry residents on a number of ethical topics, I believe that this vignette could be effectively used to illustrate not only the more obvious ethical issue of sexual misconduct but the more subtle one of abandonment. After viewing this vignette, one could pose to residents or students the following questions: (1) We all know that sexual misconduct, especially in psychiatry, is unethical in medical practice. What is the responsibility of Dr. Bowen after she had a sexual encounter with her patient, Mr. Jones? Should she have confronted Mr. Jones, explained the impropriety of their relationship, and informed him that she will find him an appropriate replacement? (2) What could she have done to mitigate the abandonment issue? Would giving reasonable notice of her termination be sufficient? (3) What was the ethical responsibility of Dr. Shaye? Should he have reported her to the appropriate authorities? For instance, the AMA's Code of Medical Ethics states clearly that a physician should report unethical conduct (where appropriate) to state licensing boards, law enforcement authorities, or "the appropriate authority for a particular clinical service."[8] Did he need to report Dr. Bowen's conduct to all three authorities? (4) Did he enable her abandonment by transferring her patient without encouraging her to speak with him first? Or, was he doing the right thing by ensuring she had zero contact with Mr. Jones? Although the ethical issue of sexual misconduct here is black and white, the issue of abandonment raises more interesting shades of gray. Hopefully, this vignette can trigger some robust discussions on this important ethical topic.

REFERENCES

1. Pellegrino, E.D. 1995. Nonabandonment: An old obligation revisited. *Annals of Internal Medicine* 122(1995): 377–378.
2. Opinion 8.115 - Termination of the Physician–Patient Relationship. *AMA Code of Medical Ethics*. Retrieved October 28, 2010 from http://www.ama-assn.org/ama/pub/physician-resources/medical-ethics/code-medical-ethics/opinion8115.shtml
3. Principles of Medical Ethics. *AMA Code of Medical Ethics*. Retrieved October 28, 2010 from http://www.ama-assn.org/ama/pub/physician-resources/medical-ethics/code-medical-ethics/principles-medical-ethics.shtml.
4. Jerrold, L. 2005. Patient Abandonment. *American Journal of Orthodontics and Dentofacial Orthopedics* 127: 265–266.
5. Schleiter, K.E. 2009. Difficult Patient-Physician Relationships and the Risk of Medical Malpractice Litigation. *Virtual Mentor*. Retrieved October 28, 2010 from http://virtualmentor.ama-assn.org/2009/03/hlaw1-0903.html
6. On Patient Abandonment. *American Occupational Therapy Association Ethics Commission Advisory Opinion on Patient Abandonment*. Retrieved October 28, 2010 from http://www.aota.org/Practitioners/Ethics/Advisory/36510.aspx
7. Sarkar, S.P. 2004. Boundary violation and sexual exploitation in psychiatry and psychotherapy: A review. *Advances in Psychiatric Treatment* 10: 312–320.
8. Opinion 9.031 - Reporting impaired, incompetent, or unethical colleagues. *AMA Code of Medical Ethics*. Retrieved October 28, 2010 from http://www.ama-assn.org/ama/pub/physician-resources/medical-ethics/code-medical-ethics/opinion9031.shtml

privacy and confidentiality: *21 grams*

nancy berlinger

21 Grams (2003). Sean Penn, Naomi Watts, Benicio Del Toro, Charlotte
Gainsbourg. Directed by Alejandro Gonzalez Inarritu. Duration: 125 minutes.

Scene: DVD Chapter 14, Scene 00:52:47 to 00:53.35

21 *GRAMS* EXPLORES THE ATTRACTIVE AND perilous idea that
human lives and fates are interconnected. Director Alejandro
Gonzalez Inarritu uses contemporary automotive culture to move
his characters into position, to show that they are connected and what they value.
One of the consequences of car culture—the car crash—functions as plot hinge,
forcing different lives into relationship with one another. While not initially situated
within a medical environment, a car crash can be of bioethical significance because
automobile accidents and other human tragedies, while the source of pain and
suffering, may also produce commodities that Western society considers good:
donated organs.

The film has a nonsequential narrative structure: the order of the scenes seems
to be random, showing lives in isolation, until the viewer begins to notice recurring
characters and references, and starts piecing together the chronology and relationships. Near the beginning of the film, we see a youngish man on a ventilator in an
ICU. We hear his thoughts: He is in "death's waiting room," in the "pre-corpse
club." Later scenes reveal that his name is Paul, a math professor. Soon after this
opening, two brief scenes show a young woman and a gynecologist who specializes
in assisted reproduction. After completing a physical exam and noting that the
patient's fallopian tubes are damaged—the purpose of the visit is to determine
whether the young woman, Mary, is able to conceive—the physician asks her if she
has ever had an abortion. Mary acknowledges that she had ended a pregnancy
while separated from her husband. She explains that she wants to become pregnant
now because her husband is dying: He's got "one month left." Subsequent scenes
establish that Paul and Mary are married, and that Paul is waiting for a heart transplant. He sneaks cigarettes, which is against the rules for transplant candidates.
While waiting for the call from the transplant center, Mary and Paul squabble
about her visit to the fertility clinic, which Paul eventually visits for semen
collection. Aware of Paul's medical condition, a physician at the clinic emphasizes
that Paul will "probably never meet" his biological child: the goal of the procedure
is to allow Mary to conceive, bear, and raise a child in the event of Paul's death.

Scenes from other lives interrupt the story of Paul and Mary. A young mother named Christina receives a phone call about a car accident. Jack Jordan, a weather-beaten man with a troubled past, arrives late to his own birthday party, telling his wife, "I just ran over a man and two girls." The viewer can guess where Paul's new heart is going to come from.

The establishment and use of neurological criteria for making a determination of death is intertwined with the development of technologies that could support the cardiopulmonary functions of a body in which the brain can no longer support these functions; of diagnostic tests for measuring brain activity; and of techniques and therapies to permit viable organs to be transplanted from one human body into another.[1,2] Clinical, ethical, and legal standards for organ donation and transplantation have evolved to protect three entities: the donor, the recipient, and the organs themselves, which constitute an extremely limited resource.[3] This is a complex area of bioethics. Ethicists and physicians have challenged the "dead donor rule," which requires that a donor be declared dead before vital organs are removed; they point out that a prospective donor with a catastrophic and irreversible neurological injury may not quite fit the neurological criteria for a declaration of brain death.[4] So long as cardiopulmonary support is maintained, this patient's body will continue to function biologically. While this patient would be expected to die if cardiopulmonary support were withdrawn, this measure would imperil the vital organs. So, is this patient really dead, or is this patient a person with a traumatic brain injury? When this patient is an organ donor—or this patient's surrogate has given consent to organ donation and to the withdrawal of life-sustaining technologies—should this patient be declared dead under the neurological criteria, or under cardiopulmonary criteria following withdrawal?[5]

21 Grams shows what it means when the beeper of a person waiting for a heart transplant goes off: Another person, a healthy person, has just had a catastrophic brain injury. Technologies are supporting this person's cardiopulmonary functions, keeping viable organs perfused with oxygenated blood. Yet, another person is being asked to make "final decisions," and is being told about another patient who is "gravely ill" and in need of a healthy heart. The film hints at the current ethical debate when a hospital staff member tells Christina that her husband has very little brain activity—it is unclear whether he fits the neurological criteria—and then quickly mentions this other patient, the one who can benefit from her devastating loss.

When Paul wakes up from his transplant surgery, he asks, "Whose heart do I have?" He is told the rules: donors and recipients are anonymous to one another, to protect their privacy.[6] Although Christina's husband is dead and therefore has no interests, Christina's own privacy is at stake, as is Paul's. While donors and recipients may have some post-transplant contact by mutual consent—Paul is told he is permitted to write an unsigned letter to his donor's family—it would be inappropriate to grant an organ recipient the right to intrude on a grieving family, or to grant that family the right to monitor the conduct of the recipient of their loved one's heart, or to suggest that the recipient owed the donor or the donor's family something in return for this gift. Bioethicists have observed that the reliance on the "gift" metaphor in organ donation is problematic. We tend to know the identity of the person who gives us a gift, and the acceptance of a gift tends to incur a reciprocal obligation. So, what do you give the (dead) person who gave you his—or, rather, your—life?[7] Rules concerning the privacy of donors and recipients follow from the principle of autonomy, which honors the status and rights of the patient, and other individuals, as persons. These rules are also efforts to manage difficult psychological issues of privacy and intimacy that are part of organ donation and transplantation.

We know Paul cheats: on his pretransplant regimen, and also on his wife. He cheats on the rules of the donor–recipient game, too, hiring a private investigator to find out where his heart came from. How did the PI get this confidential information? Clinical standards and ethics guidelines keep transplant teams separate from patient care teams, to minimize the potential for conflicts between the interests of a prospective organ donor who is still receiving care as a patient, and the interests of a potential organ recipient who is also receiving care as a patient. Hospital policy concerning patient privacy and the confidentiality of patient information extends to access to different types of records. Hospital staff have an ethical duty not to divulge the protected information they are authorized to use. Did the PI bribe a worker who had access to records linking Paul to the donor? Did he get to these records in some other way? He doesn't say.

The PI also gives Paul information about Christina, and about Jack Jordan, the driver of the truck that killed her family. These details will prove to be irresistible as Paul tries to satisfy his desire "to know who I am now." Meanwhile, Paul and Mary are trying to figure out who they are now, as a couple and as a potential family. During a celebratory dinner party with friends, Mary announces, "We are going to be parents," explaining that she is going to have an operation and then artificial insemination. When Paul asks her later why she made this announcement, given that the two of them had not yet decided whether to follow through on a plan that had been premised on the likelihood of Paul's imminent death, Mary says, "I've already made my decision."

These developments—Paul's transplant, Mary's desire to go ahead with plans to conceive a child, and Paul's assertion of a claim on private information about the family of an organ donor—set up a scene in which Paul and Mary are shown in the office of the fertility-clinic gynecologist. While explaining the surgical procedure that will allow Mary to become pregnant, the physician, in passing, mentions the "damage from the abortion." Paul asks, "What abortion, Mary?"

The ethics of this scene seem straightforward. Mary is this physician's patient. Her physician has an obligation to protect her privacy and, under physician–patient privilege, to keep confidential any disclosure of information made in the context of the physician–patient relationship, apart from specific circumstances in which breaking confidentiality would prevent imminent harm to the patient or another person.[8] Therefore, Mary's physician acted unethically in disclosing her medical history without her permission. Even if the physician assumed that a married patient who sought to become pregnant using her husband's sperm, and who needed surgery to repair an injury to her reproductive organs prior to insemination, would have shared information about her medical history with her husband, assumptions do not excuse unethical behavior. The physician should have asked Mary, in private, whether her husband knew why she needed surgery, and determined how much information Mary had disclosed or wished to disclose. A fertility medicine specialist or another medical professional working with a couple may appropriately perceive himself to be in a physician–patient relationship with the couple as a unit, as well as with one or both individuals in the relationship. The ethics literature on prenatal genetic counseling, for example, recommends that the professional in the counseling role establish a relationship with the couple and avoid suggesting that one partner is the focus of the counseling relationship. However, a couple consists of two individual persons. A professional must be mindful that each of these individuals has interests, and that the professional obligation to act in the best interests of the person in need of care is not fulfilled by treating two persons as if they are one person.[9,10]

If a physician concludes that in protecting one patient's privacy he is also concealing information from another of his patients, such that this other patient's ability to make informed choices concerning this patient's own medical treatment, including his voluntary participation in assisted reproduction, is being constrained, the physician is confronted with an ethical dilemma. In this case, the obligation to protect Mary's privacy and the confidentiality of physician–patient communications inside of the fertility specialist's ongoing treatment relationship with Mary may compete with this same physician's truth-telling obligations to Paul as a new patient. Again, Mary's physician should have anticipated this scenario and should have discussed this with Mary at the time of their initial physician–patient discussion of her medical history.

Subsequent scenes reveal the fallout from this breach of physician–patient privilege and from Paul's own breach of donor–recipient confidentiality, as he contacts Christina and becomes enmeshed in her life and her efforts to cope with the deaths of her husband and children. Mary decides to leave Paul, telling him, "I'll have surgery and I'll be inseminated with your child, with or without you." When Paul says he won't authorize this, Mary reminds him, "You already have. I have a signed copy of your authorization to use your semen."

This small, intense scene raises its own bioethical issues. Does Paul's reproductive material really belong to Mary now, making him her sperm donor rather than her spouse? Conversely, does Paul have the right to challenge or revoke his prior authorization, which was given under the presumption that he would soon die? Bioethicists and legal scholars have, in recent years, considered the ethical and legal dimensions of postmortem and post-relationship parenthood, including the procurement of sperm from a woman's recently deceased husband, and the custody and use of frozen embryos following the break-up of a relationship.[11,12,13] These real cases, like the fictional case of Paul and Mary, ask how one person's wish to become a parent should be considered with respect to interests of another person who would be the biological parent of a future child, and also with respect to the interests of this future child. And, they echo the question that this film asks, over and over: What claims does an individual have on the bodies, and the lives, of others?

REFERENCES

1. Wijdicks, E.F.M. 2001. The diagnosis of brain death. *New England Journal of Medicine* 344: 1215–1221.
2. Greenberg, G. 2001. As good as dead. *The New Yorker* August 13, 2001, 36.
3. Truog, R.D. 2008. Consent for organ donation: Balancing conflicting ethical obligations. *New England Journal of Medicine* 358: 1209–1211.
4. Truog, R.D., and Miller, F.G. 2008. The dead donor rule and organ transplantation. *New England Journal of Medicine* 359: 674–675.
5. Miller, F.G., and Truog, R.D. 2008. Rethinking the ethics of vital organ donations. *Hastings Center Report* 38(6): 36–46.
6. Cleveland Clinic. *Contacting the family of your organ donor.* Retrieved May 3, 2010 from http://my.clevelandclinic.org/services/lung_transplantation/hic_contacting_the_family_of_your_organ_donor.aspx
7. Lauritzen, P., et al. 2001. The gift of life and the common good: The need for a communal approach to organ procurement. *Hastings Center Report* 31(1): 29–35.
8. Beauchamp, T.L., and Childress, J.F. 2008. *Principles of biomedical ethics*, 6th ed. pp. 302–310. New York: Oxford University Press.
9. McDaniel, S.H. 2005. The psychotherapy of genetics. *Family Process* 44(1): 25–44.
10. Lippmann, A. 1993. Prenatal genetic testing and geneticization: Mother matters for all. *Fetal Diagnosis and Therapy* 8(1): 175–188.
11. Batzer, F.R., Hurwitz, J.M., and Caplan, A. 2003. Postmortem parenthood and the need for a protocol with posthumous sperm procurement. *Fertility & Sterility* 79(6): 1263–1269.
12. Ahuja, K.K., Mamiso, J., Emerson, G., et al. 1997. Pregnancy following intracytoplasmic sperm injection treatment with dead husband's spermatozoa: Ethical and policy considerations. *Human Reproduction* 12: 1360–1363.
13. Alghrami, A. 2005. Deciding the fate of frozen embryos. *Medical Law Review* 13: 244–256.

6

god at the bedside:
shadowlands

robert c. macauley

Shadowlands (1993). Anthony Hopkins, Debra Winger, Edward Hardwicke.
Directed by Richard Attenborough. Duration: 131 minutes.

DVD Chapter 22 Scene 1:59:41 to 2:00:45

SHADOWLANDS IS BASED ON THE true story of C.S. Lewis (Anthony Hopkins), a professor of English literature at Oxford and later Cambridge, who is perhaps best known as the author of *The Chronicles of Narnia*. In the early 1950s, he strikes up a friendly correspondence with Joy Gresham (Debra Winger), a fledgling American poet and mother of two boys. They eventually meet when Joy and her young sons visit England, and following her divorce, she moves there permanently. After agreeing to marry in name only to enable her to stay in the country, they subsequently fall in love even as Joy is diagnosed with cancer. The film details a brief period of remission, followed by a recurrence and ultimately Joy's death, which Lewis struggles to understand in light of his Christian faith.

Several times early in the movie, Lewis casually refers to pain as "God's megaphone to rouse a deaf world." But in the aftermath of his beloved wife's death, he is forced to confront loss on a more personal level than ever before. In one scene near the end of the film, Lewis reunites with the university faculty for the first time since Joy died. While several colleagues offer condolences, a clergyman proffers platitudes, such as "Life must go on." Lewis replies that he's not sure if it must, only that it does. And although Lewis implores his friends not to tell him "it's for the best," the clergyman asserts that only God the Creator can know why something like this would happen. After describing human creatures as "rats in a cosmic laboratory," Lewis summarizes his situation: "It's a bloody awful mess, and that's all there is to it."

Lewis's response is understandable. Serious illness—whether affecting oneself or a loved one—inevitably causes a person to ask, "Why me?" For those without a specific religious belief, the answer may be random occurrence or the cruelty of fate. But for those who are religious, the question takes on added significance by potentially casting doubt upon their understanding of God. They might well question how a loving God could allow something like this to happen to them, or wonder if it could be divine punishment for something they did. Illness, therefore, "is a spiritual event. [It] grasps persons by the soul and by the body and disturbs them both."[1]

At its inception nearly 50 years ago, bioethics was well-equipped to address questions such as these. As Albert R. Jonsen writes, "Theologians presided over the creation of bioethics."[2] The field could roughly be divided into Roman Catholic and Protestant camps, the former emphasizing natural law and the role of the Church *magisterium*, the latter focusing on Scriptural commands and the proper response to a loving God. Gradually, bioethics has become more secularized, thereby broadening the field's applicability and relevance. Modern bioethicists, however, may not be as well-versed in the religious traditions of patients.

This can be problematic when patients respond to serious illness based on their spiritual beliefs. Denial is a common initial reaction—indeed, Elisabeth Kübler-Ross cites it as the first stage of grief [3]—and in the case of devoutly religious patients, this may take the form of faith in miracles. "This can't be happening to me" becomes "this *isn't* happening to me," and trust in divine intervention may prompt requests for seemingly futile treatment, if only to buy more time for God to act. Physicians, trained in the scientific method, are inevitably challenged by anticipation of an event that—by definition—defies the laws of science. Faced with seemingly unreasonable treatment decisions and a breakdown in communication, they often request an ethics consultation.

Clinical ethics focuses on "the identification, analysis, and resolution of moral problems that arise in the care of a particular patient."[4] An awareness of the spiritual basis of a patient's decision is necessary to sensitively address these concerns. As an Episcopal priest, as well as a physician-ethicist, I am most knowledgeable about the Christian tradition, but am also comfortable engaging patients and families of other traditions in faith-based dialogue. In response to an expectation of a miracle, for example, I might refer to the old saying that "God answers all prayers, but sometimes the answer is 'No.'" This is illustrated in my own religious tradition—and that of C.S. Lewis—by Jesus' words on the night before he was crucified: "Father, if you are willing, remove this cup from me; yet, not my will but yours be done."[5]

Far from questioning someone's trust in miracles, I often find it helpful to take their presuppositions to their logical conclusions. After much heartfelt conversation, I often end up asking something like, "If you *really* believe what you say you believe, what would that mean for the patient's care?" I might observe that if an omnipotent deity wishes to save a person's life, He shouldn't require human creations such as ventilators to do so. Viewed in this light, requests for continued aggressive treatment might actually reflect an unconscious *lack* of faith, which raises an entirely different set of questions (and responses).

While some religious patients wait for a miracle, others reluctantly accept aggressive treatment because they believe they have no choice. This view often stems from their sense that refusing certain interventions constitutes euthanasia. A particularly complex example of this dilemma involves the use of feeding tubes in Roman Catholic patients. This issue made headlines in 2004 when Pope John Paul II stated that feeding tubes are "in principle, ordinary and proportionate and, as such, morally obligatory."[6] By contrast, the *Ethical and Religious Directives*, which guide treatment in Catholic health systems, view feeding tubes in light of the Church's longstanding emphasis on balancing benefits and burdens.[7] The burdens of artificial feeding (such as aspiration) are well-documented, and the benefit is often uncertain. For example, feeding tubes have been shown to not prolong the lives of patients with severe dementia.[8]

While some have interpreted the Pope's statement as a return to the Church's prior emphasis on the distinction between "ordinary" and "extraordinary" treatments, one which is increasingly difficult to apply to the evolving world of medical technology, others point to the fact that the Pope was referring to surrogate decision-making for patients who were not terminally ill. It is also important to note that he advocated feeding tubes "in principle," just as the *Directives* do in the absence of overwhelming burden. And, perhaps most importantly for Catholic patients wrestling with a similar decision, the Pope himself refused a permanent feeding tube when he was in the final stages of Parkinson's disease. These clarifications can empower Catholic patients to make their own decision in light of the highly nuanced teaching of their Church.

It should be clear by now that an ethicist needs to respect the importance of religion in the lives of patients and families, and be willing to engage them on that level. He or she must be able to identify the spiritual basis of a patient's concerns, and be sufficiently familiar with that particular faith tradition to put those concerns in context. This can be a significant challenge in a pluralistic, post-Christian world. Fortunately, the ethicist need not be a follower of that religion, nor is he called upon to judge whether the patient's religious beliefs are objectively "correct."[9] Rather, he is simply honoring the heartfelt beliefs of a patient struggling to make sense of a threatening present and uncertain future.

Spirituality not only plays a role in medical decisions, but also in how people cope in the aftermath of those decisions. According to Kübler-Ross, anger follows denial, and this is exemplified in Lewis's response to the clergyman's glib consolation. Yet, this emotion can be very difficult for some religious people—especially Christians—to express. Many feel that trust in God requires equanimity in the face of suffering, as if anything less would reflect an absence of faith. Not wanting to compound their grief with a sense of guilt, they might respond in a way that suggests either they don't understand their situation, or they are emotionally barred from accepting it.

Here, it can be freeing to offer those who mourn *spiritual* permission to be honest with their feelings, citing their own Scriptures in support this approach. One example in the Judeo-Christian tradition is the Psalms, which often include expressions of anger toward God, yet always with the hope of greater understand and reconciliation. My Old Testament professor in seminary went so far as to add a spiritual twist to a medical aphorism: When friends were really angry at God about something, she often advised them to "take two Psalms and call me in the morning."

C.S. Lewis was facing the loss of his faith as well as his wife, and while a bioethicist could not prevent the latter, he could bravely address the former. He could have invited Lewis—in the words of his own religious tradition—to share his anger with his God, and in so doing begin the process of grieving and transformation. Eventually, Lewis does come to the conclusion that pain, far from being a megaphone to rouse a deaf world, is the inevitable result of having loved. "The pain now is part of the happiness then," Lewis says as the movie concludes. "That's the deal." If only those around him had had the courage—and the knowledge—to walk with him on that journey.

REFERENCES

1. Sulmasy, D.P. 1999. Is Medicine a spiritual practice? *Academic Medicine* 74:1002–1005.
2. Jonsen, A.R. 1998. *The birth of bioethics*, p. 41. New York: Oxford University Press.
3. Kübler-Ross, E. 1969. *On death and dying*. New York: Macmillan.
4. Jonsen, A.R., Siegler, M., and Winslade, W.J. 1986. *Clinical Ethics*, 2nd ed., pp. 3. New York: Macmillan.
5. Luke 22:42. New Revised Standard Version.
6. As quoted by Catholic News Agency, *Pope's Rejection to Starvation and Dehydration*. Retrieved November 16, 2009 from http://www.catholicnewsagency.com/resource. php?n=421
7. United States Conference of Catholic Bishops. 2001. *Ethical and religious directives for catholic health care services*, 4th ed. Washington, DC: United States Catholic Conference.
8. Finucane, T.E., Christmas, C., and Travis, K. 1999. Tube feeding in patients with advanced dementia: A review of the evidence. *Journal of the American Medical Association* 282: 1365–1370.
9. Lindbeck, G.A. 1984. The nature of doctrine: Religion and theology in a post-liberal age. Louisville, KY: John Knox Press.

conflict of interest, the physician and big pharma: *the fugitive*

cory franklin

The Fugitive (1993). Harrison Ford, Tommie Lee Jones, Sela Ward, Julianne Moore. Directed by Andrew Davis. Duration: 130 minutes.

DVD Chapter 17 scene 1:52:52 to 1:54:44

T HE FUGITIVE IS THE EXCITING story of Dr. Richard Kimble (Harrison Ford), a prominent Chicago surgeon wrongly convicted of murdering his wife and sentenced to be executed. On his way to prison, he escapes and sets out to find the real killer, all the while being pursued by a dogged U.S. Marshal (Tommie Lee Jones). It turns out the real killer is part of a greedy scheme by a pharmaceutical company seeking U.S. Food and Drug Administration (FDA) approval for a groundbreaking new drug. The company, in partnership with a corrupt physician (Jeroen Krabbe), has falsified research on the drug to score huge profits. Because he has uncovered evidence his colleague took deliberate steps to hide serious complications of the drug, Kimble was the real target of the murderer; his wife was killed by mistake. In the film's climax, the company's research fraud is exposed, the dishonest physician is discovered, and Kimble is exonerated.

In this scene, Kimble, still the subject of an intense manhunt, interrupts his colleague's presentation to an assembled group of scientists at an elaborate dinner. Kimble publicly exposes the research fraud in no uncertain terms, shouting to the audience, "He falsified his research!" Just prior to this, his colleague, in his presentation, made a telling Freudian slip by alluding to the "dishonest, excuse me honest, open, joint ventures between academic medicine and the pharmaceutical industry." Certainly, this plotline, with the outré Hollywood touch of a murder, is extreme. But it is effective in raising legitimate and serious questions about relationships and conflicts of interest between physicians and health care companies that include pharmaceuticals and device makers. Other scenes in the movie also touch on this issue through the portrayal of lavish receptions and junkets provided for physicians by the drug company (full disclosure—I was a technical advisor for the movie and contributed ideas to some of these scenes). The corrupt physician's slip in his speech is the best starting point for a discussion of conflicts of interest between physicians and the pharmaceutical companies, since it provides some useful context. It also leads to the most crucial question: How honest or dishonest are the mutual relationships involving physicians and Big Pharma in the pursuit of research, promotion, purchasing, and investments? The question is a complex one without a simple answer, and it covers a number of relationships. Conflicts of interest, for purposes of this discussion, are defined as activities that carry personal benefit (money or equivalent emoluments) that might call into question the physician's duty to the interests of patients or society. Essentially, the issue is: Can the physician who receives money or other gifts from outside sources be trusted completely? Historically, conflicts of interest have been a source of contentious debate within the medical profession. For decades, physicians have functioned as paid spokesmen and researchers for corporate interests. In the middle of the last century, for example, it was even common for physicians to endorse cigarettes in advertisements and on TV. At the same time, an element of distaste arose in the commercialization of research. In the 1950s, famed journalist Edward R. Murrow posed the question of who owned the polio vaccine patent to the vaccine's discoverer, Jonas Salk. Salk's famous reply, "There is no patent. Could you patent the sun?"

In 1980, the editor of the *New England Journal of Medicine*, Arnold Relman, describing the medical-industrial complex, wrote, "In this medical market, physicians must act as discerning purchasing agents for their patients and therefore should have no conflicting financial interests."[1] That statement appeared during what now seems like an age of innocence; since then, conflict of interest issues have taken on a new urgency, with health care erupting into a trillion-dollar business. Coincidentally, that same year, Congress passed the Bayh-Dole law permitting physician investors from their academic home institutions to share royalties from licensing or commercializing intellectual property (the bill's purpose was also to provide greater federal oversight of conflicts of interest).[2] This coincided with an explosion in medical research and the aggressive marketing of new products (with physicians playing a crucial role), as well as with opportunities for investment in new ventures. All of these situations presented physicians with opportunities to enhance their professional reputations and/or their income by cooperating with industry, in ways previously not possible.

A recent review of studies published between 1982 and 1997 estimated that physicians met with pharmaceutical representatives at least weekly, and residents accepted six gifts per year from industry representatives.[3] Another study showed that 94% of physicians had some kind of relationship with the pharmaceutical industry, usually involving receiving food in the workplace (83%) or accepting free drug samples (78%). Of those responding to the aforementioned survey, 35% received reimbursement for attending professional meetings, and 28% collected payment for consulting, giving lectures, or enrolling patients in trials.[4] These relationships are a double-edged sword. Physicians, despite their occasional protests to the contrary, are indeed influenced by these gifts and benefits. Studies show that, as a result of these interactions, physicians' prescribing patterns change in ways not necessarily supported by the clinical literature. For example, they may choose newer, more expensive drugs over well-established drugs with equivalent effectiveness. In addition, the pharmaceutical industry seeks out locally prominent physicians to influence hospital formulary decisions, as well as hiring nationally known physicians to be spokesmen for their products. The prescribing physician receives tangible benefits and the cachet of practicing at "the state of the art," both powerful incentives for accepting a system that winks an eye at conflicts of interests. Balanced against the aforementioned risks is the fact that certain industry-promoted drugs offer improvements over older medications and may be underused by physicians. Industry-sponsored professional meetings, when not overly commercial, often provide valuable physician education. Without question, patients can and do benefit from certain relationships between medicine and industry.

When dealing with pharmaceutical companies, physicians should not ignore obvious conflicts of interest. Their primary duty is to their patients. Institutions and professional organizations must formulate guidelines for practitioners. In specific situations, limits on outside physician compensation, recusals of certain physicians from formulary committees, and voluntary restrictions by pharmaceutical companies on hospital marketing activities are measures worth considering. However, these must be considered carefully: Unduly severe restrictions run the risk of denying patients real benefits.[5] One favorable development is the new regulations drafted by professional and industrial organizations. In 2002, the Pharmaceutical Research and Manufacturers of America (PhRMA) created a code of conduct for physicians and industry emphasizing patient benefit and the advancement of the practice of medicine. The code discourages companies from giving physicians gifts and reimbursements unrelated to patient care (e.g., tickets to sporting events). The American College of Physicians and the American Medical Association have followed suit with similar codes of conduct.[6] Research conflicts of interest, like that portrayed in *The Fugitive*, present a more complicated dilemma. What is appropriate for physicians who have a financial stake in the drugs, devices, and surgical procedures they research? The physicians may be working on valuable research, but financial interests may compromise his or her objectivity. How should these be approached? Those with the most at stake— patients who become research participants—are not of a single mind on the issue. One study from the National Institutes of Health revealed that patients' reactions ranged from concern to indifference to acceptance to encouragement of investigators' collaboration with industry.[7] Patients generally did want to be notified of such collaborations and assumed the host institution monitored such interactions to prevent abuses. This suggests that patients anxious to find cures for their conditions believe research will benefit them and are willing to tolerate physician–industry relationships, as long as they receive some notification. Researchers should guarantee disclosure to patients as a "reasonable person" disclosure; that is, what a reasonable person would want to know. The academic center must have an adequate oversight process to protect patients from egregious conduct in conflict-of-interest situations involving investigators.

As the health care sector has become a major component of the American economy, the issue of physicians owning equities and possible conflicts of interest takes on added importance. Certainly, individual physician prescribing habits have no effect on most publicly traded companies. The doctor who owns stock in Merck or Pfizer is not engaging in any conflict of interest activity when he or she prescribes the company's products. However, in certain cases, physicians with specialized practices might have conflicts of interests if they prescribe expensive medications or use surgical devices made by smaller, less-diversified companies in which they own equity. Conceivably, these physicians might generate enough volume to influence the value of the stock and their own holdings. The physician who owns equity in a privately held company with a product that gains market approval (e.g., a product the physician invented) runs the risk of serious conflict of interest by using or promoting the product or device. In this case, the physician's home institution should scrutinize the issue of stock ownership carefully. The question of divestiture in these cases requires further examination. An especially serious conflict-of-interest question deserving greater scrutiny is the physician-expert assuming the role of independent reviewer for medical journals or as an authority who issues practice guidelines. The *New England Journal of Medicine*, whose editor warned about conflicts of interest back in 1980, had to concede more recently that it was no longer possible to find expert reviewers for key articles who did not have ties to industry. Because of this, the journal was forced to change its reviewer policy from "no conflict" to "no significant conflict."[8,9] A related issue is the failure of some authors to disclose their industry connections to journals where they submit their work, despite new more stringent disclosure requirements in most major medical journals. Journal editors have claimed they were caught unaware when an undisclosed conflict of interest surfaced in an article they published. At the minimum, this situation mandates that journal editors exercise greater diligence in the prepublication process and strengthen their disclosure rules for prospective authors. A high-profile conflict of interest recently occurred after a panel of nationally renowned cardiologists issued a report advocating that more people be treated with lipid-lowering drugs. It was subsequently discovered eight of the nine guideline authors received payment from companies making lipid-lowering drugs. In a statement, the coordinator of the National Cholesterol Education Program who oversaw the recommendations tried to dismiss the conflict of interest by saying, "If you excluded all the people who have any financial connections to industry, you'd exclude all the people who are most expert." His opinion went essentially unchallenged in a medical community reluctant to acknowledge the possibility of bias in guidelines such as these and how this issue might affect a large population.

A final word on disclosure. Disclosure is not a substitute for avoiding conflicts of interest, but it is one of the essential cornerstones of managing the problem. When conflicts are deemed unavoidable, physicians must be transparent about their relationships with industry and make necessary information available on the salaries, honoraria, consulting fees, and royalties they receive from companies. This information should be made accessible to the public, as well as to the physician's home institution. When in doubt, the default position should be disclosure. However, this is not universally accepted by everyone in the medical community: At least one author has criticized an overzealousness to explore conflicts of interest as "the new McCarthyism in science."[10] Consequently, the exact rules for disclosure should serve as a topic of discussion and analysis by medical faculty and students at every institution. *The Fugitive* demonstrates why conflict-of-interest questions are so difficult to pigeonhole. Simply imagine an alternative scenario in the movie: Suppose the drug the physician-villain was working on with the pharmaceutical company did not have dangerous side effects but actually turned out to be a safe, breakthrough drug. He would be the hero of the movie—except there would be no murder and no plot. The relationship between physician and industry would be of benefit to all involved, and his friend Richard Kimble would not be a fugitive but a proud colleague feting him at the head table of the medical meeting.

The current nature of conflicts of interest in medicine resists simple proscriptions and demands careful analysis. Simply banning the drug rep from bringing pizza to lunch for the residents hardly represents a sufficient response to addressing the myriad situations representing conflicts of interest today. The next generation of physicians must develop policies and management strategies for the many situations that will arise when doctors and the medical industrial complex sit down at the table together. These rules should be flexible but unambiguous—no standard legal boilerplate or hypocritical "value statements" observed only in the breach. The rules will require disinterested ombudsmen and outside scrutiny from the public. All of that is necessary but not sufficient. No matter what the situation, the medical community must strive for greater intellectual honesty and more probity. At stake is public trust in the profession. Just ask Richard Kimble.

REFERENCES

1. Relman, A.S. 2008. Medical professionalism in a commercialized health care market. *Cleveland Clinic Journal of Medicine* 75(6): S33–S36.
2. Bayh-Dole Act. Pub L 96–517, 37 CFR 401 (1980).
3. Wazana, A. 2000. Physicians and the pharmaceutical industry: Is a gift ever just a gift? *Journal of the American Medical Association* 283: 373–380.
4. Campbell, E.G., Gruen, R.L., Mountford J., Miller, L.G., Cleary, P.D., and Blumenthal, D. 2007. A national survey of physician-industry relationships. *New England Journal of Medicine* 356: 1742–1750.
5. Camilleri, M., Cortese, D.A. 2007. Managing conflict of interest in clinical practice. *Mayo Clinic Proceedings* 82(5): 607–614.
6. Studdert, D.M., Mello, M.M., Brennan, T.A. 2004. Financial conflicts of interest in physicians' relationships with the pharmaceutical industry: Self-regulation in the shadow of federal prosecution. *New England Journal of Medicine* 351: 1891–1900.
7. Hampson, L.A., Agrawal, M., Joffe, S., Gross, C.P., Verter, J., and Emanuel, E.J. 2006. Patients' views on financial conflicts of interest in cancer research trials. *New England Journal of Medicine* 355: 2330–2337.

8. Angell, M., and Kassirer, J.P. 1996. Editorials and conflicts of interest (editorial). *New England Journal of Medicine* 335: 1055–1056.
9. Drazen, J.M., and Curfman, G.D. 2002. Financial associations of authors (editorial). *New England Journal of Medicine* 346: 1901–1902.
10. Rothman, K.J. 1993. Conflict of interest: The new McCarthyism in science. *Journal of the American Medical Association* 269: 2782–2784.

the impaired physician: *drunks*

delese wear

Drunks (1997). Richard Lewis, Lisa Harris, Amanda Plummer, Faye Dunaway, Calista Flockhart, Dianne Wiest, Spalding Gray, Parker Posey, Howard Rollins. Directed by Peter Cohn. Duration 90: minutes.

DVD Chapter 5 Scene 00:50:11 to 00:55:42

DRUNKS REVOLVES AROUND AN ALCOHOLICS Anonymous (AA) meeting in a Times Square church basement. Based on Gary Lennon's play "Blackout," the film showcases an unsentimental portrait of addiction and the struggle for sobriety. The film focuses on Jim (Richard Lewis), whose sobriety is dramatically tested when he reluctantly leads the meeting for the first time in seven months. Full of feverish anger as he tells his story, he closes with a confession: He wants to get drunk, and does just that when he abruptly leaves the meeting for an all-night binge. Director Peter Cohn intercuts Jim's misadventures over the course of the night—mostly buying alcohol in convenience stores and sitting on bar stools—with stories told by the others left behind in the basement meeting: Becky (Faye Dunaway) is a divorced parent not sure how losing custody of her child will influence her sobriety; Joseph's (Howard Rollins) drunkenness behind the wheel put his child in the hospital; Debbie (Parker Posey), a narcissistic, insufferable young woman who identifies strongly with Janis Joplin.

Rachel (Dianne Wiest), a now-sober physician currently working 18 hours a day to forget the loss of her husband and children because of her addiction to Demerol and scotch, tells one of the most convincing stories. In a five-minute monologue, she relates the chronology of her addiction and recovery. Years ago, she was placed in detox in the hospital where she worked, and after rehab and life in a halfway house with other physicians, she then returned to the same institution. She began to practice again, often sleeping on the sofa in her office. "I worked, I worked, I worked... I stayed straight, stayed clean, and stayed sober," she says, but now returns to AA because of a new awareness of the similarities between her present life of unending work and her life as an addict. *Now* she isolates herself in crowds of doctors and patients who always need her; *then* she isolated herself with Demerol and scotch. "I have not done the work of AA," she says quietly, "the thing of looking at how I blew up my life. I guess that's why I'm here."

Drunks offers viewers several points of inquiry critical to the professional development of physicians at all levels. It has been estimated that 10%–15% of all

practicing physicians will at some time during their careers develop a substance
abuse disorder.[1]

Thus, on a practical level, both trainees and practicing physicians should know
the ethical and legal dimensions of physician impairment by drugs and alcohol.
Rachel describes how she was initially "caught" by the police, passed out in her car
with her children. This incident prompted her to turn herself in to the hospital,
thus escaping an intervention by a colleague. Nonetheless, the issue of turning in
a colleague is difficult for many physicians to address, even though the American
Medical Association (AMA) Code of Medical Ethics[2] is quite clear on the subject:
"Physicians have an ethical obligation to report impaired, incompetent, and/or
unethical colleagues in accordance with the legal requirements in each state." The
Code elaborates:

> Physicians' responsibilities to colleagues who are impaired by a condition
> that interferes with their ability to engage safely in professional activities
> include timely intervention to ensure that these colleagues cease practicing
> and receive appropriate assistance from a physician health program. Ethically
> and legally, it may be necessary to report an impaired physician who
> continues to practice despite reasonable offers of assistance and referral to a
> hospital or state physician health program. The duty to report under such
> circumstances, which stems from physicians' obligation to protect patients
> against harm, may entail reporting to the licensing authority.

However, among some physicians, the ethical dilemma is choosing between
protection of the privacy and confidentiality of their impaired colleague and the
safety of patients[3]; for others, there remains a real concern that a colleague's
reputation or career will be irreparably hurt because of such reporting, or that
they may be sued for defamation.[4]

Yet, under the Health Care Quality Improvement Act, physicians who offer
information about an impaired physician are immune from liability unless they consciously provide false information.[4] Others reasons for the reluctance to confront
physician colleagues is the absence of adequate standards "to identify signs of need,
difficulty in ascertaining with confidence that a colleague is experiencing serious
problems, and lack of familiarity with available resources that can offer supportive
interventions."[5] Even witnessing the passed-out Rachel in a sweltering locked car
with her two children crying in the back seat might have given some of her colleagues pause in reporting, with easily crafted explanations of Rachel just being
stretched too far, or of the incident being a one-time event, and so on. Still, a 2005
survey of physicians found that a majority of physicians would report a colleague
impaired by a drug or alcohol, and 22% of those surveyed actually had done so.[3]

Still, it was Rachel herself who realized that she needed help—or at the very
least, that it would be better to turn herself in than to wait for a colleague or
hospital authority to do so. She delivers the details of her recovery with a calm

matter-of-factness as she acknowledges how the hospital took charge and told her precisely what she must do in the sequence of detox and rehab; she does not seem to characterize the hospital's actions as stern dispensations of "punishment" or "discipline." Yet, "disciplinary action" remains the standard language used to describe the impaired physician who has been "caught" or "turned in"; indeed, drug and alcohol impairment are some of the leading causes for such action against physicians in the United States.

Still, while the "vast majority" of physicians who have substance impairment do "surprisingly well in recovery,"[1] there may be much to be gained by situating their addictions into a larger conversation about physician health and wellness. For example, Taub and colleagues[5] note that, while the problems of alcoholism and substance abuse have been given more attention than other conditions (most often in the form of discipline), "the medical profession may be more successful in achieving the required standards by fostering a culture committed to health and wellness as well as supporting impaired physicians." Rachel's most recent parking lot incident illuminates how critical this wider commitment should be to the health of physicians. What does it mean to the individual and the profession when a physician works 18-hour days, most often sleeping on an office couch?

Collectively crafting and sustaining a culture of health and wellness—that's real collegiality, not just protecting one's own, as it is often conceived. One wonders where Rachel's colleagues are since her reinstatement. We might assume that she has had ongoing drug testing; she may have had an initial mandate to continue with AA (itself co-founded by a physician, Dr. Robert Smith, in 1935) or other support groups—all part of the disciplinary aspect of her addiction[6]—but based on her five-minute story, there seems to be nothing in her current life but personal and professional isolation. She notes that she has always had her work ("It's never let me down"), but even that must be questioned, given the painful affect she displays at the meeting. We know that physicians' unrecognized emotions and attitudes can negatively affect physician–patient communication; they can also undermine physicians' abilities to "experience and convey accurate empathy; may preclude or distort meaningful discussions with patients… or may lead to underinvolvement or overinvolvement with certain patients. Unacknowledged needs can 'leak' inappropriately during the medical encounter and endanger the physician–patient relationship[7]." As we watch Rachel, we wonder where all her weariness and pain go when she is actively caring for patients. The surveillance may continue regarding her addictions, but any real support seems to be absent from her life. Now, she seeks the support offered by AA again—but what is the role of the professional culture of medicine to help her rebuild her life? Doesn't Rachel and others like her deserve thoughtful and compassionate care of the same standard provided to non-physician patients"?[5] "Physician, heal thyself" may be one of the most important precepts in medicine, but the moral landscape of the profession must be one that encourages health and wellness for all its members, not just the patients it serves.

REFERENCES

1. Gastfriend, D.R. 2005. Physician substance abuse and recovery: What does it mean for physicians—and everyone else? *Journal of the Americaon Medical Association* 293: 1513–1515.
2. Opinion 9.031– Reporting impaired, incompetent, or unethical colleagues. *AMA Code of Medical Ethics.* Retrieved June 30, 2009 from http://www.ama-assn.org/ama/pub/physician-resources/medical-ethics/code-medical-ethics/opinion9031.shtml
3. Farber, N.J., Gilibert, S.G., Aboff, B.M., Collier, V.U., Weiner, J., and Boyer, E.G. 2005. Physicians' willingness to report impaired colleagues. *Social Science & Medicine* 61: 1772–1775.
4. Liang, B.A. 2007. To tell the truth: Potential liability for concealing physician impairment. *Journal of Clinical Anesthesia* 19: 638–641.
5. Taub, S., Morin, K., Goldrich, M.S., Ray, P., and Benjamin, R. 2006. Physician health and wellness. *Occupational Medicine* 56: 77–82.
6. Holtman, M.C. 2006. Disciplinary careers of drug-impaired physicians. *Social Science & Medicine* 64(207): 543–553.
7. Novack, D.H., Suchman, A.L., Clark, W., Epstein, R.M., Najberg, E., and Kaplan, C. 1997. Calibrating the physician: Personal awareness and effective patient care. *Journal of the American Medical Association* 278: 502–509.

the boundaries of physician relationships: *people will talk*

michael farrell

People Will Talk (1951). Cary Grant, Jeanne Crain. Directed by Joseph L. Mankiewicz, based on the play "Dr. Praetorius" by Curt Goetz. Duration: 103 minutes.

DVD chapter 7 scene 00:38:18 to 00: 39:00

PEOPLE WILL TALK IS A psychologically complex movie about physician behavior and the relationships that physicians develop. The movie can be used to initiate discussion about several bioethical questions,[i] but my classes with *People Will Talk* have most often focused on issues of professionalism and the boundaries of physician relationships with patients, colleagues, family, and friends. The main character of *People Will Talk* is Dr. Noah Praetorius (Cary Grant), a highly regarded medical school faculty member whose methods are humanistic and holistic. The movie begins with an intriguing preamble:

> This [movie] will be part of the story of Noah Praetorius, M.D. That is not his real name, of course. There may be some who will claim to have identified Dr. Praetorius at once. There may be some who will reject the possibility that such a doctor lives, or could have lived. And there may be some who will hope that if he hasn't, or doesn't, he most certainly should.

Regardless of how the movie's creators originally intended the preamble to be read, for today's audiences the phrase "he most certainly should" seems to provoke discussion about the characteristics of the ideal physician. In my classes, I ask students to consider how personal physicians' relationships with patients may become, and whether a physician ceases being a physician outside of his or her professional role. *People Will Talk* uses several interwoven plot lines to explore these themes.

The major plot line in *People Will Talk* is the complicated development of Dr. Praetorius' relationship with Deborah Higgins (Jeanne Crain), a part-time student who becomes a patient and then later his wife. Dr. Praetorius meets Deborah when she interrupts a gross anatomy lecture by fainting. Dr. Praetorius evaluates her and advises her to see a physician. As Dr. Praetorius leaves the scene, Deborah gazes after him with an intensely speculative look on her face.

Later, Deborah comes to see Dr. Praetorius in his clinic and tests positive for pregnancy. In subsequent conversation, it emerges that Deborah is not married and that her child's father died in military service overseas. Deborah laments that her pregnancy will "kill" her father and that she won't be able to tell him, at which Dr. Praetorius gently scoffs. Deborah leaves his office and shortly afterwards shoots herself in the hallway. Dr. Praetorius rushes Deborah to surgery, but he seems to be powerfully affected when another character comments that she will likely try to kill herself again (DVD time 26:51).

Later that evening, he returns to Deborah's hospital bedside and tells her that the pregnancy test result had been an error, apparently so that she will be able to have what he earlier had called a "health-giving sleep." She is horrified and embarrassed at having told Dr. Praetorius about her former boyfriend, and miserably asks, "Are all your patients women?" and comments "I guess they all fall in love with you" (DVD time 38:51). Dr. Praetorius gently denies this and leaves for home, apparently intending to return in the morning to tell her that she is in fact pregnant. He is alarmed when she sneaks out from the hospital and disappears. It takes the better part of a week for Dr. Praetorius to locate Deborah's home address, and he travels there intending to inform her that she is in fact pregnant. Dr. Praetorius meets Deborah's father (Sidney Blackmer), a likeable gentleman who regards himself as a failure except for his "one accomplishment, Deborah." Dr. Praetorius finds that he cannot tell her father about the pregnancy result, any more than Deborah could have told him. He speaks with Deborah alone and confronts her about her absconding from the hospital. Deborah has trouble replying but eventually challenges Dr. Praetorius that he has come to her home because he is romantically interested in her. Dr. Praetorius is taken aback (perhaps for the only time in the entire movie), and for reasons that are never made clear, finds that he cannot inform her about the true pregnancy result. The two share a dramatic kiss and hurriedly depart to be married.

With his suave self-control reestablished, Dr. Praetorius becomes the model husband who seems devoted to his newfound love. Two weeks later, Deborah suspects that she has become pregnant by her new husband, but in a conversation that smoothly juxtaposes the communication style of a husband and a physician, Dr. Praetorius reveals to Deborah that she had been pregnant all along. Deborah voices her horror (begins at DVD time 1:21:54):

DEBORAH: You're quite a noble character, aren't you?... I've heard of doctors that were self-sacrificing and unselfish, but apparently there's no limit to yours. Were you that afraid I'd kill myself... afraid enough to marry me to keep me from it?

PRAETORIUS: Is it conceivable to you that I would?

DEBORAH: It seems obvious, doesn't it?

PRAETORIUS: You mean that as a doctor, I was faced by a situation which I could only meet by marrying you, that I did it as a remedy? Deborah, as you know I believe in using any form of therapy that will make people well, but it would be highly impractical to make marrying my patients a standard form of treatment.

DEBORAH: Why did you marry me?

PRAETORIUS: Because I was in love with you.

Deborah asks him to explain why he fell in love with her, and he answers that he "couldn't say why." Deborah scoffs that his falling in love was too convenient and asks how he could have suddenly fallen in love, "a man as exact as you, with a reason for everything." Dr. Praetorius' repeatedly insists that he loves her and their baby, enough to remove most of the doubt from Deborah and the movie's audience.

Dr. Praetorius' other relationships are also explored throughout the movie. In the second major plot line, a medical school inquiry is instigated by Dr. Elwell (Hume Cronyn) into Dr. Praetorius' previous relationships with patients and the character Shunderson (Finlay Currie). It emerges at the inquiry that, shortly after graduating from medical school, Dr. Praetorius had posed as a small-town butcher who became widely renowned for miracle cures, many of which were actually standard medical treatments because of his hidden qualifications as a licensed physician. Shunderson is a kindly but somewhat slow-witted elderly man who acts as Dr. Praetorius' valet, but whom Dr. Praetorius describes as a "friend" who "helps at whatever he can." It emerges that Shunderson had been convicted of murder under ambiguous circumstances and was thought to have been executed by hanging. Dr. Praetorius received his supposed cadaver as a donation from the hangman, but found that he had survived with anoxic brain injury. The faculty inquiry panel eventually dismisses both of Dr. Elwell's complaints as being frivolous and unjustified.

In my class sessions on *People Will Talk,* at least one student typically voices disapproval or outrage at the thought of a physician marrying a patient. In an era where professional distances are encouraged, medical students regard personal relationships outside of the official doctor–patient interchange with disapproval or alarm. Indeed, many professional codes discourage physicians from developing sexual relationships with patients. Hippocrates' oath states:

"With purity and with holiness I will pass my life and practice my Art... Into whatever houses I enter, I will go into them for the benefit of the sick, and will abstain from every voluntary act of mischief and corruption; and, further from the seduction of females or males..."[1]

In the modern perspective, a sexual or romantic relationship with a patient is regarded as problematic because of the patient's vulnerable or powerless position in the relationship.[2] Another problem can emerge if a transference situation arises, in which emotions and desires originally associated with one person, such as a parent or sibling, are unconsciously shifted to the physician.[3] In 1991, the relationship problem was considered by the American Medical Association's Council on Ethical and Judicial Affairs, with the somewhat ambiguous conclusion that "sexual contact or a romantic relationship with a former patient may be unethical under certain circumstances."[4] A more detailed theoretical framework was subsequently laid out by Farber et al. to understand love, boundaries, and patient–physician relationships.[5] A reasonable summary of these and other sources might state that romantic relationships should raise concern because of the patient's vulnerability and other complexities, but may be acceptable under certain circumstances.

When I began teaching about *People Will Talk*, I was prepared to cite professionalism codes and why they have been developed, and why they are not easy to apply to Dr. Praetorius' character. After many such discussions, I now listen calmly to participants' disapproval and proceed to ask the group to consider an unrelated question: "When does Dr. Praetorius act like a physician, and when does he act like a regular man?" In the ensuing discussion, students explore how physicians might interact with the world and where their responsibilities begin and end. As is often the case with the medical humanities, the ambiguous circumstances faced by the characters in *People Will Talk* can serve to initiate discussions about the rationale behind a bioethics decision. In my view, it seems that the creators of *People Will Talk* believed that the marriage between Dr. Praetorius and Deborah was acceptable, but wanted to leave some room for doubt because of the complicated circumstances. Similar ambiguities remain with regard to Shunderson and Dr. Praetorius' masquerade as a butcher. It seems that the Dr. Praetorius character is intended to be a masterful communicator who brings a humanistic approach to every patient's care and his physician persona into many of his non-clinical relationships. This interpretation seems easier to make because of a few exceptions in the movie, such as Dr. Praetorius' unusual lack of control when confronted by Deborah at her home, or the boyishly immature conversations he has with his friend Professor Barker (played by Walter Slezak).

An interesting teaching device that I use before the movie is to have students write down adjectives describing their concept of the "ideal physician." After the movie, I ask for reactions to the Dr. Praetorius character (which are often negative), but then point out how many of the ideal characteristics that they wrote down are present in Dr. Praetorius' character. This exercise and the discussion about boundaries have often helped students to gain a richer understanding of the bioethical complexities underlying the issues of professionalism, professional codes of conduct, and the development of individual relationships by physicians throughout their lives.

NOTES

i. In my teaching sessions with *People Will Talk,* I allow discussion to follow the interests of the group. Most of my class discussions have focused on the issues of professionalism discussed in this essay, but I was initially drawn to the movie because it illustrates various types of communication strategies (DVD times 10:45, 14:38, 17:16, 37:11). *People Will Talk* can also be used to jump-start discussion on truth-telling and disclosure of errors and results to patients. The movie also contains a widely cited monologue on the use of cadavers in gross anatomy classrooms, and how students should think of cadavers (DVD time 8:31). Finally, the movie also provides an interesting historical perspective on abortion before *Roe v. Wade* (time index 18:37), and on interactions between allopathic medicine and other medical traditions (the second plot line described in the essay).

REFERENCES

1. Hippocrates, Decorum XVI. 1923. In W.H. Jones (Ed.), *Hippocrates with an English translation*. London: Heinernann.
2. Blackshaw, S.L., and Miller, J.B. 1994. Boundaries in clinical psychiatry. *American Journal of Psychiatry* 151(2): 293; author reply 295–296.
3. *The American heritage dictionary of the English language*, 4th ed. 2006. Boston, MA: Houghton Mifflin Company.
4. Council on Ethical and Judicial Affairs, American Medical Association. 1991. Sexual misconduct in the practice of medicine. *Journal of the American Medical Association* 266(19): 2741–2745.
5. Farber, N.J., Novack, D.H., and O'Brien, M.K. 1997. Love, boundaries, and the patient-physician relationship. *Archives of Internal Medicine* 157(20): 2291–2294.

10

cross-cultural issues and medical decision-making: *worlds apart*

maren grainger-monsen and stephen murphy-shigematsu

Worlds Apart (2003). Documentary comprised of four trigger films: Justine Chitsena's Story: Lao American; Robert Phillips' Story: African American; Mohammad Kochi's Story: Afghan American; Alicia Mercado's Story: Puerto Rican American. Produced and directed by Maren Grainger-Monsen, M.D. and Julia Haslett. Cross-cultural medical advisors: Alexander R. Green, M.D.; Joseph R. Betancourt, M.D., M.P.H.; J. Emilio Carrillo, M.D., M.P.H. Duration: 48 minutes.

DVD chapter 1, scene 0:00—11:00, Justine Chitsena's Story

WORLDS APART IS A DOCUMENTARY film that tells the story of four culturally diverse patients and families faced with critical medical decisions as they navigate the American health care system. Shot in patients' homes, neighborhoods, places of worship, and hospital wards, *Worlds Apart* provides a penetrating look both at the patient's culture and the culture of medicine. The film is shot in a cinema-verité style that captures live clinical interactions as they happen, and includes interviews with patients, families, and the medical staff involved, but no narration. Like other films by Dr. Grainger-Monsen, *Worlds Apart* speaks to the need for developing cultural competence and knowledge of health disparities in health professionals.[1]

This segment of *Worlds Apart* shows the dilemma of a young Lao-American woman, Bouphet Chitsena, caught between the strong beliefs of her mother and the recommendations of her doctors regarding her four-year-old daughter, Justine, who has an atrial septal defect (ASD; a hole in the muscular wall between the two atria in her heart). The doctors believe it should be surgically repaired, but Bouphet's mother, Thn Chitsena, is opposed to the operation because she does not believe anything is wrong with Justine, who appears healthy. She also believes that the operation will leave a scar on the child's body that will be carried through life and into the afterlife for all eternity. The grandmother's opposition is based in the family's strong cultural beliefs and traditional healing practices as members of Khmu, an ethnic group in Southeast Asia that has a mistrust of Western medicine.

A previous crisis, caused when Bouphet had overruled her family and allowed two-year-old Justine to have what turned out to be a successful bone marrow transplant, hovers over the present conflict. Now, in deciding whether to have the ASD repair, Bouphet expresses her excruciatingly difficult position when she says,

"It was my decision. My family was against me. They accused me of trying to kill my child. I realized that I would be the one in the hospital with Justine if anything happened. If anything went wrong, it would be my responsibility." She realizes that if she decides to agree with surgical repair of the ASD, she risks being ostracized and separated from her family. Yet, she fears that if she does nothing, she risks losing her daughter.

Bouphet's dilemma highlights issues that arise when patients, family members, and health care professionals have different perspectives on illness, medicine, and health.[2] In cases like this, it is vital to explore the patient's explanatory model of illness and treatment—meaning their specific beliefs about the cause of their illness and its treatment. This explanatory model can have a major impact on health care decisions and outcomes.[3]

In Bouphet's family, as in many others, beliefs, values, and concerns about health are culturally based.[4] These beliefs vary greatly, not only between cultural groups but also within cultural groups and within families as they are influenced by acculturation and generational differences.[5] Bouphet, for instance, grew up in a Thai refugee camp, came to the United States as a teenager, and doesn't believe that a surgical scar will be a permanent problem for her daughter. Grandmother Thn, however, is convinced that it will. For Bouphet, the real issue is being ostracized from the family, and she feels unable to risk this devastation. Her American-born Laotian daughter, Justine, on the other hand, while not having yet formed her views on illness, will probably have a much more Westernized view of the world: When the "Make a Wish Foundation" offered to give her anything she wished for, her wish was to meet Britney Spears.

Cultural differences among family members usually mean they have diverse ways of understanding illness and health. We help patients by trying to understand what they and their families think caused their health problems and how these health problems affect their lives. By understanding their different explanatory models, medical treatments can be offered that will have the best clinical outcomes, yet might not conflict with the patient's (and family's) beliefs.[6] Asking family members what worries them most and what kinds of treatment they think would work is a major step in this process. Asking questions such as, "what do you believe is the problem with Justine's heart?" or "what concerns you most about this procedure?" elicits the patient's explanatory model and provides the health care practitioner with greater insight regarding what a family considers most important for the patient.

In Justine Chitsena's Story, the family's role in decision-making also raises another important cross-cultural issue. The assumption, often made by health professionals, that patients (or parents of a minor) are autonomous decision-makers and that family members play a more peripheral role is culturally biased. In many cultures, certain members of the family have authority and make decisions based on a hierarchy of gender, age, or birth order.[7] In Justine's Laotian family, for example, the grandmother's influence is enormous. Bouphet's dilemma is profound because when she chooses to go against her mother's wishes and does not follow her advice, she is breaking cultural traditions and risks losing connection to the rest of her family.

There are several other examples of the importance of family, religious advisors, and community attitudes on patient decision-making in *Worlds Apart*. In Mohammad Kochi's story, for example, we see his Iman advise Kochi that, while trusting that God's will is good, he must also do what he can to heal himself by following recommended medical treatment. Robert Phillips is influenced by the history of the Public Health Service Syphilis Study at Tuskegee, which makes African Americans suspicious about health care provider motives when suggesting treatment options. In these situations, it helps all concerned when health care providers show respect for cultural beliefs, understand reasons for conflict, reassure patients of their good intentions, and explain why they believe in the efficacy of the treatment being recommended.

Justine Chitsena's story also highlights the dilemma of those medical professionals who advocate surgery. They believe that early intervention is the standard of care and that the low-risk surgery is the right course of treatment. Chances for Justine's defect to close spontaneously, at her age, are small, and while there is no urgency in closing the defect from a clinical standpoint, there is a risk that permanent damage will result if surgery is postponed indefinitely. Thus, the doctors must wrestle not only with their own beliefs, but also with their opinions regarding the alternative treatments advocated by the family. They are challenged in this situation to understand and respect the family's beliefs. They must decide whether they can find a way to work with the family to incorporate their wishes without compromising the health outcome for Justine.

In this story, we witness how communication skills, important in dealing with all patients, are crucial when cultural differences in perspective are great. This is especially difficult for medical professionals who feel that scientific truth is concrete. In serving our patients, we must accept the reality that "truth" for them may be different[8] from our own. If we can see beyond narrow biomedical and legal perspectives and communicate in a way that shows understanding of the patient's and family's perspectives, we create a possibility for reaching mutually agreeable solutions. Our effectiveness as healers, in cross-cultural situations, is greatly enhanced if we can explain our perspective, maintain our flexibility, and come up with creative ways to meet the patient's needs while aiming for the best possible clinical outcome.

Numerous obstacles and dangers exist in learning to be culturally sensitive, as it is difficult to give up the security of our worldview and consider that another worldview may be equally valid for a person from a different cultural background.[9]

Rigidly held, our own cultural beliefs can be a great barrier in communicating with patients from culturally diverse backgrounds. It is therefore an ethical issue to strive for empathic relations that extend understanding to the cultural beliefs of our diverse patients.

When we screen the film, we explain that the physicians were able to offer Justine minimally invasive surgery that could repair the defect in her heart wall without causing the scarring that was the obstacle for Thn, her grandmother. Bouphet found this to be a reasonable compromise, decided to go forward with this approach, and Justine did well postoperatively. This is an important example of how, by making an effort to truly understand the real issue that was at the heart of a cross-cultural conflict, the physicians were able to come up with a compromise that addressed the families' concerns while at the same time solving the medical problem.

Justine Chitsena's story focuses on the importance of exploring the patient's explanatory model of illness and treatment by showing how patients' and families' beliefs about illness and medical procedures can have a major impact on their health care decisions. It teaches us how exploring beliefs carefully and respectfully is crucial to cross-cultural interactions, encouraging self-reflection and increased awareness of the importance of culture in health care. In today's world, culturally sensitive and respectful communication and understanding are essential aspects of high-quality medical care that can have great impact on patients' health outcomes.

REFERENCES

1. Murphy-Shigematsu, S., and Grainger-Monsen, M. Forthcoming 2010. The impact of film in teaching cultural medicine. *Family Medicine*.

2. Kleinman, A., Eisenberg, L., and Good, B. 1978. Culture, illness, and care: Clinical lessons from anthropologic and cross-cultural research. *Annals of Internal Medicine*, 88: 251—258.

3. Aidoo, M., and Harpham, T. 2001. The explanatory models of mental health amongst low-income women and health care practitioners in Lusaka, Zambia. *Health Policy and Planning* 16: 206–213.

4. Xiong, P. 2003. Painful cultural differences in a Hmong family: The mother's perspective. In K.A. Culhane-Pera, D.E. Vawter, P. Xiong, B. Babbitt, and M.M. Solberg (Eds.), *Healing by heart: Clinical and ethical case stories of Hmong families and western providers*, pp. 198–206. Nashville, TN: Vanderbilt University Press.

5. Culhane-Pera, K.A., Her, C., and Her, B. 2007. 'We are out of balance here': A Hmong cultural model of diabetes. *Journal of Immigrant Minority Health* 9: 179–190. Retrieved from http://www.springerlink.com/content/r04313332884251m/

6. Mill, J. 2000. Describing an explanatory model of HIV illness among aboriginal women. *Holistic Nursing Practice* 15(1): 42–56.

7. Cha, D. 2003. *Hmong American concepts of health, healing, and conventional medicine.* New York: Routledge.

8. Plotnikoff, G.A. 2003. Defining best interest for a Hmong infant: A physician's challenge. In K.A. Culhane-Pera, D.E. Vawter, P. Xiong, B. Babbitt, and M.M. Solberg (Eds.), *Healing by heart: Clinical and ethical case stories of Hmong families and western providers*, pp. 159–164. Nashville, TN: Vanderbilt University Press.

9. Murphy-Shigematsu, S. 2002. *Multicultural encounters: Case narratives from a counseling practice.* New York: Teachers College Press.

part four

communication and provider–patient relationships

the deleterious effects of insensitivity: *range of motion*

jay m. baruch

Range of Motion (2000). Rebecca De Mornay, Henry Czerny, Barclay Hope, Charlotte Arnold, Kayla Perlmutter, Kim Roberts. Directed by Donald Wrye. Duration: 100 minutes.

DVD chapter 2 scene 00:09:14 to 00:09:50

THE FRAGILE AND UNPREDICTABLE BRAIN, the seat of our conscious awareness of the world and the people in it, serves as the central plot device in *Range of Motion*, a made-for-television movie. Rebecca De Mornay plays Lainey Berman, the wife of the handsome Jay (Henry Czerny) and mother to two beautiful young daughters. Her dreamy life in an old house of polished wood and sun-dappled windows gets shaken beyond comprehension when her husband falls in a freak running accident and sustains a head injury that leaves him in a coma. With her once athletic, sexy, and loving husband now in a second-rate convalescent home, Lainey rails against the pessimism of unfeeling doctors and hard-hearted nursing home staff. She faces threats to her own faith, love, and vision of family. Hoping one day he'll wake up and their lives will resume as before the disastrous accident, she devotes herself to his care, only to discover the pain associated with holding out for miracles.

In this scene, Lainey rushes to the hospital and is confronted with news that her husband had surgery to remove fluid from around his brain. He's unconscious, intubated, connected to a ventilator. Then, a few weeks later, we see that he's breathing on his own, but in a state of unconsciousness, unresponsive to his environment. The doctors inform Lainey of the still sizable swelling of the brain and that this difficult news is "painful for all of us." Lainey is instructed to be realistic. There is an 80% chance her husband will never wake up, and if he did, a strong possibility of speech impairment, memory loss, and crippling disability. The chief of neurology brings down the paternalistic hammer on the conversation. He declares that nothing more can be done for her husband. "Good luck," he says to Lainey, then abruptly stands and leaves.

"Good luck, is that it?" screams Lainey as the chief of neurology recedes down the corridor. The doctor who first broke this news to her recommends counseling. A woman armored in a business suit informs Lainey that her husband can't stay where he is. It costs $5,000 a week, and her insurance won't cover it. Other, more salvageable, patients need the bed. "You call yourself healers?" Lainey asks these women as they, too, walk away down the hallway, abandoning her at this moment of unbearable grief. "My husband is not a statistic," she cries out to them. "He's my husband."

In this troubling scene, physicians trample slipshod over the foundational precepts of medical ethics. They disregard patient autonomy, seem disinterested in beneficence, and with the snarky comment about resource allocation, take a shot at justice as well. But disturbing, unethical conduct by physicians can make for fascinating entertainment and discussion, especially when the scene plays its pro-vocative melodramatic hand with insensitive medical professionals who make decisions using suspect knowledge and dangerous logic. I'd like to focus on the following ethical questions: Who decides what information and values are valid and deserving of respect in medical decision-making and using what criteria? Does respecting patient autonomy and dignity require physicians to participate in treatment they believe ineffectual? If not, what does it mean to be a healer?

The neurosurgical literature states that recovery of consciousness from a post-traumatic persistent vegetative state is unlikely after 12 months in adults and children.[1] In this scene, the physicians throw up their arms after only a few weeks, which is presumably too early for reaching this conclusion. Even if 80% of patients in this situation at this point in their illness never wake up, that means 1 in 5 regain consciousness, odds that some—providers and family—might find sufficient cause for optimism. The physicians reveal biases by framing data in the negative. They conclude that nothing more can be done. In other words, any treatment from this point forward would be ineffectual or futile.

The futility debate of the 1990s centered on whether there are treatments, interventions, or goals that aren't worth pursuing, and if health care providers could then limit, or refrain from, continuing treatment. It was a battle framed around both ethics and economics. The high-profile case of Helga Wanglie con-cerned an 86-year-old, ventilator-dependent woman who had been in a persistent vegetative state for over a year. The doctors at Hennepin County Medical Center wanted her removed from the ventilator, regarding continued treatment as non-beneficial and failing to serve Mrs. Wanglie's best interests. The courts decided in favor of the family, but didn't address the appropriateness of intensive care, only that Mr. Wanglie, as her husband, was uniquely situated to make decisions on her behalf.[2]

Such heated conversations typically take place in hospitals at the end of life, with different parties holding varying opinions about the appropriateness and goals of treatment. The literature in the early 1990s demonstrated the bioethical and medical community struggling, and failing, to achieve consensus. Treatments were considered futile if they merely preserved permanent unconsciousness or could not end dependence on the intensive care unit, or if empirical data demon-strated that treatment has less than a 1% chance of benefiting the patient.[3] Medical futility was also conceptualized as treatment that will not accomplish its intended goals, when burdens or costs of treatment far exceed any benefits, or the benefits themselves are uncertain or controversial.[4] This scene doesn't involve end-of-life care, but the health care team decides to stop aggressive medical care, a unilateral decision that infuriates Lainey.

The decision that goals aren't worth pursuing isn't a question of futility, but a conflict of values, and a plurality of values impedes reaching consensus on the issue.[5] Such dilemmas pit patients and families against physicians, breeding antagonism and mistrust, moods that infiltrate throughout this movie. Patient autonomy and the right to self-determination do not obligate physicians to sacrifice professional integrity and the commitment to do no harm by applying treatments they consider hopeless, harmful, or not medically indicated. But medical professionals, I feel, are required to make decisions that are sensitive to the patient's wishes and needs, and reasoned from a firm grasp of the medical literature.

The treatment team misuses empirical data to substantiate their decision regarding what is in Jay's best interests. Physicians can't assume data derived from meticulously designed and implemented studies involving large numbers of patients will apply with absolute certainty to a particular patient with particular variables.[6] Lainey has every right to insist that her husband is not a statistic. When the physician lists potential disabilities that might greet Jay if he wakes up, she appears to be intuiting that life with these disabilities wouldn't be worth living. That opinion is founded on her professional and personal values. Some patients with limited life expectancy secondary to chronic obstructive pulmonary disease, congestive heart failure, and cancer fear the burdens of severe functional and cognitive impairment as worse than death,[7] but we don't know whether Jay shares these same fears.

The physicians never ask Lainey to consider what her husband would want if he could appreciate his circumstances. Such questions would not only demonstrate respect for his autonomy and dignity, but might make for a better scene. Would Lainey know his wishes, make a decision *as* him, and not *for* him? Good ethical decision-making, just like good story-telling, depends on backlighting the characters' pasts to better appreciate their present. Autonomous choice is a right of patients,[8] but the doctors never address Jay as a person. They refer only to his condition, his prognosis.

Even if their paternalistic arrogance and insensitivity are difficult to stomach, the doctors' decision to transfer Jay might not be unreasonable. He isn't dependent on a ventilator to breathe. He requires tube feedings, rehabilitation, and time, all of which doesn't require hospital-level care. Maybe resource allocation motivates the move as well. They need the bed, and his care could be carried out elsewhere.

Do the physicians have to be so rude and cold? Is this behavior evidence of character deformity, or is it perhaps a protective defense built over time in response to regular doses of medical catastrophe and devastated families? Did previous personality conflicts with Lainey occur? Was she a family member with unrealistic expectations who made undue demands on staff? We don't know what motivates the physicians' inability to empathize with Lainey's traumatic experiences. The decision is "painful for all of us," they say. How selfish and delusional, equating their "pain" with a wife's torment. They turn their backs when she refuses to comply; she is offered counseling, as if her feelings and beliefs count as pathological. This scene provides a glaring tutorial on the perils of poor communication skills for medical providers. Why didn't the physicians emphasize the rehabilitation services and treatments available to Jay? How should physicians respond when faced with situations in which treatment is nonbeneficial, harmful, or won't accomplish their intended goals?

From my own experiences, I believe that patients and their families should never feel abandoned. My discussions with families in the emergency department center on the patient's values and wishes. I try to explain the medical facts clearly, in terms the family will understand, and then place the anticipated goals of treatment in light of the medical situation. I never say there is "nothing we can do." Indeed, there is much we can do. We can provide aggressive end-of-life care, or we can offer conscientious and compassionate comfort care. Either way, the care continues.

REFERENCES

1. The Multi-Society Task Force on PVS. 1994. Medical aspects of persistent vegetative state—first of two parts. *New England Journal of Medicine* 330: 1499–1508.
2. Angell, M. 1991. The case of Helga Wanglie: A new kind of "right to die" case. *New England Journal of Medicine* 325: 511–512.
3. Schneiderman, L.J., Jecker, N.S., and Jonsen, A.R. 1990. Medical futility: It's meaning and ethical implications. *Annals of Internal Medicine* 112: 949–954.
4. Ethics Committee of the Society of Critical Care Medicine. 1997. Consensus statement of the Society of Critical Care Medicine's Ethics Committee regarding futile and other possible inadvisable treatments. *Critical Care Medicine* 25: 887–891.
5. Truog, R.D., Brett, A.S., and Frader, J.S. The problem with futility. 1992. *New England Journal of Medicine* 326: 1560–1564.
6. Prendergast, T.J. 1996. Futility and the common cold. How requests for antibiotics can illuminate care at the end of life. *Chest* 107: 836–844.
7. Fried, T.R., Bradley, E.H., Towle, V.R., and Allore, H. 2002. Understanding the treatment preferences of seriously ill patients. *New England Journal of Medicine* 346: 1061–1066.
8. Beauchamp, T.L., and Childress, J.F. 2009. *Principles of biomedical ethics*, 6th ed. New York: Oxford University Press.

2

interprofessional relationships:
the hospital

deirdre neilen

The Hospital (1971). George C. Scott, Diana Rigg, Barnard Hughes, Richard Dysart. Directed by Arthur Hiller. Duration: 103 minutes.

DVD Chapter 2 Scene 00:10:55 to 00.14:30

T*HE HOSPITAL* IS PADDY CHAYEFSKY'S bleak yet funny satire on hospitals and modern medical treatment (or rather maltreatment) in the 1970s. The film records one day in the life of Dr. Herbert Bock (George C. Scott), medical director of a public New York City hospital, as he contemplates the wreckage of his life and career. His hospital is imploding from political, racial, and economic tensions; on this day, three staff members will die there as well. When the film opens, Bock has left his wife and is living in a ratty hotel room; he is drinking heavily enough that others have mentioned it to the hospital's CEO; he is ignoring his rounds and actually contemplating suicide.

This scene has three parts: the discovery by the nurses of the death of Dr. Schaefer; Bock's learning by telephone of his resident's death; and Bock's confrontation with Mrs. Christie, the head nurse, at the bedside. In each part of the scene, and throughout the film, patient care standards, professionalism, and beneficence are violated. Nurse Perez seems indifferent as she reports to the charge nurse that Dr. Schaefer is dead in a patient's bed. The charge nurse does not even look up from her paperwork to give her response, "What the hell are you talking about? I don't know what the hell you're talking about." When the very hung-over Bock reaches the hospital and realizes that two different nurses have given Schaefer medication and treatment meant for a patient, thus killing him, he tears into the Chief Nursing Officer (his counterpart) in a verbal assault that is brutal, unremitting, and unforgiving. She is not allowed to answer him; his sarcasm explodes in a fusillade of violent images ending with, "Where do you train your nurses, Mrs. Christie, Dachau?"

Although more than 30 years have elapsed since the film appeared, viewers may not be overly shocked by Bock's outburst or Christie's stoic silence in the face of it. The inequality of power between medicine and nursing continues to resonate today. What has changed somewhat is the recognition that the results of such an imbalance can be stressful, harmful, and even deadly for both health care professionals and patients.[1] Medical errors can kill, and when Mrs. Christie says, "These things happen," Bock is right to find both her statement and her staff's errors appalling and inexcusable. Yet, so is his borderline contempt for her and her profession. He publically dresses her down in front of a hospital administrator, members of her staff, and passersby in the hospital corridor. As Storch and Kenny note in their essay on moral work, "many other health providers are part of [the health care] team, but, as the original health professionals, physicians and nurses must lead by example. Their inability to do so constitutes an ethical failure."[2]

In the context of the film, Bock's outburst is considered neither a breach of courtesy nor a lapse in professional ethics but rather the hallmark of a driven, dedicated physician. He is merely marking his territory and reminding the nurses that they are subordinates. Today, however, this scene can elicit an important discussion about physicians' professional responsibilities and ethical behavior. As the American College of Physicians says in its ethics manual, "power imbalances that can be abusive," such as those between a physician and a nurse, go against medical ethics.[3] Despite the medical profession's awareness and the Accreditation Council for Graduate Medical Education (ACGME)'s continued emphasis on advancing education in medical professionalism, disruptive behavior such as that depicted in the film still occurs in hospitals and during medical training today. The costs of such behavior are serious and can be seen in high staff turnover, burnout, and increased risk for ineffective or substandard care of patients.[4] Thus, there are pragmatic reasons as well as moral ones for examining and improving the professional behaviors that physicians and nurses display during their workdays.

Nursing has widely advanced both its role and its knowledge base since this film, yet in a hospital setting, a nurse may still be viewed by a physician as primarily a subordinate. Nurses today perform "highly specialized tasks and administrative responsibilities," yet often have to prove their competence with physicians each and every time.[5,6] The converse for the physician remains true: Competence is assumed until otherwise demonstrated. Few dare to question the physician's behavior or decisions.

These ongoing tensions may be part of the reason for the current nursing shortage, and hospitals and physicians need to examine what role their attitudes and behaviors may be playing in the nurses' flight from the profession. In one national survey, "as many as two-thirds of nurses say they've been abused by physicians at least once…" [such abuse ranged from verbal to physical and sexual harassment].[7] Another researcher looked at several surveys done with medical residents and found abuse among housestaff significantly correlating to suboptimal care and unprofessional behavior.[8] In other words, we may be teaching clinical staff by daily example that abusive behavior is part of the training, part of what must be endured. And thus begins a self-perpetuating cycle that allows behavior that directly contradicts principles of compassion and respect. The physician who berates a nurse, the nurse who then berates a resident—exactly where do we expect empathy for the patient to begin? It makes little sense to write down codes of conduct if we are going to allow certain individuals to violate them under the rubric of their being brilliant, demanding, or (most ironically) highly principled.

Nursing has created a new approach for hospital care called the *magnet program*; it identifies benchmarks to measure the quality of care being provided by its credited institutions. Not surprisingly, two of the key requirements for a magnet hospital are workplace empowerment and collaborative nurse–physician relationships.[9] These attributes are seen to increase job satisfaction and to influence patient safety. Other researchers look at expanding the opportunities for nurse–physician collaborations through education, training, and open forums. Not surprisingly, the articles and research data about such collaborations are found almost exclusively in the nursing literature. Nurses understand that their relationship to physicians does impact patient care and their ability to carry out their duties.[10] Physicians who have participated in some of these surveys do not seem to place as high an importance on the collaborative aspect between themselves and nurses. They explain away their occasional disruptive behavior as a reaction to their orders not being carried out correctly or in a timely manner. The implication is that if nurses do what physicians tell them, all will be well.

In the film, we see the effects of poor communication between professionals, chronic understaffing, and the disrespect that has filtered down from the top administrators to the ranks. When Bock attacks the nurses' womanhood ("And every time one of your nurses has her period, she disappears for two days!"), the audience is supposed to laugh, but such remarks today are not funny. They demonstrate a lack of professionalism and an abuse of position. They reflect an unacceptable ignorance about what understaffing of nurses means to patient care. And, they are responsible for helping to create a dispirited, dysfunctional staff that is delivering poor patient care much more akin to maleficence than beneficence.

If more collaboration occurs between medicine and nursing during education and clinical training, we can assume relationships between practitioners will also improve. If physicians do not understand the extent of responsibilities and time demands made on the nursing staff, they will continue to underestimate the benefits that a competent and collegial staff brings to their patients, as well as to the medical profession. Although *The Hospital* is meant more as entertainment than education, its narrative provides examples of dubious professional behavior, malpractice, moral dilemmas, and damaging stereotypes that persist within the medical profession. Discussion of this scene can lead to intense examination of one's own behavior and attitudes toward other professionals. Hierarchies in medicine and hospitals, for example, can be analyzed to see how they affect patient care and medical professionalism.

REFERENCES

1. Institute of Medicine. 2004. *Keeping patients safe: Transforming the work environment of nurses.* Washington, DC: National Academies Press.

2. Storch, J.L., and Kenny, N. 2007. Shared moral work of nurses and physicians. *Nursing Ethics* 14(4): 478–491.

3. Snyder, L., and Leffler, C., for the Ethics and Human Rights Committee. 2005. Ethics Manual, 5th ed. *Annals of Internal Medicine* 142: 560–582.

4. Pfifferling, J.H. 1999. The disruptive physician. *Physician Executive* 25(2): 56–61.

5. Fagin, L., and Garelick, A. 2004. The doctor-nurse relationship. *Advances in Psychiatric Treatment* 10: 277–286.

6. Rothstein, W.G., and Hannum, S. 2007. Profession and gender in relationships between advanced practice nurses and physicians. *Journal of Professional Nursing* 23(4): 235–240.

7. Rosenstein, A.H. 2002. Nurse-physician relationships: Impact on nurse satisfaction and retention. *American Journal of Nursing* 102(6): 26–34.

8. Mareiniss, D.P. 2004. Decreasing GME training stress to foster residents' professionalism. *Academic Medicine* 79(9): 825–831.

9. Lake, E. 2002. Development of the practice environment scale of the nursing work index. *Research in Nursing and Health* 25: 176–188.

10. Armstrong, K., Laschinger, H., and Wong, C. 2009. Workplace empowerment and magnet hospital characteristics as predictors of patient safety climate. *Journal of Nursing Care Quality* 24(1): 55–62.

3

"difficult" patients?: *passion fish*

carl lundstrom

Passion Fish (1992). Mary McDonnell, Alfre Woodard, Vondie Curtis-Hall, David Stathairn. Directed by John Sayles. Duration 135: minutes.

DVD Chapter 3 Scene 00:11:30 to 00:16:00

PASSION FISH TELLS THE STORY of an actress, May-Alice (Mary McDonnell), who is hit by a car and becomes paraplegic. Remaining in shocked disbelief about her condition throughout the initial rehabilitation sessions in New York, she rejects professional help and finally returns to her family home in Louisiana. Her homecoming to her neglected Louisiana abode is marked by the notable lack of success of a number of agency "nurses" assigned to her. Eventually, the arrival of Chantelle (Alfre Woodard), a young black woman from Chicago trying to recover her life after drug addiction, leads to some stabilization of the situation. The two women initially clash but eventually come to understand each other in a mutually beneficial interaction.

The designated scene succinctly deals with two people whose aims and ideas never merge. It takes place immediately after May-Alice arrives at the old home place and is assisted by her first nurse, a determined Russian woman (Marianne Muellerleile). May-Alice, still shocked by her injury and her situation, remains adamantly uncooperative, lashing out at anyone who dares to help her. Her nurse is very determined to fulfill her role as she sees it: keeping everything clean and, in an orderly fashion, tending to the needs of her charge. Inevitable friction results, and the two are constantly battling back and forth over May-Alice's behavior, which consists of endless alcoholic drinks and apathy. The end result is a stalemate: One morning at breakfast, May-Alice throws egg on the newly cleaned, beautiful wooden wall of her room, resulting in the abrupt departure of the Russian nurse.

In this example, the caregiver (the Russian nurse) is preoccupied with her own point of view—to give the kind of care she thinks appropriate. The patient, unimpressed by the nurse's care plan, pushes back, with neither appreciating the other's position. A standoff results, with the nurse giving way and losing all chance to benefit her patient. May-Alice quickly descends into deeper despair, following the arrival (and rapid departure) of a succession of increasingly self-absorbed nurses.

Five principles of patient–caregiver relationships are illustrated—autonomy, beneficence, empathy, collaboration, and power—first in the vignette, and then expanded upon in the film. The details governing each of these principles are not exclusive to the patient–caregiver relationship, and disregarding any of them may derail the relationship-forming process and stop progress. Although many other issues complicate the process, relationships ultimately are about connection, and within this two-way process the details are vitally important.

First, we review the sometimes-competing principles of *autonomy* and *beneficence*. Autonomy refers to the ability of persons to govern themselves, while beneficence has to do with promoting good and withholding evil.[1,2] We can instantly see how these two ethical principles may compete. In *Passion Fish*, the patient has some right to her own decision making, regardless of the outcome. However, her injury, by its very nature, forces May-Alice to give up some of her autonomy. In addition, her self-destructive tendencies, fed by her injury and her discouragement over lost career dreams, clashes with any objective outsider's attempt to promote her own good. Clearly, perspective is needed to resolve this clash, and perspective usually takes time. A very strong sense of "doing good" may, as in this scene, result in a failure to do anything, often due to a power struggle between caregiver and patient. Here, beneficence may well appear to the patient to be a negative quality, if she is pressured to make some move toward a goal. This is where alignment—having a common interest and a common goal— is essential. If both parties view autonomy and beneficence as moving together in the same direction, they become joined in therapy. To facilitate this, several other relationship principles must be brought into play.

The next important principle in the patient–caregiver relationship is *empathy*: the ability to experience vicariously the feelings, thoughts, or attitudes of another person.[3,4] Connecting two people, particularly two dissimilar people, requires that an effort be made to understand another viewpoint and to have flexibility in thought. This flexibility may be a natural quality for some people, or it may be a learned experience. Empathy is critical to alignment. A well-known expert in this field has suggested a number of ways in which a caregiver might promote empathy.[4] The first is to be aware of one's own feelings about any given situation. This need to be objective—to step back and see the realities as the other person sees them— must happen fairly quickly. An objective view allows one to self-correct unilateral positions on an ongoing basis.

Caregivers must learn to be curious about their own negative emotions,[4] because self-reflection may provide insight into the patient's attitudes. This helps the caregiver bridge the gap with the patient's feelings. Listening for the patient's hidden emotional concerns follows, as does observing nonverbal cues. The goal is to better understand the patient and to respond appropriately to that understanding. Finally, the caregiver must accept and assimilate feedback from the patient, especially if it is negative. Accepting feedback without defensiveness promotes empathy. Using such a framework, the caregiver may utilize conflict to significantly enhance the therapeutic relationship.[4] Certainly, self-awareness is a major factor here. Empathy may be practiced and taught through role-playing exercises or reflection on the scene and the film under consideration.

The fourth principle is *collaboration*. As the conscious implementation of empathy, collaboration is the intentional coordination of concerns and goals. If patient and caregiver work together to define problems and undertake treatments, progress becomes tangible.[5] Collaboration also refers to teamwork and may involve coaching.[5] A degree of shared decision making is essential. In this scene from *Passion Fish*, a destructive lack of these qualities resulted in failure and disconnection: "I am leaving!" Later in the film, a different dynamic appears. There, two very different individuals discover the healing that comes with aligning goals and working together. Each has a sense of making a positive contribution to a common good. Actions that subvert collaboration include ignoring problems, abdicating responsibility, and being manipulative.[5] This leads to consideration of another principle—that of power and its use.

Power may be the most effective tool, as well as the most dangerous, in any relationship. Power struggles are common between individuals. Demands are often met with negative responses, and it's not uncommon for one party to hold more power than the other.[5] When this person is the caregiver, this imbalance in power may lead to retaliation from the patient. If this reaction is unexpected, the caregiver may see this as an affront or even a professional insult. In this context, the issue of boundaries may come up.[6] Again, it's time to step back and reevaluate. How can power be used for good purpose? Although empathy and collaboration may help resolve an impasse, being too close can be overpowering. Sometimes one has to back away in order to allow connections to resume, as seen later in the film. The balance of power becomes critical to the eventual therapeutic outcome.

Putting all these principles together successfully is truly an amazing accomplishment and requires trial and error, which in turn takes more time. The major portion of the film *Passion Fish* is devoted to illustrating the development of the real therapeutic relationship between May-Alice (the patient) and Chantelle (the nurse). Here, both come to recognize a mutual need for each other. This recognition of a bidirectional relationship must occur before progress can be made.[6] People just don't respond well to one-sided directions. Understanding and empathy rule supreme when it comes to moving forward in complex situations like this. In this case, the patient requires time to adjust to very unexpected circumstances. This is when patience and empathy are required by the caregiver. But relating personally to the situation does not happen without boundary setting.[6] Both parties must eventually recognize what is best for the patient, as is demonstrated by May-Alice and Chantelle by the end of the film.

In *Passion Fish*, the situation started with a natural conflict, driven by the shock and loss of the patient. A stalemate ensues, until both caregiver and patient can align their goals and aspirations. When that happens, therapeutic results appear. Very appropriate amounts of the three essential principles—collaboration, power, and empathy—are put into action for the benefit of both parties.[5] Collaboration involves a degree of shared decision making. Power also must fit the occasion, with each side recognizing when to exert power. Finally, empathy ideally will be a shared experience.[3] When these come together appropriately, we see a good example of what it means to achieve healing rather than simply a cure.

REFERENCES

1. Edge, R.S., and Groves, J.R. 2006. *Ethics of health care: A guide for clinical practice*, 3rd ed. New York: Thomson Delmar Learning.
2. Loewy, E.H., and Loewy, R.S. 2004. *Textbook of healthcare ethics*, 2nd ed. Dordrecht, The Netherlands: Kluwer Academic Publishers.
3. Larson, E.B., and Yao, X. 2005. Clinical empathy as emotional labor in the patient-physician relationship. *Journal of the American Medical Association* 293: 1100–1106.
4. Halpern, J. 2007. Empathy and patient-physician conflicts. *Journal of General Internal Medicine* 22: 696–700.
5. Elder, N., Ricer, R., and Tobias, B. 2006. How respected family physicians manage difficult patient encounters. *Journal of the American Board of Family Medicine* 19(6): 533–541.
6. Thompson, C.A. 2008. The difficult patient. *Journal of Clinical Oncology* 26(24): 4035–4036.

4

challenges faced by informal caregivers: *the hours*

david h. flood and rhonda l. soricelli

The Hours (2002). Nicole Kidman, Julianne Moore, Meryl Streep, and Stephen Dillane, Ed Harris. Directed by Stephen Daldry. Duration: 114 minutes.

DVD Chapter 6 Scene 01:24:50 to 01:27:29

BASED UPON MICHAEL CUNNINGHAM'S PULITZER Prize–winning novel of the same name, *The Hours* follows a day in the life of three women united by the thread of Virginia Woolf's stream-of-consciousness novel *Mrs. Dalloway*. At the center is Virginia Woolf (Kidman) writing *Mrs. Dalloway* in 1923. Interwoven with her story are those of Laura Brown (Moore), a desperate 1950s Los Angeles housewife reading *Mrs. Dalloway*, and Clarissa Vaughn (Streep), who, in 2001 New York, is living Mrs. Dalloway's life (a connection emphasized by the shared first name of the two characters) by preparing a celebratory party for her gay friend Richard (Harris). Richard, a writer and poet, is about to receive a major literary prize for his body of work. In their late teens, he and Clarissa shared a torrid relationship that neither can (nor wants) to forget—and he is seriously ill with AIDS.

The now middle-aged Clarissa has arrived early in the morning at Richard's dingy apartment, bearing an armload of flowers. Initially, his mind is still clouded by the hallucinations he experienced during the night. As Clarissa helps to reorient him, it becomes clear that she is Richard's closest friend, the one who fills in as family (informal) caregiver where the meager social support systems leave off. The scene at hand begins as Clarissa is about to leave, planning to return at 3:30 p.m. to help Richard dress for the awards ceremony and later party. Richard stops her to ask, "Would you be angry?" When Clarissa chooses to interpret the question narrowly—that he might not show up for the party—Richard pushes: "Would you be angry if I died?" The ensuing dialogue is tense and filled with revelation, as the two parties conduct the conversation at the levels that fit their respective needs.

Richard is tired of living with AIDS, but Clarissa will hear none of it, thus denying him any chance to address what he sees as an unacceptable quality of life, let alone the topic of the death that would be a release from his suffering. Seeking to reveal to Clarissa the underlying motivation for her care and attention, Richard asks, "Who is this party for?" Still she refuses to engage in the discussion, forcing Richard to push further: "I'm saying… I think I'm only staying alive to satisfy you." For Clarissa, however, this makes perfect sense. After all, "that is what people do.

They stay alive for each other." Since he can likely be kept alive in his present state for years, that is what he should want, must want. Her need for his presence in her life far outweighs his horror at the thought of living for years in his present AIDS-ravaged condition. Richard continues to plead his case, trying to push Clarissa to evaluate her own life and the forces that drive her caregiving, but to no avail. In a flurry of energy and metaphor, Clarissa gathers up the trash in the apartment and stuffs it (and Richard's concerns and insights) into the overflowing garbage can. Empowered by this act, Clarissa negotiates what she believes is Richard's eventual agreement to attend the party and leaves.

While physicians are frequently inept at talking about death and dying with patients and their families, the problem is even more pronounced in the homecare situation, in which a family member or other intimate, such as Clarissa, provides the majority of patient support.[1] In this setting, multiple confounding factors potentially inhibit these most important discussions between caregiver and patient: love of the patient that interferes with the ideal of "detached concern"; guilt that he is the sick one, or that care is given out of duty, not love; fear of failure in providing adequate care; and conflicting agendas, as we see with Richard and Clarissa. In addition, the caregiver may be uncomfortable with her own mortality. The end result is that the patient is denied the opportunity to talk about his fears, anxieties, and even hopes about death and dying, while the person on the other end of the dialogue is often left with a sense of inadequacy and the feeling that the patient has been let down. The patient's needs are met with denial and avoidance instead of compassion and understanding, and he is denied the opportunity to choose "the right time to die,"[2] get his house in order, and bid farewell.

As patient care increasingly moves into the home setting, with informal care-givers providing the majority of care,[3] educational strategies need to be developed to assist the informal caregiver in end-of-life discussions. One might argue that home hospice workers are so trained, but the majority of patients at home are not in a terminal condition. Richard, for example, can "live like this for years" if he takes his medications and is willing to tolerate a life of isolation, hallucinations, and fear. Informal caregivers need professional assistance in identifying their own hopes and fears, what motivates their care, and in what ways their value system may be at odds with that of their patient. For Clarissa, it is a given for people to "stay alive for each other," while the suffering Richard struggles for self-determina-tion. In his debilitated state of dependency, Richard fully realizes the power Clarissa wields over him, and that understanding will eventually lead him to suicide as the only way out of the situation.[4]

Discussions with informal caregivers frequently lead to considerations of dignity, and indeed, many caregivers are motivated by the desire to preserve the dignity of their loved one. But do they understand what gives dignity to another? Edmund Pellegrino writes that "intrinsic human dignity is expressive of the inherent worth present in all humans simply by virtue of being human... .

[e]xtrinsic or imputed dignity… is the assessment of worth or status humans assign to each other or to themselves.… . [it] can be gained or lost simply by one's own self-judgment or by the judgment of others."[5] Rebecca Dresser further states: "Dignity is promoted when others honor the patient's ordeal and look up to the person enduring the assaults of illness and treatment… [o]rdinary activities fall by the wayside and relationships are no longer the same."[6] *The Hours*, then, is particularly instructive on the issue of imputed dignity. Richard is shamed by his predicament and Clarissa's enduring attention, feels unworthy of the literary award that he fears is being made out of sympathy for his illness rather than the quality of his work, and is in no way physically or mentally capable of attending the awards ceremony or party. Clarissa compounds his loss of dignity by denying the authenticity of his experience and rejecting his pleas to be heard. Richard's utter despair is captured in the sarcasm of a single word—"Wonderful"—that he repeats at the end of the scene.

Of course, *The Hours* encourages discussions about quantity versus quality of life, the right to die, and overall end-of-life care.[7] It challenges us to consider what an "acceptable" quality of life is, and by whose criteria. It begs the questions of whether suicide is ever justified, comprehensible, or inevitable. And, it raises the perennial issue of patient autonomy. Even though Richard suffers from hallucinations that may be a by-product of HIV-associated dementia or drug toxicity, his discussion with Clarissa is clear and concise, suggesting that he is still mentally competent, albeit depressed. It would be hard to argue that Clarissa's viewpoint should prevail or that societal values alone should guide his care.

Finally, in bringing to such vivid life (and death) a patient with AIDS, *The Hours* is a valuable film for our time. We have become complacent about this disease in the United States even though as many as 55,000 new diagnoses of HIV infection are made each year and 14–15,000 deaths from AIDS still occur annually.[8] Moreover, the suicide rate for male AIDS patients is estimated to be 17 to 36 times greater than that for the healthy population.[9] While dementia, drug toxicity, and depression may all play a part, we must consider whether there is something unique about living with HIV or the prolonged anticipation of dying with AIDS that contributes to this statistic. We must ask if the informal caregiver to someone with AIDS, who knows her patient is not "terminal" by the usual criteria, walks a more perilous path than her caregiving peers as a result.

When one compares Michael Cunningham's novel with David Hare's remarkable screenplay, it is evident that, while staying true to the original work, Hare also underscores the complex relational and medical ethical issues in *The Hours*. He represents both sides of the dialogue in painfully realistic ways, bringing to the fore the ambiguity inherent in so many family caregiving situations rather than presenting pat answers, as Hollywood is prone to do. A thoughtful viewing of this scene raises questions relevant not only to homecare but to medical education and national medical policy in general.

REFERENCES

1. Staton, J., Shuy, R., and Byock, I. 2001. *A few months to live: Different paths to life's end*, pp. 23–56. Washington, DC: Georgetown University Press.
2. Hardwig, J. 2009. Going to meet death: The art of dying in the early part of the twenty-first century. *Hastings Center Report* 39(4): 37–45.
3. Retrieved September 19, 2009 from http://www.thefamilycaregiver.org/who_are_family_caregivers/care_giving_statstics.cfm
4. *The Hours*. DVD chapter 15, scene 01:30:55 to 01:34:00.
5. Pellegrino, E.D. 2008. The lived experience of human dignity. In *Human dignity and bioethics: Essays commissioned by the president's council on bioethics*, pp. 513–537. Washington, DC: The President's Council on Bioethics.
6. Dresser, R. 2008. Human dignity and the seriously ill patient. In *Human dignity and bioethics: Essays commissioned by the president's council on bioethics*, pp. 505–512. Washington, DC: The President's Council on Bioethics.
7. Jennings, B., Kaebnick, G.E., and Murray, T.H. (Eds.). 2005. Improving end of life care: Why has it been so difficult? *Hastings Center Report Special Report* 35(6): S1–S60.
8. Retrieved September 19, 2009 from http://www.avert.org/usa-statistics.htm
9. Kaufman, D.M. 2007. *Clinical neurology for psychiatrists*, 6th ed., pp. 135. Philadelphia: Saunders.

5

benevolent deception: *send me no flowers*

catherine belling

Send Me No Flowers (1964). Rock Hudson, Tony Randall, Edward Andrews, Paul Lynde. Directed by Norman Jewison. Duration: 100 minutes.

DVD chapter 4 scene 00:13:58 to 00:22:00

THE PROTAGONIST OF THIS ROMANTIC comedy, George (Rock Hudson), lives in mid-1960s American suburbia with his wife, Judy (Doris Day). George, a hypochondriac, suffers from a comic stereotype of anxiety about illness and depends on a vast cabinet full of medications. In the film's opening sequence—after an epigraph from William Osler, "The desire to take medicine is probably the greatest feature which distinguishes man from animals"—he dreams about television commercials for prescription medications, giving a thought-provoking sense of how much—and how little—has changed since the 1960s regarding pharmaceutical advertising. Misunderstandings ensue, until the happy ending when the confusion is resolved and George is liberated from his now empty medicine cabinet.

In the selected scene, George visits his primary care physician because he is worried by chest pain. The doctor, a caricature of a certain kind of mid-century American family doctor, is unashamedly more interested in his income and golf game than in his patient. He examines George, dismisses the pain as indigestion, and provides some pills. George goes into the bathroom to take his medication right away, and while there, overhears the doctor talking on the phone about someone else's electrocardiogram, which apparently reveals a fatal problem. He also hears the doctor say that he does not plan to tell the dying patient his prognosis. George, sure that he is that patient, tries to confront the doctor who, unaware that he has been overheard, makes things worse by saying that if George *were* terminally ill, he would probably not tell him the truth. George leaves in despair, certain that he is dying.

The scene provides a vivid instantiation of medical paternalism. The physician makes largely well-intentioned (if not very thoughtful) decisions on the patient's behalf without the patient's fully informed consent. The focus here is especially on benevolent deception—when a physician actively withholds information about diagnosis or treatment from a patient, or even provides misinformation, with the intention of protecting the patient. The scene reveals the danger of deception, even in the guise of benevolent medical paternalism, and vividly demonstrates the effects of such deceptions: the patient can no longer trust his physician and is left isolated in his fear. In a different genre, or a different culture, this visit could lead to tragedy.[3,4] (The Kurosawa film, *Ikiru*, presents a dramatic corollary for this scene.)

This scene in *Send Me No Flowers* represents the doctor as more interested in his own status and income than in his patient's well-being, and depicts the patient as a nervous back-seat driver who questions the doctor's every statement. In doing so, the scene provides thought-provoking images of a less-than-ideal patient–physician interaction, and facilitates a discussion both about the historical context (Do scenes like this take place today? What has changed and what has not?) and about conditions in the practice of medicine likely to promote paternalism and patient anxiety. An interesting historical and disciplinary subtext is this primary care doctor's explicit resentment of specialist physicians who, in his view, earn more money for less work, and how his antipathy translates into disdain for the very real needs of his patient: He observes that most of his patients are not sick—and if they were, he would refer them to a specialist.

The doctor also disregards confidentiality, discussing the dying patient by name (although George misses this part of the conversation). Since 1996, the Federal Health Insurance Portability and Accountability Act (HIPAA) has enforced the ethical duty to respect patient confidentiality, in particular the HIPAA Privacy Rule, but a patient's right to limit the sharing of information they give their doctors is as old as Hippocrates. The scene presents not only the doctor's disregard for privacy, but also the complex and harmful unintended consequences of such carelessness.

This film was made at about the time when informed consent was emerging as a patient's legal right and, with it, the need for full disclosure of the diagnosis, and the options and implications of treatment.[1,5] When George asks about the pills he is prescribed, his doctor replies, "You wouldn't know if I told you, just take them." By making into a comic figure a physician who disregards these ethical developments, the film suggests that audiences were already expected to question his high-handed authority and disregard for the truth, although they might not yet fully recognize the harmful effect such deception could have or generalize from his behavior to the assumptions held by most in the medical profession at the time.

The scene presents the effects of this paternalistic deception on the patient. When George asks about his condition and his medication, his need for information marks him not as a modern, autonomous patient, but as the classic difficult hypochondriac.[7] His attentiveness is presented as comic paranoia. George gives everything a sinister subtext, getting in the way of the doctor's effort to reassure him quickly and alleviate the "indigestion" he fears is heart disease. He is all too ready to assume the worst. George's unarticulated sense of having a right to be informed and to be allowed to participate in diagnosis and decision-making is now considered the ethical standard, although in practice wide variations exist.

The scene immediately following this one reinforces the film's exploration of benevolent deception. George's wife, Judy, is in her kitchen "making his sleeping pills," as she explains to a friend. George relies on Seconal capsules to sleep, but Judy has realized that a placebo works just as well, so she refills the capsules with sugar. Both scenes of medicalized lying set the stage for the poor communication and harmful confusion that follows. Despite the film's comic and romantic happy ending, it remains a cautionary tale about the harm that can be done by even the most well-intentioned disregard of another's right to accurate information on which to base his autonomous decisions. This scene can serve, then, as a good starting point for discussions on the emergence of, and reasons for, our current medical ethics of patient autonomy and informed consent, as well, perhaps, as the unintended effects of the new responsibility it places on patients.[2]

REFERENCES

1. Faden, R., Beauchamp, T., and King, N. 1986. *A history and theory of informed consent.* New York: Oxford University Press.
2. Veatch, R.M. 2009. *Patient, heal thyself: How the new medicine puts the patient in charge.* New York: Oxford University Press.
3. Numico, G., Anfossi, M., Bertelli, G., Russi, E., et al. 2009. The process of truth disclosure: An assessment of the results of information during the diagnostic phase in patients with cancer. *Annals of Oncology* 20: 941–945.
4. Innes, S., and Payne, S. 2009. Advanced cancer patients' prognostic information preferences: A review. *Palliative Medicine* 23: 29–39.
5. Hirsh, B.D. 1961. Informed consent to treatment. *Journal of the American Medical Association* 176: 436–438.
6. U.S. Department of Health and Human Services. Health Information Privacy. Retrieved October 26, 2009 from http://www.hhs.gov/ocr/privacy/
7. Barsky, A.J. 2001. The patient with hypochondriasis. *New England Journal of Medicine* 345: 1395–1399.

6

team dynamics and ethics
of responsibility:
whose life is it anyway?
and *bringing out the dead*

anne h. jones

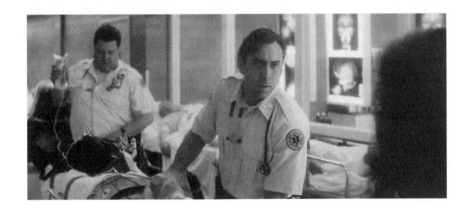

Whose Life Is It Anyway? (1981). Richard Dreyfuss, John Cassevetes, Christine Lahti, Bob Balaban, Kenneth McMillan. Directed by John Badham. Duration: 119 minutes.

DVD Chapter 16 Scene 1:00:25 to 1:03:34

Bringing Out the Dead (US, 1999). Nicolas Cage, Patricia Arquette, John Goodman, Marc Anthony. Directed by Martin Scorsese. Duration: 121 minutes.

DVD Chapter 2 Scene 00:08:46 to 00:10:30

ADAPTED FROM THE 1978 BRITISH play by Brian Clark, *Whose Life Is It Anyway?* relates the story of Ken Harrison (Richard Dreyfuss), a vibrant and successful 32-year-old sculptor who has become paralyzed below the neck (quadriplegic) as the result of an automobile accident. Faced with the prospect of living many more years in such a dependent condition, Harrison decides he would rather die. To do so, he must hire an attorney (Bob Balaban) to force his doctors and hospital to discharge him, so that he can go home, where he will die without the regular treatment and dialysis that he needs.

In this scene, Dr. Michael Emerson (John Cassevetes) has called in a psychiatrist, Dr. Sandy Jacobs (George Wyner), to ask him to see Harrison. Emerson wants Jacobs to declare Harrison clinically depressed and therefore mentally incompetent to make decisions about his own care, so that Emerson can have Harrison involuntarily committed until he decides to live. When Jacobs reminds Emerson that two psychiatrists will have to see Harrison and concur that he is clinically depressed, Emerson asks if Jacobs can find some other "old bastard" who "believes in something better than suicide." Jacobs tells him there is a psychiatrist at St. Joseph's who is a "staunch Catholic," and Emerson thanks him. While they have been talking, Dr. Clare Scott (Christine Lahti) has come in. Angry that Emerson would disregard Harrison's wishes and resort to such tactics, Scott tells Emerson that she is not sure she would have the courage to live in Harrison's condition, with "no privacy," and "no sense of dignity." When she asks Emerson whether he would want to live that way, Emerson responds, "We're doctors. We're committed to life. I'm a physician, not a judge." As Scott turns to leave his office, Emerson warns her that if Harrison should suddenly die, he will order an autopsy and "act on whatever is found."

Based on the 1999 autobiographical novel by Joe Connelly, *Bringing Out the Dead* focuses on Frank Pierce (Nicolas Cage), a burned-out paramedic working in the early 1990s on the streets of the neighborhood in which he grew up, New York City's Hell's Kitchen. As he begins a three-day weekend shift on a night full of "heat, humidity, and moonlight," Pierce reflects while he drives the ambulance that he has been "losing control" in the last year and that he hasn't "saved anyone in months." Paired with a different partner each night of his long weekend and haunted by the hopelessness and futility that surround him, Pierce struggles to maintain his concentration.

In this scene, Frank and his partner Larry (John Goodman) arrive at the emergency room (ER) of Our Lady of Perpetual Mercy Hospital, bringing in Old Man Burke, who has suffered a heart attack and cardiac arrest. Even though Burke had gone too long without breathing by the time the paramedics arrived at his family's apartment, Frank eventually got his heart restarted. As Larry and Frank push Burke's stretcher into the ER, the security guard, two nurses, and a physician tell them that the hospital is on "diversion," not accepting any more patients because things are so backed up that there are no available beds or rooms. The place is chaotic, with patients on gurneys lining the hallways, and more trying to break in past the security guard. Greeted by Nurse Crupp (Aida Turturro) with "Don't even think about it," Frank tells her that Burke had said that he wanted them to bring him there because "the nurses at 'Misrey' are the best." Hearing this, Nurse Crupp relents, goes to steal a stretcher from X-ray, and returns saying they can put Burke in room three. Meanwhile, Dr. Hazmat (Nestor Serrano) sees Burke, whom he has pronounced dead over the phone, and demands to know why they bothered to transport. Told that Burke now has a pulse, Dr. Hazmat looks at Burke's fixed and dilated pupils and calls him "plant food" that doesn't belong in the hospital. Having delivered the brain-dead Burke, Frank and Larry leave.

Although the medical settings and details in these scenes differ significantly, both feature conflict among members of a health care team about ethical responsibilities for their patients. In the older movie, *Whose Life Is It Anyway?* (1981), the senior physician disregards not only the patient's wishes but also the ethical concerns of the team's junior physician because, in the rigid medical hierarchy of the time, he is the "captain of the ship," holding final authority and ultimate responsibility for the patient; therefore, he expects everyone—including all members of the medical team—to follow his orders. Although the concept of senior doctor as captain of the team and ultimate decision maker was contested in American law as early as 1949, the belief and practice still persists in some clinical settings and in some countries.[1] In the era of paternalistic "macho" medicine,[2] the "captain" often failed to address the ethical concerns and distress of team members who disagreed with him, and the patient's only protective recourse might well have been to seek legal intervention. In a similar ethical conflict today, a senior physician would be expected to engage patient and team members in open discussion of the medical and ethical issues and confer about the best course to take in a particular circumstance.[3,4] If such a discussion reaches no resolution, a team member might request an ethics consultation.[5,6] The power dynamics displayed so effectively in this scene exacerbate the conflict and provoke an angry confrontation, one that might have been avoided had the senior physician engaged in respectful listening and exchange. Even if medical options and ethical stances do not change as a result of open communication, treating the patient and all members of the health care team with empathy and respect helps create an environment that encourages healing (not necessarily a cure) for those who experience or witness intractable suffering as a result of medical circumstances they cannot change.[7] Team members can support each other professionally and emotionally—even if they disagree.

Conflicts over ethical issues in patient care often occur between doctors and nurses,[8,9] but in this film they are intergenerational rather than interprofessional: the most powerful senior doctor and nurse are both "committed to life," as Dr. Emerson avows, and the most prominent junior doctor and nurse, who interact more often and more personally with the patient than do their elders, gradually become supportive of his wish to die. This generational difference in attitudes toward patient autonomy reflects the social changes under way in medicine and medical ethics at the time. Yet, Dr. Emerson's finest moment comes after the legal hearing in which the judge affirms Ken Harrison's competency and right to refuse treatment. Instead of angrily discharging him, Emerson promises to accept the verdict and stop treatment but pleads with Harrison to stay in the hospital, so that, should he change his mind and decide for life, the medical team would be nearby, ready to help him.

The scene from the more recent movie, *Bringing Out the Dead* (1999), shows a far less hierarchical and somewhat more collegial health care team. In the chaotic ER setting, the lack of time and space coalesce to make an extended discussion among team members or an ethics consultation extremely difficult. Both sides of this team are working hard to fulfill their responsibilities to their patients as best they can: The two paramedics resuscitate their patient and bring him to the hospital for further care; the overwhelmed members of the ER staff try to turn away additional patients to use their limited resources for the patients they have already accepted. Those responsible for the individual patient thus stand in direct conflict with those trying to care for the many. Although the institutional resolution is the policy of diversion, team members remain susceptible to pleas from their colleagues to take just one more patient; so, they do. In this kind of highly stressful environment, personal appeal and persuasion counters and undermines established policy. Even though team members may be in conflict with each other, they remain trapped between their professional duty to help patients and the futility of their efforts in the violent and chaotic world around them.

Anything more than an improvised and temporary solution to the intractable conflict presented by lack of resources falls beyond the capacities of individual team members to achieve. It depends upon societal will and political action to provide more resources for health care. Although the traditional ethical mandate is for health professionals to do their best for the individual patient before them, situations that require them simultaneously to ignore other patients in need of care can be emotionally devastating.

Frank Pierce's need to find meaning in his work by saving lives, which he has not been able to do in months, causes him to disregard the medical evidence before him and work desperately to restart Burke's heart, even though he knows that Burke is already brain dead. Frank invokes music, spirits, and miracles in his futile efforts to save Burke—and the world around him. No one on his team has the power to do anything more.

REFERENCES

1. Van Norman, G. 1998. Interdisciplinary team issues. In *Ethics in Medicine*. Seattle: University of Washington School of Medicine. Retrieved January 20, 2010 from at http://depts.washington.edu/bioethx/toics/team.html

2. Klass, P. 1987. Macho. In *A not entirely benign adventure: Four years as a medical student*, pp. 76–79. New York: G. P. Putnam Sons.

3. American College of Physicians. 1998. Conflicts among members of a health care team. In *Ethics Manual*, 4th ed. *Annals of Internal Medicine* 128(7): 576–594. Retrieved January 20, 2010 from http://www.annals.org/content/128/7/576.full sec-77

4. American Medical Association. 2008. Opinions on interprofessional relations. In *Code of medical ethics*. Chicago, IL: American Medical Association. Retrieved January 20, 2010 from http://ama-assn.org/ama/pub/physician-resources/medical-ethics/code-medical-ethics.shtml

5. DuVal, G., Sartorius, L., Clarridge, B., Gensler, G., and Danis, M. 2001. What triggers requests for ethics consultations? *Journal of Medical Ethics* 27(1): i24–i29.

6. Orr, R.D., and de Leon, D.M. 2000. The work of the clinical ethicist in conflict resolution. *Journal of Clinical Ethics* 11(1): 21–30.

7. van Soeren, M., and Miles, A. 2003. The role of teams in resolving moral distress in intensive care unit decision-making. *Critical Care* 7(3): 217–218. Retrieved January 20, 2010 from http://www.ncbi.nlm.nih.gov/pmc/articles/PMC270673/

8. American Nurses Association. 2001. Relationships with colleagues and others. In *Code of ethics for nurses with interpretive statements*. Washington, DC: American Nurses Association. Retrieved January 20, 2010 from http://www.nursingworld.org/ethics/code/protected_nwcoe813.htm. Also downloadable from http://www.nursingworld.org/MainMenuCategories/EthicsStandards/CodeofEthicsforNurses.aspx. Retrieved December 4, 2010.

9. Yates, E.M. 2010. Nurses and the medical team. *Virtual Mentor* 12(1): 1–65. Retrieved January 20, 2010 from http://virtualmentor.ama-assn.org/site/current.html

7

professional boundaries: *waitress*

douglas s. diekema

Waitress (2007). Keri Russell, Nathan Fillion, Cheryl Hines, Jeremy Sisto, Andy Griffith. Directed by Adrienne Shelly. Duration: 108 minutes.

DVD Chapter 8 Scene 00:32:52 to 00:37:45

JENNA (KERI RUSSELL), A SMALL-TOWN waitress who creates delicious pies for Joe's Diner, remains trapped in an unhappy marriage to her controlling, immature, and emotionally abusive husband, Earl (Jeremy Sisto). Slowly accumulating cash from her tips and hiding the money from Earl, she hopes to win a pie-baking contest and use the prize money to start a new life. When she discovers that she is pregnant with Earl's baby, she feels even more hopeless. When Jenna goes to her first prenatal visit, she finds a new physician, Dr. Jim Pomatter (Nathan Fillion), covering for the woman who has been her long-time physician. At a second visit, Jenna impulsively kisses the doctor, and the two begin an illicit affair. While complicated by the fact that both are married, the relationship gives Jenna renewed hope and confidence. The movie reaches its climax when Jenna goes into labor and her husband, her friends from the diner, Jim Pomatter, and Jim's wife (a medical resident at the hospital) all converge at her bedside.

The scene featured in this chapter occurs after Jenna's first visit with Dr. Pomatter. Jenna has experienced some spotting and calls Dr. Pomatter, who tells her to come to the office before she goes to work (and before the office opens). Jenna arrives and offers the doctor a bag of her homemade tarts. After Jenna changes into a gown, Dr. Pomatter enters the exam room, asks her a few questions, says he won't need to examine her, and asks her to get dressed and meet him in his office. Back in the office, Dr. Pomatter tells Jenna that spotting is "a perfectly normal symptom in early pregnancy," leading to an awkward exchange with Jenna about why it was necessary to have her come to the office for that information. She tells the doctor that he makes her uncomfortable, storms out of the office, and then realizes she has forgotten her purse. As she returns to the front door, Dr. Pomatter is holding her purse. Without saying anything, she kisses him, thus beginning the romantic relationship between them.

This scene raises questions about appropriate boundaries between a physician and his or her patient. In the movie, these boundary issues present themselves in two ways. First, Jenna brings a gift for the physician to each of her visits, an act that may or may not fall outside of the appropriate boundaries of the relationship.

Second, Jenna and Dr. Pomatter develop a mutual attraction that progresses to a romantic relationship. This clearly represents a boundary violation.

Patients may give gifts to their physicians, especially in the context of a long-term relationship. Under most circumstances, these gifts possess more symbolic than material value.[1] Jenna brings a pie to each of her physician visits and presents it to the doctor. On her first visit with Dr. Pomatter, she reluctantly gives him the pie, since it was intended for her usual physician. By the end of that visit, she presents him with the pie, and when she returns for a second visit, she comes bearing her "peachy-keen" tarts. For most physicians, accepting a modest gift does not involve a serious conflict, while refusal of a gift may be perceived as an affront by the patient. Dr. Pomatter appropriately accepts this modest gift from his new patient. As the monetary worth of a gift increases, however, it may become more difficult to maintain appropriate boundaries in the professional relationship. Gifts of significant value can alter the professional relationship, potentially affecting the physician's judgment. They may also be given with the expectation that the gift will somehow be reciprocated in ways that may not be appropriate, thus placing the physician in an uncomfortable position. When a physician feels uncomfortable with a gift, he or she should share these concerns and graciously refuse the gift.[2]

This scene also illustrates a second, more concerning, boundary violation. Jenna's connection with her new physician rapidly evolves beyond the professional relationship to a personal and romantic entanglement. Dr. Pomatter's willingness to pursue a personal liaison with a patient while remaining her physician clearly violates existing ethical codes,[3,4] and would qualify as sexual misconduct under many state regulations. One of every 200 physicians in the United States is disciplined for sexual misconduct with a patient at some time during his or her career, with violations ranging from sexual intercourse to inappropriate comments.[5,6]

While Jenna initiates the physical dimension of this relationship, the elimination of a boundary between the personal and professional relationship with her physician/obstetrician remains troubling for two important reasons.[7] First, within the unavoidably asymmetric physician–patient relationship, there always exists an inherent risk for patient exploitation, especially when the health care being delivered may include some degree of personal or physical intimacy. The success of the doctor–patient relationship depends on the ability of the patient to trust the physician completely. Patients should feel physically and emotionally safe with their physicians. If there is one clear ethical line, it is that patients should not feel vulnerable to romantic or sexual advances while receiving medical care. While Dr. Pomatter does not make any romantic or sexual overtures toward his patient, Jenna's own feeling (perhaps recognizing that the physician feels similarly) becomes clear when she tells Dr. Pomatter, "I'm not sure I want you to be my doctor anymore. You make me feel uncomfortable." Dr. Pomatter responds appropriately, apologizing and acknowledging that he shouldn't make her feel uncomfortable. Minutes later, she kisses him and he responds by asking her if they can meet somewhere outside of the professional context.

Up to this point, one could argue that Jenna has acted on her own feelings and initiated the relationship without any encouragement from Dr. Pomatter. But a second concern remains. Patients may develop feelings of gratitude, affection, or dependence toward their physicians—all of which may result in efforts to initiate a relationship with the physician that extends outside of the professional realm. Even concern expressed by a caring physician may be misinterpreted by a patient as a reflection of interest in a personal relationship. Physicians must remain alert to this possibility and moderate their own behavior in a way that does not encourage this misperception. It is also worth pointing out that many ethical codes and state regulations would explicitly reject patient consent or initiation as a justification for pursuing a romantic relationship with a patient.[3,4] According to Washington State's administrative code, for example, "it is not a defense that the patient... initiated or consented to the conduct, or that the conduct occurred outside the professional setting."[8]

A second important issue arises once a personal intimate relationship exists. Maintaining an effective therapeutic relationship between two parties who have an intimate personal relationship can be a significant challenge. The clinical judgment of physicians who become intimately involved with a patient may become clouded. Under these circumstances, the physician should end the professional relationship after ensuring the transfer of the patient's medical care to another appropriate practitioner. This concern would presumably include decisions by physicians to care for family members (especially spouses and children) and close friends. While termination of the physician–patient relationship represents a minimal ethical duty, the physician must also recognize that sexual contact with a former patient, although less clearly proscribed, may also be unethical, especially if the patient may be influenced by the previous therapeutic relationship or the relationship exploits trust, knowledge, emotions, or influence derived from that relationship.[3,4]

This scene offers an effective tool for teaching sessions. Most physicians and medical students know it is wrong for them to initiate a romantic relationship with a patient, especially in the context of a medical visit. However, the issues become more subtle when the patient, not the physician, initiates the contact, thus leading to a more nuanced discussion. This scene also raises three additional issues worth discussing in teaching sessions because they illustrate the difficulties and subtleties of an absolute prohibition on personal relationships between physicians and patients.[9]

First, Jenna and Dr. Pomatter live in a small town. While single physicians who practice in urban areas can easily meet friends and potential partners who seek medical care from other physicians, those who practice in the rural or small town context may find that nearly everyone they encounter in nonmedical settings receives medical care from the physician's office. This becomes more acute when there is only one physician in town. While boundary issues remain problematic and must be managed, it is also naïve to expect a small-town physician not to make friends with neighbors and potentially develop a romantic attraction to someone in the community. It may be that the only way to manage this situation is for single physicians not to practice in rural areas, but then one must also ask whether it is better for a rural area to remain without a physician if one who is in a long-term relationship cannot be found.

Second, Dr. Pomatter agrees to meet Jenna before the office opens in order to accommodate her work schedule. While this may be a generous and kind gesture, meeting his patient with no one else present in the office shows poor judgment. It clearly made Jenna feel uncomfortable, as she expresses in this scene. Furthermore, given his feelings of attraction toward Jenna, agreeing to meet her in the office without anyone present suggests intent to act unethically. Finally, what happens in the office without anyone present can be perceived differently by the patient and physician, potentially leading to allegations of misconduct that may be difficult to defend. Physicians should develop and follow clear and consistent office policies about the presence of a chaperone during parts of the physical examination, taking into account context, local customs, families' religious and cultural traditions, and the need for patient privacy. The presence of a chaperone should be noted in the patient record.

Finally, one aspect of this issue has not been adequately explored in the literature. Boundary issues are almost always discussed with certain assumptions about gender—i.e., that the physician is a male. In exploring this issue with medical students and residents, I frequently switch that stereotype to help them explore how much of the concern about boundaries is related to the professional relation-ship versus more traditional concerns about the power differential between men and women being exacerbated within a professional relationship. Would they feel the same way about what happened in this scene if the physician were female and the patient was male? While it is frequently the case that students and residents feel differently when the physician is a female, it should be recognized that sexual mis-conduct with female physicians and male patients does occur, that it can be just as exploitive and harmful to the patient, and that the crucial issue is the power imbal-ance that exists in the physician–patient relationship.[10]

The movie assists in illustrating some clear recommendations for clinicians. First, all physicians should consider having a chaperone present when they examine areas of the body that might be considered sensitive. Second, clinicians must readily acknowledge that they may occasionally develop feelings of sexual attraction toward a patient, recognize those feelings when they arise, and be prepared to discuss them with a trusted colleague. Third, physicians should never act on feelings of sexual attraction toward a patient, and should be pre-pared to transfer the care of a patient to another health care provider when those feelings persist. Fourth, physicians should be cautious about special arrange-ments that increase the likelihood of an inappropriate encounter with a patient, such as special scheduling or meeting the patient alone, outside of the office, or at the patient's home.[4] Finally, when a patient shows signs of being interested in a relationship with the clinician, the clinician should be particularly cautious about being alone with the patient and consider transferring care.

REFERENCES

1. Drew, J., Stoeckle, J.D., and Billings, J.A. 1983. Tips, status and sacrifice: Gift giving in the doctor-patient relationship. *Social Science and Medicine* 17: 399–404.
2. American Academy of Pediatrics, Committee on Bioethics. 1999. Appropriate boundaries in the pediatrician-family-patient relationship. *Pediatrics* 104: 334–336.
3. Council on Ethical and Judicial Affairs, American Medical Association. 1991. Sexual Misconduct in the Practice of Medicine. *Journal of the American Medical Association* 266 : 2741–2745.
4. American College of Obstetricians and Gynecologists, Committee on Ethics. 2007. Sexual misconduct: ACOG committee opinion no. 373. *Obstetrical Gynecology* 110: 441–444.
5. Dehlendorf, C.E., and Wolfe, S,M. 1998. Physicians disciplined for sex-related offenses. *Journal of the American Medical Association* 279: 1883–1888.
6. Enborn, J.A., Parshley, P., and Kollath, J. 2004. A follow-up evaluation of sexual misconduct complaints: the Oregon Board of Medical Examiners, 1998 to 2002. *American Journal of Obstetrical Gynecology* 190: 1642–1653.
7. Bolland, G., and Darken, R. 2000. Sexual relationships between doctors and patients: Ethical issues towards the new millennium. *Monash Bioethics Review* 19: 43–55.
8. Medical quality assurance commission standards for professional conduct. *Washington Administrative Code*, Title 246, 246–919–630, effective 9 February 2006.
9. Weiner, J. and Tolle, S.W. 2005. Sex and the Single Physician. In L. Snyder (Ed.), *Ethical choices: Case studies for medical practice*, 2nd ed. pp. 99–106. Philadelphia: American College of Physicians Press.
10. Webb-Pullman, J. 1996. Consent revisited: Sexual abuse by health care practitioners. *Law Institute Journal* 70: 26–29.

8

integrity and boundary setting:
antwone fisher

sherry l. braheny

Antwone Fisher (2002). Denzel Washington, Derek Luke, Joy Bryant, Sally Richardson. Directed by Denzel Washington. Duration: 120 minutes.

Scene: DVD chapter 12 scene 00:38:55 to 00:39:05

ABUSED AS A CHILD, SEAMAN Antwone Fisher (Derek Luke) is easily provoked into repeated fist fights by taunting shipmates. Navy psychiatrist Dr. Davenport (Denzel Washington) is given only three sessions to evaluate Antwone in order to make a recommendation as to whether he is fit to stay in the Navy. Reluctant even to talk at first, Antwone is expertly coaxed to tell his story through the patient, compassionate professionalism of Dr. Davenport. Eventually, Dr. Davenport becomes so empathetic with Antwone that the physician–patient relationship blurs into that of father and son, one he always longed for but never was able to have. Dr. Davenport guides Antwone through his first romantic relationship and convinces him to seek out the family that he never knew in order to resolve his inner conflicts. Because Dr. Davenport has his own personal issues, he, as much as Antwone, is struggling to balance his own particular inadequacies with his professional life.

This scene begins when Dr. Davenport gives his patient his home phone number and says, "Call me anytime, day or night [whenever you need me]." General boundary setting in the physician–patient relationship is not always as straightforward as it may seem, and one may question what and where are the "rules" or guidelines establishing an ethical physician–patient relationship. Hidden in the American Medical Association's "Principles of Medical Ethics"[1] is the line, "A physician shall uphold the standards of professionalism... ." However, these standards are not defined. The Oath of Hippocrates reads, "I will... abstain from whatever is deleterious and mischievous [and] will abstain from every voluntary act of mischief and corruption; and, further, from the seduction of females or males... ."

What exactly does this mean for physicians? There appears to be a pretty clear consensus that we should not engage in sexual relationships with our patients, but the details of acceptable behavior in establishing the physician–patient relationship are not codified.[2] Although much has been written about setting the boundaries of physician–patient relationships,[3–5] I don't recall ever taking a course on "boundary setting" in medical school. Yet, setting boundaries clearly is important to think about prior to meeting patients in any medical practice, and it should be a part of the standard curriculum.

A physician's giving out a personal phone number or his or her personal address of residence to a patient, for example, is probably not appropriate because it sets the stage for false expectations. If patients are told that they may call "anytime," some will definitely expect to be able to call *anytime,* even for frivolous reasons. For example, I had a patient call me at 3:30 a.m. for an "opinion" about something that was bothering her. She had been told that I was "on call" and therefore expected me to be awake and working all night and available to chat. While most patients are reasonable and appreciate being told ahead of time when physicians won't be available and their alternatives in case of emergencies, this patient didn't know that the general rules of "on call" meant working the day before, as well as all night and twice as hard the next day "post call," and fitting in sleep somewhere between emergency night calls. One quickly learns that clear communication is key to setting appropriate patient expectations.

Not only is there the possibility of significant misunderstanding as to how and when to use a health care provider's personal demographic information, there are times when providing such information may actually be dangerous. Reports cite that physician stalking may be increasing.[6] With the present economic depression, robbery has become much more frequent, even in suburban neighborhoods. In areas where drug abuse is significant and judgment is clouded, there may be frivolous lawsuits for false expectations gone awry. All the more reason for physicians not to give a patient their home addresses.

Should physicians allow or encourage patients to call them by their first name? Is this a boundary violation? Actually, it depends on the local culture. In Switzerland, for example, first names can be the norm.[7] In the United States, however, it is usually not considered appropriate. Yet, physicians almost invariably address patients by their first names, in order to put them at ease. Even nurses will call a patient sitting in a waiting room by his first name. (Interestingly, at a Veteran's Administration hospital, on more than one occasion, vets had a difficult time calling me Dr. Braheny, preferring Mrs. Braheny or even Mrs. Dr. Braheny, although I was not married at the time.)

Mention is made in the literature of differentiating between major boundary "violations" and minor boundary "crossings."[8,9] Examples of boundary violations would be entering into a sexual relationship with a patient or accepting an expensive gift, whereas boundary crossings might be calling the doctor by her first name, or accepting a small gift with every visit. Many, but certainly not all, American physicians would consider it ethical to accept an occasional gift of small monetary value. Personal standards among physicians differ as to what value makes a gift unethical to accept. As Dr. Edmond Pelligrino reminds us, physicians have an ethical obligation to care for all patients with beneficence, nonmaleficence, and confidentiality.[2] The virtuous physician also cares for patients with empathy. Sometimes, however, conflicts arise between empathy and confidentiality. Let's take the following example.

In a hospital where I practice, a new program is being taught to nurses and other health care team members (including physicians) that encourages more personal initial contact with hospital patients to make them feel more comfortable. Nurses are told to introduce themselves, then say, for example, "I want to get to know you better before we start our day together." Personal questions such as "Who brought you those flowers?" or questions about some personal bedside item or piece of clothing are encouraged. Nurses are, of course, also taught to be sensitive to clues from patients who might not want such personal questioning about subjects unrelated to their immediate health care needs. To date, the program has reportedly prompted more immediate positive feedback from patients than ever before. Showing empathy and compassion are attributes of a good physician, but one must be careful that clear boundaries are set to prevent false expectations of the patient, especially if the physician takes for granted boundaries that the patient doesn't understand.

Some patients welcome the asking of personal questions and rate this very high on the bedside manner scale. Others definitely do not, and wish to keep even routine personal information private—even from their physicians. One sensitive patient expressed great resentment at my routine question asking her level of education. She felt compelled to defend why she had to quit grade school to support her family and didn't have the opportunity to continue school. This is obviously a very relevant question for any physician, but not for her. Another patient admonished that it was none of my business to ask about the health of her sister, since she was not my patient. These are obviously not unethical questions taken in this context, but they demonstrate some of the extreme boundaries of personal confidentiality that some patients place upon their physicians.

From a health care professional's perspective, one might wonder whether there are preset individual developmental boundaries that help maintain the status of certain relationships. Anne Scott discusses, from the nursing point of view, how individuals establish personal boundaries and how they develop as a person ages.[10] She lists examples of behaviors in people with "open" and "closed" boundaries, and how these traits might affect relationships with others. The discerning empathetic physician during a first interview will consciously or subconsciously take note of these traits to decide which boundaries need to be emphasized and which ones may or may not be taken for granted. The basic expectations and responsibilities of a physician–patient relationship may be outlined briefly in an introductory pamphlet handed to the patient at the first visit. The outline may be useful at that or future visits to stimulate further discussion of boundaries that do not seem to be understood.

In this movie, the overstepping of ethical boundaries is illustrated in a variety of fashions, and Dr. Davenport's empathetic involvement with his patient clouds his judgment in setting clear boundaries for an appropriate patient–physician relationship. Throughout the movie, both patient and physician repeatedly cross these boundaries. Antwone's personal questions of Dr. Davenport are inappropriate, but Dr. Davenport encourages some and rebukes Antwone for others, thus confusing the boundaries even more. Dr. Davenport is not sure of the boundaries himself. He repeatedly refers to Antwone as "son," strongly encouraging a father-son relationship. Yet, when Antwone shows up unexpectedly at his doorstep just to share some good news, Dr. Davenport, who happens to be in the midst of a serious family discussion with his wife, coldly receives him, showing his resentment at his unannounced visit to his home. They both agree that uninvited visits will not happen again. By trial and error, mistakes are made and forgiven, conflicts are defined and worked out, and eventually there is a satisfying resolution for both physician and patient. In real life, however, this is not always the case.

REFERENCES

1. Principles of Medical Ethics. Adopted by the AMA's House of Delegates June 17, 2001. 1995–2009 American Medical Association. Retrieved from http://www.ama-assn.org/ama/pub/physician-resources/medical-ethics/code-medical-ethics.

2. Pelligrino, E.D. 1998. The metamorphosis of medical ethics: A 30-year retrospective. *Journal of the American Medical Association* 269(9): 1158–1162.

3. Linklater, D., and MacDougal, S. 1993. Boundary issues. What do they mean for family physicians? *Canadian Family Physician* 39: 2569–2573.

4. Farber, N.J., Novack, D.H., Silverstein, J., Davis, E.B., Weiner, J., and Boyer, E.G. 2000. Physicians' experiences with patients who transgress boundaries. *Journal of General Internal Medicine* 15:770–775.

5. Nisselle, P. 2000. Danger zone. When boundaries are crossed in the doctor-patient relationship. *Australian Family Physician* 29(6): 541–544.

6. Manca, D.P. 2005. Woman physician stalked. Personal reflection and suggested approach. *Canadian Family Physician* 51: 1640–1645.

7. Hansel, A., Nubling, M., and Langewitz, W.A. 2008. do patients respect the line? Transgression of boundaries reported by Swiss general practitioners. *Patient Education and Counseling* 72: 424–428.

8. Shaili, J., and Roberts. L.W. 2009. Ethics in psychotherapy: A focus on professional boundaries and confidentiality practices. *Psychiatric Clinics of North America* 32: 299–314.

9. Goldberg, A. 2008. Some limits of the boundary concept. *Psychoanalytic Quarterly* 77(3): 861–875.

10. Scott, A.L. 1998. Human interaction and personal boundaries. *Journal of Psychosocial Nursing* 26(8): 23–27.

9

respect for persons: *the death of mr. lazarescu*

ignacio maglio

The Death of Mr. Lazarescu (2005). Ion Fiscuteanu, Luminata Gheorghiu,
Gabriel Spahiu. Directed by Cristi Puiu. Duration: 150 minutes.

DVD chapter 6 scene 01:00:17 to 01:06:26

MR LAZARESCU, A 60-YEAR-OLD MAN, lives with his three cats in a humble and gloomy Bucharest apartment. With a sister in a far-away city and a daughter who has moved to Canada, the lonely widower has no one to help him when he suddenly starts having headaches and stomach pains. He calls for an ambulance. When it arrives, a very unsuccessful search for a hospital begins. Mioara, a nurse who tries to alleviate his suffering during visits to four different medical institutions, accompanies Mr. Lazarescu during his travels from one hospital to another. During the next two hours, the viewer witnesses Mr. Lazarescu's sufferings from a lack of adequate medical assistance, depersonalized medical care, and inhumane treatment. Ultimately, Mr. Lazarescu's emergency room experiences, whose personnel fail to provide him with appropriate care, hasten his death.

During this ultimately fatal journey, Mr. Lazarescu's dignity and autonomy are continuously ignored. Some surgeons, for example, try to obtain judicial immunity by requesting a signature of consent under falsified circumstances, thus demonstrating minimal levels of respect for autonomy. Members of the medical team care for him in a haphazard manner, moving about in the emergency room, succumbing to stress and increasing fatigue as they care for a number of incoming victims from a traffic accident. General remarks about his alcohol addiction and urinary incontinence seem to justify negative moral reproaches. Thus, conflicts are evident between the work of health care providers and the situation of the unfortunate Lazarescu, conflicts that are sordid and difficult to understand. His health care providers are worried about the marriage of a partner, make personal telephone calls, and are busy preparing coffee while Lazarescu needs someone to relieve his pain. The social context is consistent with the lack of medical care offered to Mr. Lazarescu; the precarious situation of a community in an underdeveloped health care system perpetuates the misfortune, illness, and suffering of the patient.

This film promotes discussion of a central core of medical practice: respect for individual dignity in the doctor–patient relationship and participation of the patient in the medical discussion by means of informed consent intended to preserve the best interests of the patient. The protection of dignity is an essential pillar of medical ethics. Every individual must be considered an end in himself, never a means; each patient must be treated as unique and unrepeatable. Each patient is a human being with essential rights.

Mr. Lazarescu's dignity, however, is ignored in every hospital. He is systematically disregarded and neglected. Because his decreasing health is, in part, related to his unhealthy lifestyle, doctors feel justified in their lack of proper assistance. The unacceptability of such behaviors is founded in the first right of every individual, which is to be considered as a *judicial person*.[1] The basic premise of mutual respect[2] must also be sustained, especially in a patient–provider clinical relationship. We must consider the other individual as a person, as a fellow creature, avoiding any form of domination and humiliation through our behaviors and attitudes.

The hospitals visited by Lazarescu ignored the dimension of dignity carried by him as an ill human being. They treated him as an anonymous object, whose identity was reduced to a disordered classification of symptoms (headache, vomit, radiographs, clinical studies, computed tomography scans). Respect for the individual lies in that individual's intrinsic value. It is manifested in conscious autodetermination,[3] the free and unrestricted responsibility of each person for the design of his or her own life project. Lazarescu's beliefs and preferences, however, remain constantly disregarded. In his contact with physicians, differential relations of power show a tragic asymmetry, one in which health care personnel blame the "sick one" for his condition. This film thus depicts the aberrant behavior exemplifying a medical system in crisis, the human miseries of selfishness, and cruel treatment by a health team whose innocent victim[4] is Lazarescu. In caring for this patient, the characteristic values of each person in relation to his own sickness is never taken into account, and there is a nonexistent attitude of caring among the doctors who look after Lazarescu. The conceptual difference between *sickness*, as defined by the biomedical model, and *illness*, as a cognitive and affective experience that people perceive of their own suffering, is totally ignored.

Access to information and to available medical alternatives is also a fundamental right of patients. In the doctor–patient relationship, the right to manage one's own body is achieved by means of respect for an essential rule of medical responsibility: the process of informed consent. The origin of the informed consent doctrine doesn't appear in biomedical tradition, but rather in a legislative construct of those duties inherent to the practice of the profession. "Information and consent... . have no historical roots in the medical practice."[5] Lately, a practical and conceptual framework has been constructed for the informed consent process. This framework emphasizes a process that is more operative and respectful of the wishes and preferences of patients. It conceptualizes autonomy by means of *informed election*, whereby each patient can choose freely among a number of therapeutic offering proposed by doctors. Independent individuals without conflicts of interest could make these offers.[6]

Some experts raise the idea of *informed participation*, a process by which a patient participates in the decision-making process to determine his or her treatment. The keys to successful informed participation are mutual agreement on responsibilities, a configuration of the problem from the patient's point of view, a definition of alternative therapies, and a decision on the control of any chosen alternative.[7] However, "juridicalizing" the informed consent process, with the legitimate intent of "demedicalizing" it, may bring about an undesirable effect: Sticking to the rules, no matter what, provoked by the paralyzing fear of malpractice.

This scene, in which Lazarescu is compelled to sign an informed consent, shows one way to evade potential litigation. Contrary to what is shown in this scene, in which Lazarescu is told that everything will be fine, that the proposed surgery is without complications (other than occasional paralysis), informed consent must be an instrument of participatory interchange, one in which the doctor informs clearly and the patient demonstrates comprehension, confidence, and truthfulness. Throughout the process, the doctor not only selects and transfers adequate and appropriate information, but also listens to the patient. This interactive model places equal importance on the opinions of both participants: The doctor knows about the sickness, the patient knows about his own needs.[8] Doctors must understand and accept, therefore, how patients perceive and evaluate the risks and advantages of clinical medicine.[9]

The appalling route of Mr. Lazarescu shows one of the most tragic faces of inequality: the absence of adequate medical assistance in poor, emerging countries, and even more unjust, among vulnerable groups in rich countries. In contrast to the idea of euthanasia, the film proposes "mistanasia," the unhappy death produced by inadequate medical assistance and near-total social abandonment. Despite the social inequities and human miseries shown in this film, however, *The Death of Mr. Lazarescu* offers hopeful signs for the human condition: from the solidarity and support of his neighbors, to the care and worries of Mioara, the dedicated nurse who shows that the purest and kindest acts occur when the person receiving care has no power at all. The attitude of this nurse should mark a new direction in our need to rehumanize medical practice. The understanding of ethical practice in medicine, therefore, starts with the awareness that not everyone is the same, no one is an object, not everything is bought, and not everything has a price. Maybe this is the best moral lesson of the film.

REFERENCES

1. Campos, B., and German, J. 1991. *Teoría general de los derechos humanos* (p. 20). Buenos Aires: Editorial Astrea Buenos Aires.,
2. Larenz, K. 1985. *Derecho justo. Fundamentos de ética jurídica*. Madrid: Civitas Madrid.
3. Mateo Martín, R. 1987. *Bioética y derecho*. Barcelona: Publisher Ariel.
4. Parsons, T. 1976. *El sistema social*. Madrid: *Revista de occidente*.

5. Katz, J. 1978. Informed consent in therapeutic relationship: Legal and ethical aspects. In W.T. Reich (Ed.), *Encyclopaedia of bioethics*, Vol. 2. New York: Free Press.

6. Veatch, R.M. 1995. Abandoning informed consent. *Hastings Center Report* 25(2).

7. Lidz, W.C., Appelbaum, P.S., and Meisel, A. 1988. Two models of implementing informed consent. *Archives of Internal Medicine* 148: 1385–1389.

8. Kraut, J. A. 1992. Deber de información y derecho a la información. *JA* II 834.

9. Eraker, S., and Politser, M. 1982. How decisions are reached: Physician and patient. *Annals of Internal Medicine* 97: 262.

10

speaking truth to power: *pan's labyrinth*

lois l. nixon

Pan's Labyrinth (2006). Ivana Baquero, Sergi Lopez, Maribel Verdu, Alex Angulo, Doug Jones Gil, Ariadna. Directed by Guillermo Del Toro.
Duration: 119 minutes.

DVD Chapter 17 scene 1:23:42 to 1:24

IRECTOR GUILLERMO DEL TORO SETS *Pan's Labyrinth* in Spain during 1944, a time when determined insurgents are rebelling against the Franco-imposed fascist regime. The film begins with a young girl, Ofelia, and her sick, pregnant mother, Carmen, traveling through dense woods in a chauffeur-driven car. The difficult relocation of the near-term mother and her daughter to a remote military outpost has been arranged by Carmen's new husband, Captain Vidal. He has insisted that his child be born where he and his forces are stationed—in spite of his wife's difficult pregnancy and the dangers imposed by ongoing rebel attacks. The audience soon learns that Captain Vidal, Ofelia's stepfather is cold, ruthless, and dangerous. This essay will examine two concrete illustrations relating to the idea of *speaking truth to power* by the courageous physician in del Torro's elaborate and multidimensional story, and consider how that idea is of essential value in medicine.

The camp doctor, a caring and ethical person, personifies someone willing to question unwarranted decisions, *to speak truth to power* in two specific instances. The first and less disturbing example occurs when Dr. Ferreiro expresses immediate concern about his new patient, Vidal's wife, and the wisdom of the difficult journey she has endured. Although he advises the captain that his wife is unwell and frail, the soldier dismisses the physician's concern by noting that his "son" must be born here, in the camp. The doctor's response about the unpredictability of the baby's gender clearly infuriates the captain. Puzzled and alarmed by the Captain's foolish remark and bullying attitude, the physician provides compassionate care for Carmen, whose condition requires confinement to bed. When Ferreiro tells the captain of his serious concern for her life, the captain commands that, should a choice occur, his "son's" life is to take precedence.

The second example of *speaking truth to power* occurs when an injured rebel is taken prisoner and brought to the angry captain for questioning. Vidal interrogates the man using excruciating methods of torture. Badly beaten, the brutalized man passes out in pain. The captain orders Ferreiro to revive his chained prisoner so that torture can continue. When Vidal steps outside for a moment, the severely abused man pleads for the doctor to end his suffering. Now, fully apprised of the captain's brutal nature, aware of the array of torture instruments he sees before him, and disturbed deeply by what he is witnessing, Ferreiro complies with the abused man's request.

Situated between the captain's direct order and the request of the tortured and dying man, Ferreiro is pushed to the ultimate level of risk. Within minutes of providing euthanasia and with full knowledge that his intervention will not go unnoticed, he speaks truthfully to the furious oppressor:

VIDAL: "Why did you do it?"

FERREIRO: "It was the only thing I could do."

VIDAL: "No. You could have obeyed me."

FERREIRO: "I could have, but I didn't."

VIDAL: "It would have been better for you. You know it. I don't understand. Why didn't you obey me?"

FERREIRO: "To obey—just like that—for the sake of obeying without questioning—that's something only people like you can do."

Without any thought about the doctor's singular role as care provider to both his ill wife and vulnerable soldiers, the enraged captain aims his pistol and shoots the resigned physician in the back.

When a person with power demonstrates aberrant, tyrannical behavior, the risks associated with speaking against him, even in truth, can be very dangerous. The soldiers who witness Captain Vidal's brutality throughout the story clearly remain uncomfortable with the abuses of power, yet have learned to remain silent. We suppose that such circumstances are not uncommon in the military: Leaders do not expect to be challenged, and soldiers are trained to follow orders. In medicine, however, the standards and expectations should be very different.

In their discussion about speaking truth to power, Papadimos and Murray note that Foucault's "analysis of free speech is relevant to the mentoring of medical students. This is especially true given the educational and social need to transform future physicians into able citizens who practice a fearless freedom of expression on behalf of their patients, the public, the medical profession, and themselves in the public and political arena."[1]

Perri Klass, for example, raises the issue about *speaking* (or not) *truth to power* in a seemingly gentle and amusing short story entitled "Baby Poop." When the narrator, a medical student member of an attending team of neurologists, approaches the patient, a newborn in a bassinet, she observes out loud that the baby smells "poopy" and needs to be changed. An uncomfortable silence followed. "None of us," wrote the student, "admitted in any way that there was anything to smell except the standard aroma of disinfectant. We stood tall. We were doctors... . And finally we finished our exam and marched out; as we left the room, a nurse came hurrying over to the bassinet, carrying a paper diaper."[2]

This consideration of *speaking truth to power* to those higher in the medical hierarchy reveals not just an unexpressed dismissal of an observed problem that could be corrected easily, but also some potentially disturbing questions: Might it be unwise to speak truth to those more powerful? Could students, interns, or junior colleagues suffer career-related consequences if they dare speak out from within the medical hierarchy? Just as Captain Vidal's soldiers understood the importance of their code of silence, the lesson for the young medical student in this story is potentially the same.

Silence, however, may also be self-defeating in other ways. In "Touching," a short story by physician-writer David Hellerstein, a third-year student is assigned to Dr. Snarr, a clumsy and insensitive gynecologist. The student-narrator's interest in this specialty evaporates during his month-long clerkship with his would-be mentor whose vaginal exams result in patients "screaming" and "writhing" on the examination table. Snarr, he observes, reaches in "pushing so hard her hips rise from the table; and she is crying, grabbing the table with her hands. I feel sick just watching. I have no way of knowing what, if anything, Snarr is finding, since he does not explain."[3] When the student-narrator notes that if "Dr. Snarr had been a better teacher, I might conceivably have gone into his field," readers recognize how such forces of power can dim enthusiasm and redirect student interests.

Thankfully, speaking truth to power by physicians is not uncommon. Physician groups might advocate for patients in Washington, as well as in their own health care institutions. Others join national and international organizations, such as the World Health Organization, the International Committee of the Red Cross, Amnesty International, or Doctors Without Borders, among others, to help observe, identify, and speak out on behalf of injustices affecting abused, vulnerable, and largely unrepresented and otherwise invisible populations. Frequently, their vital messages are buttressed and made even more compelling by *visual* storytellers whose narratives bring situations to life, generate interest, and arouse support.

The scene in *Pan's Labyrinth* in which Dr. Ferreiro meets his death, represents an extreme point in the "fearless freedom" position, one that most physicians never want or need to confront and fulfill. The medical humanities provide many other stories and narratives to health sciences students regarding role-modeling, values, and appropriate attitudes and behaviors, as embodied in Foucault's writings and in contemporary medical standards. Works by Ariel Dorfman (*Death and the Maiden,* film), Athol Fugard (*Tsotsi,* film), Eddie Adam (*Speak Truth to Power,* photographs), Fernando Botero (*Abu Ghraib 50,* paintings), and Ari Folman (*Waltz with Bashir,* film) provide accounts that similarly inspire, influence, and underscore the tenets of conviction, and, of speaking truth to power.

Many filmmakers, photographers, and artists—the record keepers for very real social problems—thus demonstrate a willingness to write about or portray legitimate differences that beg for discussion and debate. Unfortunately, as with the dispute between Captain Vidal and Dr. Ferreiro, the stakes can occasionally be deadly for those who would confront egregious forces of oppression. These and other narratives, however, define who we are both separately and collectively. As Christopher Isherwood has noted, "Story allows for a distance—a way of observing, experiencing from afar. Often it's the way to get a truth."[4]

REFERENCES

1. Papadimos, T., and Murray, S.J. 2008. Foucault's "fearless speech" and the transformation and mentoring of medical students. *Philosophy, Ethics, and Humanities* 3: 12.
2. Klass, P. 1987. Baby Poop. In *Not an entirely benign procedure*, p. 162. New York: G.P. Putnam's Sons.
3. Hellerstein, D. 2001. Touching. In *On doctoring*, pp. 354–357. New York: Simon & Schuster.
4. Isherwood, C. May 6, 2005. Stories that tell vs. storytelling. *New York Times*.

part five

health care policy and social responsibility

individual rights versus the public interest: *outbreak*

sarah r. lieber and alan wertheimer[i]

Outbreak (1995). Dustin Hoffman, Rene Russo, Morgan Freeman. Directed by Wolfgang Petersen. Duration: 125 minutes.

DVD Scenes 17–19 00:56:14–00:58:40

A DEADLY VIRUS THAT ORIGINATES IN Motaba River Valley, Zaire, infiltrates the United States. Carried by an African monkey shipped to California, the virus spreads when an unwitting Customs employee tries to sell the animal; when he cannot find a buyer, he releases it. The seller travels to Boston, where he dies, and people in the town of Cedar Creek, California (pop. 2,600), where the monkey is released, begin to die at an alarming rate. Unlike the first strains of the virus, the new strain becomes airborne and has a mortality rate of 100%. To contain the epidemic, the government sends officials of the United States Army Medical Research Institute of Infectious Diseases (USAMRIID) and the Center for Disease Control (CDC) to Cedar Creek. The town is put under tight quarantine, while Colonel Sam Daniels of USAMRIID (Dustin Hoffman) struggles to find the source of the infection and create a serum.[1] In this essay, we address scenes that involve the quarantine of the town. Military vehicles roll in, and the bewildered residents are forbidden to leave. Some assert their rights by trying to escape the tight cordon placed on the town, and military personnel use deadly force to prevent them from leaving.

Outbreak raises numerous ethical issues. For example, the film questions whether it is justifiable to lie, steal, and disobey orders in order to serve a good cause. The film's most important *medical ethics* issue concerns the apparent conflict between protecting public health versus respecting the rights of the individual. At one point, it appears that it may be necessary to obliterate the entire town—"Operation Clean Sweep"—in order to prevent the virus from escaping and endangering the entire population of the United States. The film casts the virus as an agent of war, justifying the use of force and citing that the flu pandemic of 1918 killed more people than did World War I. The film asks, in effect, if it is morally acceptable to use force against those who carry the virus even when they are essentially innocent victims. In less dramatic terms, the movie raises issues about the moral importance of public health concerns as opposed to the rights and well-being of individuals.

To put the previous point in more philosophical terms, *Outbreak* raises the age-old tension between *utilitarianism* and *deontology*.[2] Utilitarianism tells us to maximize the well-being of all, whereas deontology argues, among other things, that individuals may have obligations and rights that cannot be violated for the sake of the greater good.[3,4] Utilitarian philosophers, such as John Stuart Mill, have argued that an individual's liberties and rights can be overridden to prevent harm or to benefit others.[5] So, in a typical philosopher's example, utilitarianism might ethically permit the killing of one healthy person if his organs can be redistributed to save five others. By contrast, deontology would say that such an action remains inherently wrong, even if doing so would promote the greater good.[6]

This basic theme regularly appears in our lives, as well as in movies and on television. In contemporary times, nations have engaged in the wholesale slaughtering of chickens in a (perhaps misguided) effort to contain avian flu, and herds of healthy cattle have been slaughtered to contain mad cow disease. The threat of terrorism made particularly salient on September 11, 2001 has given rise to heated discussions of the "ticking time bomb" arguments for the use of torture to protect the public.[8]

Outbreak raises an important and general principle about ethical reasoning. In the final analysis, however, the film does not directly confront the tension between public health and individual rights because the hero locates the source of the virus and (with help) generates a serum. So, the infected people can be treated, and the town need not be obliterated. But, what should be done if the infected people could not be treated and saved because a serum could not be generated? Let us assume that this virus has infected this town and that government officials are all acting in good faith. They understand the value of individual rights. They are sensitive to the values underlying the United States Constitution. At the same time, these officials are genuinely concerned about the health and lives of other innocent persons who may become infected with this lethal virus if it is not contained. What then? Would it be wrong to detain the entire population of Cedar Creek? Would it be justifiable to use force to keep people from leaving town—even killing them if necessary? When do the interests of the many justify sacrificing the interests of the relatively few? Public health situations often pose real but less dramatic conflicts between the interests of some and the interests of others.[9,10] On a less dramatic level than that evident in *Outbreak*, mandatory vaccination proposals raise the conflict between protecting public health and respecting individual rights. Many states have mandatory vaccination requirements, although some parents believe that they should not be required to have their children vaccinated.

Let us consider the case of quarantine. During the severe acute respiratory syndrome (SARS) epidemic, for example, Canada used quarantine for the first time in many years.[11] It has also been discussed as a strategy for responding to a flu pandemic, should it occur. When would it be justifiable to confine an individual or all the members of a community to prevent the spread of a disease? Although reasonable people may disagree, several ethical criteria should guide our thinking. First, there should be good reason to think that others will be harmed if they become infected.[12] Certainty that an infection will spread may not be required. If we adopt what is sometimes called the *precautionary principle*, we might be justified in quarantining those with tuberculosis (TB) if there were a reasonable likelihood—say 50%—that they would spread TB by coughing. Second, we should always use the least-restrictive alternative available in attempting to protect the public. In some cases, we might try to rely on voluntary isolation or tracing mechanisms, rather than forced confinement.[12] But what would be justified if less-restrictive alternatives are not feasible or effective? Third, we must communicate to the wider society that those quarantined are being isolated for the good of society and not because they have done anything wrong. Those forced into quarantine should be treated as well as possible. This includes providing them with adequate housing, food, and access to other essential goods. In doing so, government officials acknowledge that the individual is giving up her liberties to protect the public's health; therefore, the state should reciprocate by providing care for that individual. Unlike criminals, it is not through voluntary and intentional actions that they pose risks to others; they are morally innocent carriers of a dangerous infectious agent.

The previous paragraph raises another interesting ethical question about individual responsibility. Suppose that John Doe tests positive as a carrier of a highly contagious disease. Doe is not to blame for acquiring the disease, but he now knows that he has it. The state asks Doe to isolate himself voluntarily and avoid all contact with others until he is no longer dangerous. Doe refuses. Is Doe now morally innocent? It could be argued that, even if one is not to blame for becoming a person who is dangerous to others, it may be wrong to endanger the health of others nonetheless through voluntary actions, that doing so constitutes "reckless endangerment."[13]

Outbreak asks the viewer to question how much the individual owes society, and what rights society possesses to force the individual, for the public good, to give up some of his or her fundamental rights. In so doing, the film offers a dramatic, if perhaps far-fetched example of the conflict between protecting public health versus respecting the rights of the individual. Even more importantly, the movie questions the extent to which the government may go to protect its citizens, even from each other, by positing the morally innocent victims. Some would call this murder, while others might well label it self-defense. In less dramatic terms, the movie raises issues about the moral importance of public health concerns as opposed to the rights and well being of individuals.

NOTE

i. The views expressed in this essay are those of the author. They do not necessarily reflect any position or policy of the National Institutes of Health or the Department of Health and Human Services.

REFERENCES

1. *Outbreak*. Petersen, W. 1995. USA: Punch Productions, 127 minutes.
2. Beauchamp, T.L., and Childress, J.F. 2009. *Principles of biomedical ethics*, 6th ed. New York: Oxford University Press.
3. Smart, J.J.C., and Williams, B. 1973. *Utilitarianism: for and against*. Cambridge: Cambridge University Press.
4. Darwall, S. 2002. *Deontology*. Oxford: Blackwell Publishing.
5. Parmet WE. 2008. J.S. Mill and the American law of quarantine. *Public Health Ethics* 1(3): 210–222.
6. Kamm, F.M. 2007. *Intricate ethics: Rights, responsibilities, and permissible harm*. New York: Oxford University Press.
7. Brecher, R. 2007. *Torture and the ticking bomb*. London: Blackwell Publishing.
8. Callahan, D., and Jennings, B. 2002. Ethics and public health: Forging a strong relationship. *American Journal of Public Health* 92(2): 169–176.
9. Childress, J.E., Faden, R.R., Gaare, R.D., Gostin, L.O., Kahn, J., Bonnie, R.J., et al. 2002. Public health ethics: Mapping the terrain. *Journal of Law, Medicine, and Ethics* 30(2): 170–178.
10. Upshur, R. 2003. The ethics of quarantine. *Virtual Mentor* 5(11): 1–3.
11. Upshur, R. 2002. Principles for the justification of public health intervention. *Canadian Journal of Public Health* 93: 101–103.
12. Harris, J., and Holm, S. 1995. Is there a moral obligation not to infect others? *British Medical Journal* 311(7014): 1215–1217.

consumer awareness: *the rainmaker*

paul d. banick

The Rainmaker (1997). Matt Damon, Danny DiVito, Claire Danes, Jon Voigt, Mary Kay Place, Mickey Rourke. Directed by Francis Ford Coppola. Duration: 135 minutes.

DVD Chapter 2 Scene 00:06:34 to 00:07:30

I N THE RAINMAKER, RUDY BAYLOR (Matt Damon), a young, novice attorney, goes to work for a corrupt, ambulance-chasing lawyer in Memphis, Tennessee by the name of J. Lyman "Bruiser" Stone (Mickey Rourke). As a new employee, Baylor's efforts focus on two cases: putting together a will for an old woman who becomes his new landlady and a case of insurance bad faith. In the insurance case, Baylor represents a poor family, Dot (Mary Kay Place) and Buddy Black (Red West), whom he met through a law workshop. He filed suit on behalf of the Blacks, whose son Donny Ray (Johnny Whitworth) faced certain death from leukemia without a bone marrow transplant. The payment of the bone marrow transplant had been denied eight times by their insurance company, Great Benefit. When "Bruiser" Stone's office was about to be raided by the police and FBI, Baylor and Deck Shifflet (Danny DiVito), a former, unscrupulous insurance assessor, set up their own law practice and continue preparing for trial. Baylor, having just passed the bar exam, has never argued a case before a judge and jury. As Baylor prepares for trial, the Black's son dies. Additionally, he uncovers a scheme Great Benefit ran to deny payment to every insurance claim submitted, regardless of its validity. During the trial, he confronts a group of experienced and callous corporate attorneys from the large insurance firm, headed by Leo F. Drummond (Jon Voight). Baylor ultimately wins the case. But Great Benefit files for bankruptcy and avoids paying the judgment.

In the selected scene, Deck Shifflet says that "there is nothing more thrilling than nailing an insurance company." For Baylor, this prophetic, comment foretells the results of his efforts. The scene sets the stage for the conflict and subtly provides visual symbols of key issues surrounding the insurance industry today. The insurance contract embodied by the stack of papers in Baylor's briefcase represents a metaphor of the impersonal system that surrounds access to health care. The denial of benefits, an emotionally powerful theme, resonates in discussions pertaining to health care reform. *Pre-existing condition*, one of the most contentious issues in the private insurance industry today, serves as the focal point of controversy in the movie. The most recent health care reform bill[1] before Congress addresses the removal of pre-existing conditions. The disparities in health care implied in Shifflet's remarks have also been the focus of targeted legislation.[2,3] Finally, Shifflet's reference to the "debit insurance scam" raises one of the most important issues in health care today: *consumer awareness.*

In contrast to mainstream health insurance, the industry distinguishes debit insurance from other types of insurance in that the policy is of small value and sold by a door-to-door salesperson. When the policyholder gives the agent money, the agent is trusted to take the money back to the company and credit it to the policyholder's policy. The policyholder must also trust that the insurance company will pay for medical needs as they arise, as defined by the policy. In this manner, the insurance company and the agent are viewed as professional entities by the consumer. However, it is apparent that neither measure up to this definition in *The Rainmaker.* Indeed, watching *The Rainmaker,* viewers identify with a sense of violated trust and injustice when the insurance company reneges on paying for the bone marrow transplant that directly results in Donny Ray's death. Most unsettling is to discover that Great Benefit has features similar to legitimate professional insurance carriers in business today.

The ethical dilemma in *The Rainmaker* is framed by consumer expectation that the most important dimension of any "professional" responsibility should be based upon a moral consensus for professional ethics and behavior having a common goal greater than simply profit for the company.[4] Despite the obvious fact that the insurance company runs as a business, most citizens would assume a common goal to be for a greater good of the individual, society as a whole, or both. Even Adolphus Green, the founder of Nabisco acknowledged in 1898, that "the officer of every corporation should feel in his heart, in his very soul, that he is responsible, not merely to make dividends for the stockholders of his company, but to enhance the general prosperity and the moral sentiment of the United States."[5] Great Benefit fails to demonstrate behavior with a societal purpose other than profit. Because health care insurance companies like Great Benefit occupy positions of authority over vulnerable consumer-patients, this attitude is particularly reprehensible. They possess knowledge not generally available to or readily understood by those outside of their profession and, as such, some bioethicists view this unique dynamic as a potential danger to the health care consumer.[6] Additionally, this danger can be intensified as a result of the high allocations of societal resources into health care, the potential for profit, and the potential conflict of interest between obligation to patient and obligation to shareholder. The extreme outcome of this threat was the death of Donny Ray Black. In viewing this tragic situation, the film encourages the consumer to exercise a heightened level of awareness and understanding of *caveat emptor* (let the buyer beware) during interactions with health care professionals at all levels. This does not propose or validate a removal of a free market system within health care, but rather emphasizes the need for the consumer-patient to be an educated buyer. It also assumes that the health care professional and the open market function in an ethical manner.

Then, what is a health care professional in this system and what is an ethical manner? *Webster's Family Dictionary* defines a professional as a person with a vocation that requires extensive education and training.[7] Health care professionals possess specialized education, skills, or resources that patients lack. Ideally, these skills and resources benefit patients.[8] Providers of health care at any level fall into the definition of a professional. Whether obtaining profit conflicts with the goal is a matter for intense debate. But society expects health care professionals to conduct themselves appropriately as they work in an evidence-based and service-oriented environment. To detail their legal responsibilities, real and implied contracts are used. The consumer expects the professional to base his or her scope of service on the latest and most accurate medical evidence. Additionally, health care professionals at all levels are expected to behave in an ethical, responsible, and predictable manner, based upon these principles. Thus, the visceral response that the viewer experienced when Donny Ray dies supports this expectation.

In response to the greater, societal expectation, health care professions specify and enforce moral obligations in the form of professional codes. Whether spoken or written, a professional code articulates statements of moral behavior on the part of the health care professional. The Hippocratic Oath, Oath of Amatus, Oath of Maimonides, and the Oath of a Muslim Physician taken by physicians are examples of professional codes carried down through the ages. The Declaration of Geneva after World War II, the American Medical Association Code of Ethics for Physicians, and the Nightingale Pledge taken by nurses are more recent versions, but inclusive of the same principles. Professional codes distinguish the moral behavior of professionals from the standards imposed by regulatory bodies such as state and federal agencies[8] and explain, in part, the mechanism by which health care professionals are held to a higher standard in a complex health care and medico-legal system. From a consumer standpoint, insurance companies are not exempt from these codes or biomedical ethics, as they are intimately involved in health care delivery.

Over the past 30 years, four key principles in biomedical ethics have been extensively utilized as a guide in codes of conduct: *beneficence, nonmaleficence, autonomy,* and *justice.*[9] Beneficence obliges the professional to restore health. Nonmaleficence refers to the duty of *primum non nocere* (first, do no harm). Autonomy enjoins the health care worker to respect the individuality and independence of others. Justice, a health policy principle, supports the fair allocation of medical resourses.[9] Although the definition of "fair" remains subject to debate, the lack of justice and all other key principles defined in the bioethics vocabulary appears evident in *The Rainmaker.*

For the complex system of health care to work, the consumer must have trust at multiple levels. As such, this unique paradigm can place consumers in a vulnerable position if they are not educated about the system. The ethical dilemma in *The Rainmaker* is much more systemic as there is a noticeable absence of a physician or nurse advocate for the patient. Trust was violated at both the payer (insurance company) and provider (physician, nurse, social worker, etc.) level. However, my personal experience reveals that patient advocates for the terminally ill are much more prevalent than the movie suggests. As such, we should not be made cynical toward health care professionals who provide hands-on care for patients. Additionally, this movie should not prejudice the observer against the many legitimate and ethical health insurance companies in business today. Instead, *The Rainmaker* should serve as a lesson to the consumer about the need for personal responsibility in learning as much as possible regarding their health care in a complex market. For medical providers, it should emphasize advocacy for patients in need. By doing this, providers function as consumers on behalf of their patients.

Although Great Benefit's refusal to pay for a bone marrow transplant was denied in the face of medical evidence and necessity, we are not privy to the actual terms of the contract that the Black's signed. The filmmakers imply that Great Benefit had a legal obligation to pay the claim, but the movie does not elaborate if any of the corporate personnel were liable for criminal prosecution or professional sanctions. It is not even certain if the outcome would have been different if the Blacks had sought counsel *before* they signed the debit insurance contract. To make this more complex, the movie never fully addresses the lingering ethical issue of Great Benefit's suppression of this information. But clearly, Great Benefit contributed to Donny Ray Black's death and violated all four of the key bioethical principles that frame moral behavior in health care. Knowledge of the mechanical and ethical issues as part of consumer awareness may not be sufficient to prevent the tragic outcome experienced by the Blacks, but this understanding forms the first necessary step to prevent this type of outcome. The second step is that this knowledge is known a priori, with ample market choices for consumers other than companies like Great Benefit. How all of this is to be obtained is a societal question yet to be answered.

The question of a conflict of interest between the duties to shareholders versus patients is the final societal issue in this story. In *Metropolitan Life Insurance Company v. Glenn*, the United States Supreme Court ruled that a company that both administers and funds a benefit plan operates under a conflict of interest that must be considered as a factor in a court's review of claim denials.[10] Although this case concerned withdrawn disability benefits, similar questions will be asked as the United States continues the health care reform debate. Equally contentious will be the role of government in these issues, which may not guarantee success. Nonetheless, the lesson from *The Rainmaker* remains clear: *caveat emptor.*

In *The Rainmaker*, Baylor assumes the role of a health care advocate. His actions serve as a reminder to those at any level in the health care system of the ethical and moral obligation to support the moral order that propagates justice, humanity, and equity, as provided for by Natural Law.[11] This is also a call for those in the profession to be advocates for their patients, as consumers on behalf of their patients. To the consumer-patient, the tragedy of Donny Ray Black serves as a reminder that consumer awareness is essential to assure attainment of this goal.

REFERENCES

1. H.R. 3200. To provide affordable, quality health care for all Americans and reduce the growth in health care spending, and for other purposes. Sec. 111. *Prohibiting pre-existing condition exclusions.* Retrieved August 15, 2009 from http://thomas. loc.gov/
2. H.R. 676. United States National Health Insurance Act (or the Expanded and Improved Medicare for All Act) (introduced in House) Sec 403. *Reduction in Health Care Disparities.* Retrieved August 15, 2009 from http://thomas.loc.gov/
3. H.R. 3200. To provide affordable, quality health care for all Americans and reduce the growth in health care spending, and for other purposes. Sec. 201. *Establishment Exchange; Outline of Duties; Definitions.* Retrieved August 15, 2009 from http:// thomas.loc.gov/
4. Camenisch, P.F. 1983. *Grounding professional ethics in a pluralistic society.* New York: Haven Publications.
5. Burrough, B., and Helyar, J. 1990. *Barbarians at the gate,* p. vii. New York: Harper Perennial.
6. Illich, I., et al. 1977. *The disabling professions.* Salem, NH: Marion Boyars Press.
7. *Webster's American Family Dictionary.* 2008. New York: Random House, Inc.
8. Frankel, M.S. 1996. Guidelines/codes of ethics: Merging process and content. *Science of the Total Environment* 184(1–2): 13–16.
9. Beauchamp, T.L., and Childress, J.F. 1983. *Principles of biomedical ethics,* pp. 7–9. New York: Oxford University Press.
10. *Metropolitan Life Insurance Co., et al. v. Glenn.* Retrieved August 15, 2009 from http://www.supremecourtus.gov/opinions/07pdf/06–923.pdf
11. Burke, E. 1997. *Selected writings and speeches.* P.J. Stanlis (Ed.).Washington, DC: Gateway Publishing/Regnery Publishing, Inc.

3

the psychological ethics of the whistleblower: *the insider*

bradley olson and dan aalbers

The Insider (1999). Al Pacino, Russell Crowe, Christopher Plummer, Diane Venora, Philip Baker Hall, Lindsay Crouse, Debi Mazar. Directed by Michael Mann. Duration: 158 minutes.

DVD chapter 16 scene 01.12:07 to 01.15:32

THE INSIDER PROVIDES A DRAMATIZED account of whistleblower Jerry Wigand's decision to go public with one of Big Tobacco's closely held secrets—that they have been manipulating nicotine levels to keep their customers addicted to their product. What makes this dramatic retelling worthwhile is its grounded, unromantic view of whistleblowing—the film's narrative is neither entirely heroic nor tragic; it has much to tell about the serious impediments whistleblowers face.

Wigand (Russell Crowe) arrives home to his family and affluent lifestyle to announce being fired from his research position with the nation's third largest tobacco company. He is soon contacted by Lowell Bergman (Al Pacino), a producer for the CBS show *60 Minutes*. Bergman tries to persuade Wigand into an interview. Both protagonists struggle with weighty moral questions—Bergman must constantly monitor himself to avoid exploiting Wigand, and Wigand must struggle to choose between paths of security or morality. If Wigand remains silent, he allows a lie to stand and becomes complicit in activities he knows to be immoral. If he talks, he breaches a contract, breaks the law, and loses his affluent lifestyle and the medical care needed for a daughter with asthma—he would never again find work anywhere within the reach of Big Tobacco.

In the focus scene (DVD scene 16), Wigand gives a preliminary interview to Mike Wallace for *60 Minutes*. A fuller understanding emerges of what Wigand knows, what has guided his past decisions, and what will guide his future. From Wigand's standpoint, the heads of Big Tobacco have, in televised testimony, perjured themselves, clearly misstating what was common language inside corporate culture: tobacco companies were (are) in the nicotine delivery business. The companies escalated the addictive properties of cigarettes through a lung-specific carcinogen, amplifying the nicotine's effect, while ostensibly conducting research to replace the ingredient. When tests showed its removal would affect the "taste"—and would reduce sales—the company decided it must remain until a substitute was found. Wigand refused the plan, and pressed the CEO, demanding the ingredient's removal. The CEO fired Wigand for poor "communication skills"—a euphemism for "strenuously opposing an immoral act."

Whistleblowing is a British term, originating with police officers (i.e., bobbies) who would alert the surrounding neighborhood by blowing a whistle when a crime was discovered in progress. In a society that values secrecy over transparency, institutional whistleblowers inevitably face protracted, alienated battles with governmental, military, and private bureaucracies. Wigand's story alerts us all about the need to speak truth to power.

The viewer will never know definitively what "compelled" Wigand, but a series of intriguing hints are given. With his daughter's asthma, Wigand may have come to empathize with respiratory sufferers, including smokers. He may have conjured the image of a vulnerable exemplar, a lung cancer victim. He may have instead told himself: "Regardless of the outcomes, the chemical's presence is wrong." Wigand has internalized his discipline's scientific ethics, placing a high value on truth and transparency. He may have acted according to a universal principle, questioning, "What if no one else ever took this risk?" Or asked, "What are the benefits and costs to myself, former colleagues, and family compared to others?" For whistleblowing, some form of all these questions may be asked, and the answers may tend to fall in line. There is no royal road to moral movement—action can be inspired by the epistemological assumptions of Kant's categorical imperative, utilitarianism, or Rawl's veil of ignorance.

The film delivers an implicit message of moral pluralism. As antifoundationalists have long argued, no single Archimedian point outside of history exists from which to survey the moral landscape, no simple set of rules to follow, no ethical checklist to consult, no absolute metric by which to measure the moral universe.[1–3] Wigand is facing a true dilemma—if he veers in one direction, he will do well by his family; in another, he will do well by society. Should he do the greatest good for the greatest number, as the utilitarian demands, or should he care for his family first, as tradition dictates?

When, in a critical scene, Wigand must decide whether or not to testify against Big Tobacco—a decision carrying the risk of arrest—we see the subjectivity involved. It begins with a wide-angle panorama of Wigand surrounded by attorneys, police cars, and the seaside and returns to a close-up of Wigand. Bergman appears. Wigand—with his characteristic logical-scientific style—searches for the formula:

WIGAND: "I don't know what to do…I can't seem to find the criteria to decide. It's too big of a decision to make without being resolved in my own mind."

BERGMAN: "Maybe things have changed."

WIGAND replies: "A lot's changed."

BERGMAN is confused, worried of Wigand's retreat: "You mean since this morning?"

WIGAND: "No, I mean since whenever." He waits, and then: "Fuck it…Let's go to court."

Emotion, will, impulse may be as important for whistleblowing as any deep, specific, internal philosophical calculation of cost and benefit.

Wigand's story is one of depth and pathos. Wigand wins, but his victory comes at a heavy cost: he loses his family, his lifestyle, and his reputation. At the same time, a redemption follows contamination[4]: The man fired for poor "communication skills" wins the best high school teacher award in the state of Kentucky. Wigand's comment "a lot has changed" hints at the becoming of a new, better person with a new moral sensibility. Wigand undergoes a role change, but also a character transformation as he moves from Big Tobacco researcher to high school science teacher.

Erich Fromm[5] might say that Wigand has moved from a *marketing* and/or *exploitative* character or type (and social group), epitomized by tobacco company executives and the company itself, to a *productive* character, as a high school teacher in an educational institution. The marketing character for Fromm represents a person focused on selling oneself and one's wares without substance, whereas the exploitative character finds primary satisfaction in taking from others. The productive character is Fromm's humanistic figure. The productive character focuses on creative development, not necessarily in the production of tangible objects, practical endeavors, or even art, but through one's efforts or practice; one engages in activities that affirm life and faith in humanity.[6]

Being a high school teacher within this framework, despite the pay scale, is not a diminished status. Regardless of the teaching award, the move can be seen as an ideal shift from the marketing/exploitative character to the productive[5] or socially generative one (McAdams, 2006). This semitragedy, this antihero myth, provides an inspiring, romanticized moral model. And yet, as romantic as the antihero myth may appear (and as real of a moral guide it may be), the story equally illuminates a very practical lesson. Beyond myth, the message suggests a real need to protect society against unadulterated corporate greed through stronger government policies. No one should be forced down Wigand's path to provide truth for the public good, and thus the story makes a powerful argument for more expansive federal whistleblower protections. If such lessons are learned, the necessity of such future journeys can be prevented, so that suffering is not a typical prerequisite for the voicing of important public truths.

REFERENCES

1. Lyotard, J. F. 1984. *The postmodern condition: A report on knowledge.* Translated by G. Bennington, and B. Massumi. Minneapolis: University of Minnesota Press. (Original work published 1979.)
2. Herzog, D. 1985. *Without foundations: Justification in political theory.* Ithaca, NY: Cornell University Press.

3. Rorty, R. 1980. *Consequences of pragmatism: Essays 1972–1980*. Minneapolis: University of Minnesota Press.

4. McAdams, D. 2006. *The redemptive self: Stories Americans live by.* New York: Oxford University Press.

5. Fromm, E. 1947. *Man for himself: An inquiry into the psychology of ethics*. New York: Holt, Rinehart, and Winston.

6. Fromm, E. 1962. *Beyond the chains of illusion*. New York: Credo Perspectives.

4

the ethics of withholding care: *as good as it gets*

donald a. barr

As Good As It Gets (1997). Jack Nicholson, Helen Hunt, Greg Kinnear, Cuba Gooding Jr. Directed by James L. Brooks. Duration: 139 minutes.

Chapter 13 scene 00:52:12 to 00:56:06

A WAITRESS, A WRITER, AND HEALTH care in New York City. This is about *As Good As It Gets*.

Her name is Carol (Helen Hunt); his is Melvin (Jack Nicholson). She works for minimum wage plus tips; he gets million-dollar advances on his books. She is a single mom, sharing an apartment in Brooklyn with her son and her own mom. Her son has asthma, as do so many kids in low-income, single-parent families in New York and other big cities. When her son gets sick with asthma, she has to miss work to take him to the ER. This is how it goes for thousands of kids and moms in Carol's situation.

Somehow, Carol has obtained health insurance coverage for her son, enrolling him in a health maintenance organization—an HMO. How a low-wage waitress got health insurance we are not told. Perhaps it is from the boy's father; perhaps it's a Medicaid HMO; perhaps (although unlikely) the restaurant offers its employees affordable health coverage. Melvin has different issues. He can afford all the health care he wants. His problem is not asthma; it's mental illness. His obsessions are about as compulsive as they come. He has (presumably) one of the best psychiatrists in Manhattan, yet it seems to do him little good. When he goes into the restaurant for lunch (the same restaurant every day, the same table, the same chair, bringing his own plastic fork to avoid germs) and finds a waitress other than Carol serving him, he flips out.

Set the scene: a sidewalk in Brooklyn. Carol, walking home from some errands, sees the license plate of the car parked in front of her apartment building. It says "MD." Fearing the worst for her son, she dashes up the stairs to her apartment. There she finds a strange man. "What? Please tell me!" Has her son died from his asthma while she was gone?

Her son has not died. He seems fine. Walking into the living room, the son asks his mom, "Did you know there are doctors who come to your house?" The man turns out to be Dr. Martin Betts, a doctor who makes house calls in New York City. He also gives his patients his home number to call—all for a considerable price, of course. He is a concierge physician; one of a new breed who bring the best medicine has to offer to people's doorstep, so long as they can afford his price. He has been sent by Melvin to get her son well, so she can go back to work.

Commenting to his mom on how he has been treated by Dr. Betts, the son says, "He's good—I'm an expert on doctors." Dr. Betts has examined the son, drawn blood for lab tests (you have to be good to get blood from the arm of an eight-year-old), and sits down with Carol to get more history on her son's asthma. The son has had the asthma since he was six months old. Carol has stacks of receipts for the medicines she has purchased, and a log of her son's symptoms day by day.

DR. BETTS asks CAROL: "Have they done blood tests on him?"

"Yah…"

"Only in the emergency room, or when he was well?"

"Emergency room only!"

"How about skin testing for allergies?"

"No. I asked and they said that my plan didn't cover it, and that it wasn't necessary anyway…. Why? Should they have?"

DR. BETTS hesitates: "Well…." he adds questioningly.

Carol suddenly gets it. Her son has been repeatedly sick with his asthma because her HMO wouldn't approve the type of comprehensive, preventive care that keeps asthmatic kids well, keeps them out of the ER. She can't help herself: *"Fucking HMO bastard pieces of shit!"*

Seemingly nonplussed, Dr. Betts replies, "Actually, I think that is their technical name." Dr. Betts goes on: "I promise you—from now on, your son is going to feel a great deal better." Sensing a physician who understands her situation, her frustrations—a physician who can empathize with a low-wage waitress single mom—Carol reaches over and hugs Dr. Betts. Who is going to pay Dr. Betts' bill? Dr. Betts confirms that there will be a bill. "The costs are going to be considerable." Carol needn't worry, though. Melvin has agreed to pay the bill, so long as Carol comes back to work in the restaurant in Manhattan and serves him lunch.

In 1997, when I saw *As Good As It Gets* in a theater, the crowd around me let out a cheer when Carol exploded with her expletives. That one line seemed to have captured the mood of the entire country when it came to HMOs shortchanging people on care. Writing in the *Boston Globe*, Ellen Goodman reported, "At this outburst—with none of the expletives deleted—audiences all over America spontaneously burst out in applause. It was one of those moments when you know the tide has turned… Managed-care companies are rapidly replacing tobacco companies as corporate demons… the HMOs are taking the place of the Russkies as the bad guys."[1] Giving the Canadian perspective, Matthew Rees wrote in the *Ottawa Citizen* that, "the story of how movie audiences erupt in cheers when HMOs are berated by Helen Hunt in the film *As Good As It Gets* has become the stuff of legend in Washington political circles."[2]

Prior to the 1980s, HMOs were generally seen in a positive light. When Congress passed the HMO Act of 1973, giving federal subsidy and policy support for the national expansion of HMOs, Kaiser-Permanente and other similar HMOs were cited as optimal models of care. To qualify for federal support, however, HMOs had to have a number of characteristics, one of which was that they had to be operated on a not-for-profit basis. That all changed in the 1980s. President Reagan revoked the nonprofit requirement, opening the health care system to a rapid expansion of investor-owned, for-profit HMOs. By the 1990s, when Carol was serving Melvin his lunch, the vast majority of HMOs were for-profit businesses.

Managers of for-profit businesses, including health care businesses, owe a fiduciary duty to their shareholders. Part of this duty is to optimize the return on shareholder investment. Since HMOs must provide health care to their members within the constraints of a fixed budget, every dollar spent on providing care is a dollar not available to shareholders. For much of the 1990s, managers of for-profit HMOs focused their attention on minimizing what is referred to as the "medical loss ratio"—the percentage of revenues spent on providing care to members.

Should an asthmatic child be referred to an allergist for specialized assessment and testing? For many of the early for-profit HMOs, referral to specialists was to be discouraged. In some cases, primary care physicians were penalized financially every time they referred a patient to a specialist. In others, such a referral required prior authorization from the HMO. News reports began to proliferate of unreasonable refusals of prior authorization requests. Physicians began to complain both bitterly and vocally that their medical practice was being taken over by HMO bureaucrats. Rather than rationalized systems of care that balanced cost with effectiveness (the basis of nonprofit HMOs such as Kaiser Permanente), this new model of HMO was seen in a much more negative light. Thus, when Carol (and her audience) realized that her son's HMO had been shortchanging his care, presumably in an effort to increase shareholder profit, she erupted in expletives and the theater audience into cheers. It seems clear that the American public will not put up with abusive corporations or self-interested entrepreneurs being given responsibility for allocating otherwise scarce health care resources. As Congress and the President grapple with how to form or reform our system of health care, this lesson will remain central to the discussion.

However, our story is not yet over. What are we to think of Dr. Betts? He seems to provide the best that medicine has to offer—but for a price, and a very high one at that. From an ethical perspective, how do we distinguish between an HMO that uses profit considerations in allocating care and a physician who does the same? Dr. Betts never withholds care from his patients selectively based on profit considerations; rather, he denies all care from patients unable or unwilling to pay his high price.

From one perspective, the concierge physician—the physician who provides optimal care to a select few patients willing to pay top dollar—reflects the core ethical principles of medical practice, doing whatever he or she can to serve the needs of the patient. From another perspective, the concierge physician morphs into a self-interested entrepreneur, attempting to maximize financial return on his or her educational investment.

The striking irony of the scene with Carol, her asthmatic son, and Dr. Betts is that, while the HMO is derided as representing a fundamental ethical conflict in the delivery of health care, Dr. Betts is not. Is there an ethical link between HMOs withholding care and concierge physicians withholding care? Perhaps *As Good As It Gets–The Sequel* (*As Good As It SHOULD Get*) should explore this issue.

REFERENCES

1. Goodman, E. March 29, 1998. The HMO horror show. *The Boston Globe.*
2. Rees, M. July 2, 1998. Will Helen Hunt save U.S. health care? *The Ottawa Citizen.*

5

racial and sexual identity in health care and research: *philadelphia*

kirsten ostherr

Philadelphia (1993). Tom Hanks, Denzel Washington, Jason Robards, Antonio Banderas, Joanne Woodward. Directed by Jonathan Demme. Duration: 125 minutes.

DVD chapter 3 scene 00.15:20 to 00.19:54

PHILADELPHIA HAS BEEN WIDELY RECOGNIZED as the first feature-length Hollywood film about the AIDS crisis. Released a full decade into the pandemic, the film presents many of the injustices suffered by HIV-positive gay men in a mainstream, nonconfrontational style. The sympathetic protagonist, Andrew Beckett (Tom Hanks), a rising but closeted star at a corporate law firm, is promoted to partner, awarded a major, multimillion dollar case, and then suddenly fired for incompetence. Beckett believes the partners had noticed the visible Kaposi's sarcoma (KS) lesions on his face and fired him for having AIDS; in response, he seeks representation to file a lawsuit and defend his civil rights, as guaranteed by the Americans with Disabilities Act since 1990. However, the local prominence of his former employers scares off all the other law firms in town, until Beckett finally partners up with Joe Miller (Denzel Washington), an ambulance-chasing attorney who advertises on television and voices homophobic reactions to his contact with Beckett, but ultimately wins the case and develops a sympathetic attitude toward his dying client. While much of the film takes place in the courtroom, important scenes also occur in Beckett's loft apartment (shared with his partner Miguel (Antonio Banderas), at an AIDS clinic, a hospital, a law library, and a family reunion: Rhese settings provide opportunities for the film to present various ethical issues, as well as a depiction of the community solidarity needed to fight AIDS discrimination.

In this scene, Andrew is rushed to the hospital emergency room after nearly collapsing from abdominal pain at home. Moments earlier, Andrew had been surrounded by helpful friends, including an amateur makeup artist who attempted to camouflage the KS lesions on his face. Andrew's partner Miguel rushes to meet him at the hospital, and then confronts the attending physician over a proposed—and in Miguel's view, painful and unnecessary—colonoscopy. The exchange escalates rapidly, and the doctor threatens to remove Miguel from the ER because he is "not a member of [Andrew's] immediate family." The friendly, diplomatic Tom Hanks character defuses the situation, and the scene shifts focus when his office pages him for the third time that day. Returning the call from a hospital payphone, Beckett chuckles at a television advertisement for Joe Miller's law practice, until the seriousness of the situation sinks in: The statute of limitations for filing the complaint in the case he was awarded as a new law partner is about to run out, and the document he prepared has gone missing from the office. As the tone of the scene becomes more intense, we see an exposed lesion on the back of Andrew's neck in close-up, intercut with a shot of the other occupants of the waiting room staring uncomfortably at this obvious stigma of AIDS.

Philadelphia presents a complex case for considering the ethical treatment of racial and sexual minority identities in the health care context. In the early years of the AIDS pandemic in the United States, the disease disproportionately affected sexual and racial minority groups, whose historical experience of coercion, exploitation, and neglect by health authorities led to mistrust and antagonism between these groups and medical professionals.[1] While this power imbalance raised important issues of informed consent, the ethics of research and vaccine trials, patient autonomy, privacy and confidentiality, and global health care equity, my discussion will focus on the ethical treatment of same-sex partners in medical decision-making, and the role of minority identity in health care research.

The hospital sequence highlights the institutionalized homophobia that occurs when the social and legal status of domestic partners is questioned in the medical setting. The failure of health professionals to recognize same-sex partners as legitimate family members, entitled to make medical decisions and be present at the patient's bedside, remains an ongoing ethical issue that affects patient care directly and indirectly, often despite official hospital policies that protect these rights.[2,3] Emotional support from loved ones has been widely recognized in the medical literature as playing an important role in the healing process,[4-6] and preventing a patient's access to support by denying visitation rights to a same-sex partner might thus produce a negative health outcome. Additional consequences include risk to the therapeutic relationship, as the patient might justifiably feel that a physician who does not respect the patient's same-sex partnership also does not respect the patient's basic rights.

The very notion of "minority" identity has functioned historically to pathologize difference from the white, heterosexual, middle-aged male norm that long constituted the invisible but universal standard for medical research studies.[7] Until recently, findings from these studies were assumed to be relevant for the rest of the population, without being specifically tested for broader application. This practice of generalizing research findings resulted in significant numbers of fatally inaccurate diagnoses and administration of toxic drug dosages.[8,9] From the mid-1980s to the present, the U.S. government mandated that federally funded medical research must include consideration of sex, gender, race, ethnicity, and age in clinical research, in order to correct the ethical problems produced by the historical exclusion of these groups. However, scholars such as Steven Epstein argue that the categorical inclusion of minority identities often turns social difference into biological difference, and thus produces misleading results that can restigma-tize bodily difference.[10] In *Philadelphia*, the fact that Andrew "passes" as a straight man in public and at his law firm, until the KS lesions appear in visible places on his body complicates the issue of gayness as minority identity. The character who recoils from the sight of the KS lesion in the waiting room serves as a reminder of the often-unconscious stigmatization that occurs when we are faced with unexpected signs of visible bodily difference. Similarly, the physician's abrupt rejection of Andrew's same-sex partner highlights that acknowledgment of a patient's difference from the norm can produce feelings of exclusion, not inclu-sion in the health care setting.

The role of race further complicates all of these issues. Just as the heterosexual nuclear family often functions as a normative ideal at the expense of gay relationships, whiteness often appears as the unmarked, universal skin tone from which others diverge.[11] The federal mandate to include racial and ethnic difference in research studies may redress the historical exclusion of nonwhite patients from scientific studies (except in cases of exploitation such as the Tuskegee syphilis studies),[12,13] but scientists have long disputed the biological basis of racial difference. And yet, these mandates may unintentionally reaffirm the legitimacy of viewing nonwhite people as fundamentally different from whites.[14] Similarly, some recent studies have attempted to identify a biological basis for homosexuality.[15,16] While some commentators view this hypothesis as beneficial for potentially resolving the moral and religious debates surrounding homosexuality (it is no longer a "sinful lifestyle choice" but rather an involuntary consequence of genetics), others recog-nize that historically, the notion of essential difference was often invoked to justify unequal treatment.[17] Thus, the politics of inclusion in medical research continues to raise complex ethical issues.

As the hospital scene demonstrates, *Philadelphia* opens multiple interpreta-tions, a valuable quality for generating classroom debate. While some viewers applaud the film for humanizing people with AIDS and encouraging more main-stream support for this marginalized community, others note that the clean-cut, all-American protagonist, with his unequivocally supportive extended family and friends, his social privilege as a highly educated professional, his access to health care, and his sanitized sex life, is yet another stereotypical Hollywood fantasy of AIDS, not a realistic portrayal. Adjudicating between these different perspectives on the film is critically important for considering how to increase students' sensi-tivity to the ways in which verbal and visual information can function differently in the clinical setting. Still, *Philadelphia* provides numerous opportunities for assessing the varied sources of information that come into play in any interper-sonal encounter, including between physician and patient. Racial and sexual minority identities are further complicated by class, education, religion, gender, nationality, and other aspects of identity, some of which may be visible, some invisible. The meanings one might attribute to the visible differences come from personal experiences with formal and informal educational settings such as church, school, military service, popular culture, and elsewhere. It is essential for physicians to acknowledge that, despite their scientific training, they are not immune to outside influences as they form impressions of their patients.[18] This awareness may help refine doctors' ability to recognize when they are basing important medical decisions on assumptions rather than facts, and thus may improve physician–patient communication and lead to more positive outcomes from the clinical encounter.

With each new class of medical students, the memory of the irrational, visceral fear of AIDS that led to unthinkable forms of discrimination, quarantine, and humiliation in the early years of the pandemic continues to fade. *Philadelphia* provides an important opportunity to remind students of the extreme prejudice that characterized medical institutions, including doctors, nurses, hospital cafeteria staff, janitors, health insurance companies, and others, in their dealings with people with AIDS. Poor treatment at the hands of trusted caregivers contributed greatly to the physical and emotional suffering of AIDS patients, and the complex dynamics of racial and sexual identity both fueled the panic response and furthered many patients' experiences of social ostracism.[19–21] Same-sex partners continue to face these obstacles in many health care settings today. From the present vantage point, students may find it hard to believe that well-educated scientists could treat a medical condition so emotionally and irrationally; the lesson of this film is that unconscious fears of racial and sexual contamination continue to shape personal reactions to patients, even in professional settings. Students can work to mitigate their own prejudices by practicing their analysis of verbal and visual representations of patients whose bodies deviate from the assumed norms of whiteness and heterosexuality.

REFERENCES

1. Bayer, R. 2004. AIDS. In S.G. Post (Ed.), *Encyclopedia of bioethics*, 3rd ed., p. 122. New York: Macmillan.
2. For recent accounts of these practices, see: Human Rights Campaign Foundation and the Gay and Lesbian Medical Association, 2009. *The health care equity index 2009: Creating a national standard for equal treatment of lesbian, gay, bisexual and transgender patients and their families.*
3. Parker-Pope, T. May 12, 2009. How hospitals treat same-sex couples. *New York Times.* Retrieved from http://well.blogs.nytimes.com/2009/05/12/how-hospitals-treat-same-sex-couples/
4. Ahern, D.K., Gorkin, L., Anderson, J.L., Tierney, C., Hallstrom, A., Ewart, C., et al. 1990. Biobehavioral variables and mortality or cardiac arrest in the Cardiac Arrhythmia Pilot Study (CAPS). *American Journal of Cardiology* 66: 59–62.
5. Gorkin, L., Schron, E.B., Brooks, M.M., Wiklund, I., Kellen, J., Verter, J., et al. 1993. Psychosocial predictors of mortality in the Cardiac Arrhythmia Suppression Trial-1 (CAST-1). *American Journal of Cardiology* 71: 263–267.

6. Mitchinson, A.R., et al. 2008. Social connectedness and patient recovery after major operations. *Journal of the American College of Surgeons* 206.2: 292–300.

7. Gaines, A.D. 2004. Race and Racism. In S.G. Post (Ed.), *Encyclopedia of bioethics*, 3rd ed., p. 2250. New York: Macmillan.

8. Bowles, D. 2004. A radical idea: Men and women are different. *Cardiovascular Research* 61(1)5–6.

9. Sharfstein, J.M., North, M., and Serwint, J.R. 2007. Over the counter but no longer under the radar: Pediatric cough and cold medications. *New England Journal of Medicine* 357(23): 2321–2324.

10. Epstein, S. 2007. *Inclusion: The politics of difference in medical research.* Chicago: University of Chicago Press.

11. Dyer, R. 1997. *White.* New York: Routledge.

12. Jones, J. 1993. *Bad blood: The Tuskegee syphilis experiment.* New York: Free Press.

13. Reverby, S.M. (Ed.), *Tuskegee's truths: Rethinking the Tuskegee syphilis story.* Chapel Hill: University of North Carolina Press.

14. Marks, J. 1995. *Human biodiversity: Genes, race, and history.* New York: Aldine de Gruyter.

15. LeVay, S. 1997. *Queer science: The use and abuse of research into homosexuality* Cambridge, MA: MIT Press.

16. American Psychological Association. *Answers to your questions for a better understanding of sexual orientation & homosexuality.* Retrieved from http://www.apa.org/topics/sorientation.html.

17. Proctor, R. *Racial hygiene: Medicine under the Nazis.* Cambridge, MA: Harvard University Press.

18. Zita Grover, J. Visible lesions: Images of the PWA. In C.K. Creekmur and A. Doty (Eds.), *Out in culture: Gay, lesbian, and queer essays on popular culture,* pp. 354–381. Durham, NC: Duke University Press.

19. Treichler, P. 1999. *How to have theory in an epidemic: Cultural chronicles of AIDS.* Durham, NC: Duke University Press.

20. Epstein, S. 1996. *Impure science: AIDS, activism, and the politics of knowledge.* Berkeley: University of California Press.

21. Fee, E., and Fox, D.M. 1988. *AIDS: The burdens of history.* Berkeley: University of California Press.

6

social needs of persons with disabilities: *the waterdance*

gretchen a. case

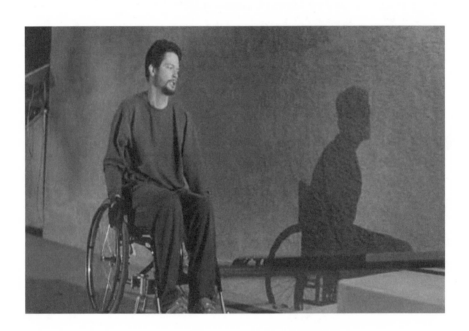

The Waterdance (1992). William Forsythe, Helen Hunt, Wesley Snipes, Eric Stoltz. Written and Directed by Neal Jimenez. Directed by Michael Steinberg. Duration: 106 minutes.

Chapter 25, 1:32:53–1:35:44

T*HE WATERDANCE*[i] FOCUSES ON THE experience of Joel Garcia (Eric Stoltz), a writer rendered paraplegic in a hiking accident, during his six-month stay as a patient in a physical rehabilitation ward at the fictional Holbrook Medical Center. Joel struggles to establish his own place in this miniature society, with particular attention to his romantic relationship with Anna (Helen Hunt), which predates his injury. Joel's is not a simple story of recovery, or of overcoming disability, but of an unsettled phase between medical crisis and stable health, between institutional routines and everyday life, between weaknesses and strengths.

In this climatic scene, Joel and fellow patient Bloss (William Forsythe), whose paraplegia resulted from a motorcycle accident, display their growing physical strength and returning sense of social identity. Throughout the film, patients in the rehab repeatedly express extreme frustration with the callous attitude the telephone operators show toward their requests. Patients constantly suffer dropped calls, long waits on hold, and wrong numbers that seem to be intentional on the part of the "phone people." Because the patients cannot dial direct, all communication with the world outside of Holbrook Medical Center depends on the cooperation of the phone people. At this point in the film, Raymond (Wesley Snipes), another Holbrook patient, has been discharged to a long-term care facility. Late one night, drunk and threatening suicide, he calls Bloss from a pay phone on a city street corner. When the phone people disconnect the call in the middle of Bloss' pleas for Raymond to identify his location, Bloss reports the emergency to a nurse and begs to be taken on a rescue mission to find Raymond.

Joel, having heard Bloss' end of the phone conversation, takes matters into his own hands. Quickly realizing where Joel is going, Bloss is right behind him to join the fight. They leave the rehab building and speed across campus in their wheelchairs to the formidable bunker housing the phone people. Joel gains entry by building an ad hoc wheelchair ramp and delivers corporal punishment for the weeks of cruelty. Joel and Bloss form only the uneasiest of alliances, as do all the

men on their ward. Connected only by the effects of their injuries and their search
to adapt to new and permanent disabilities, these men could not be more different.
Yet, they must find a way to coexist with little privacy or personal space, in beds
only a few feet apart. Conflicts among patients and between patients and staff
continue throughout this film, usually centering on issues revolving around
identity and autonomy.

The Americans with Disabilities Act (ADA) of 1990[1], passed into law just two
years before The Waterdance premiered, codifies the rights of persons with disabilities in the United States. The ADA remains an important document for a
disability ethics that recognizes impairment as not only a medical condition but
also a social circumstance. By addressing the social inequalities often encountered
by persons with disabilities alongside necessary physical accommodations, the
ADA emphasizes that successful life with a disability requires more than just medical attention. The United Nations Convention on the Rights of Persons with
Disabilities further emphasizes the importance of recognizing persons with disabilities as autonomous individuals, fully vested in their societies. The Convention
came into force in 2008, and boasts more than 140 signatories and a growing
influence on the perceptions of persons with disabilities around the world.[2]

Today, the contrast between at least two prevalent understandings of disability
drives ethical considerations[3]: the medical model and the social model. The medical
model defines disability in regard to a physical norm: a given set of abilities is
expected for a human being, and any deviation constitutes disability. The medical
model seeks a return to this established norm, and so focuses on rehabilitation,
treatment, and cure. The social model defines disability in regard to the physical
and social environment: disability is present when a person cannot perform daily
activities because of barriers external to the individual's body. These barriers may
be physical, such as the lack of a wheelchair ramp, or attitudinal, such as the idea
that paraplegic men do not have sexual needs.[4] Neither the medical model nor the
social model alone sufficiently describes the experience of living with a disability,
but comparing these two models raises important questions about paradigms
often employed without reflection.

In The Waterdance, the medical model of disability is readily apparent in
Holbrook's mission to restore the patients' health and mobility. However, the film
reflects the social model of disability as well, by insisting that these men possess
social identities in need of support and with desires for autonomy that go beyond
driving a wheelchair or accessing a building. The Waterdance also portrays incidents
of racial prejudice and frustrated sexuality that illustrate the social complexity of
rehabilitation after acquiring a disability.[i] Many films depict the medical aspects of
disability, but The Waterdance is one of the first and few films that address difficult
social issues, such as race and sexuality in the context of disability.[5] Showing only
the selected scene without the context of the entire film risks emphasizing the
physical conditions of the patients—and Joel's triumph over a physical obstacle—
and losing the social aspects of their lives. Instructors should resist reducing the

selected scene to a moment of *physical* triumph, just as they should resist reducing disability to a solely medical condition that must be overcome.

Rehab is a rarely considered but crucial period of time in which patients make great social transitions in addition to the more obvious physical adjustments.[6] While making these transitions, Joel and the other patients are humanely but surely institutionalized, with very little control of their daily experiences. When Joel and Bloss take revenge on the phone people, they are advocating for themselves as social beings, with full rights and needs rather than passive victims. Joel's determination to enter the windowless, inaccessible phone center and his ingenuity in creating a wheelchair ramp make him an active protagonist, fighting through obstacles rather than being crushed by them. In this moment, Joel represents the interests of all the patients who depend on others for daily wants and needs. He advocates for them by making physical contact with the ephemeral forces that have controlled them all. The humor and surprise of this scene come from the unexpected power with which Joel attacks and his success at subduing the phone people, followed by the recognition of his limits in a battle with a nondisabled person.

The patients in *The Waterdance* are wildly imperfect and inconsistent, contradicting widespread portrayals of persons with disabilities as saints, martyrs, or victims, especially in the context of a hospital or rehabilitation center. The most common narratives depict a person made sacred by his unfortunate circumstances who proceeds to save himself (or be saved by saintly others) through humility, hard work, and strong moral fiber. Joel, Bloss, and Raymond curse unrepentantly and at times, behave reprehensibly. Their visitors and the rehab staff are flawed, too: complaining and acting selfishly as often as comforting and acting compassionately. Just as Holbrook is not an alternate universe, and worldly concerns are not left at the door, nor are the people in Holbrook transformed into ciphers without human desires.

Instructors should turn their students' attention to why this scene marks the climax of the story. Joel's fierce reaction to the interruption of a phone call makes sense only in the context of the many frustrations he has experienced during his time at Holbrook. The phone people represent institutional obstacles to the social needs of the patients. Given that a medical institution will focus primarily on physical care, what are the possibilities for attending to social needs? What are the unintended effects of institutional procedures and rules? How can patients and staff best identify and respond to these problems?

Students also should discuss the physical violence in this scene, which exemplifies the corporeal focus of *The Waterdance*. We are following the story of men who have lost significant physical sensation and are working to establish new functionality in permanently changed bodies. Why does Joel's show of strength matter? How does it reflect a certain idea of heterosexual masculinity, one that is prominent throughout the film, as the men compete in sports, throw objects in anger, and visit strip clubs? How would this story differ if the main characters were women? If the protagonist were engaged in a nonheterosexual romance?

Imagining new story lines and new characters for this film could quickly stray off topic. Guide the students by reminding them that *The Waterdance* follows disabled people with particular, personal needs, rather than a set of paralyzed bodies that follow interchangeable paths to recovery. The great usefulness of this film is in its insistence that Joel, Bloss, and Raymond remain distinct individuals, even when their comparable bodily crises seem to resign them to the same condition. These men share a ward, but not a fate, and the disabilities they acquire do not erase their human strengths and frailties.

Both the medical profession and society at large often consider persons with disabilities, especially those with easily discernible impairments such as paraplegia, only in terms of physical condition. At Holbrook, a place where bodies are brought back to a functional status, social rehabilitation remains a distant second priority to more immediate physical needs. *The Waterdance* reminds us that the social needs of a person do not disappear in the midst of a medical crisis, and that acquiring a disability does not erase all previous experiences and desires. Indeed, attention to *social* personhood is of primary and abiding concern to each of the characters in this film.

NOTE

i. Although *The Waterdance* is an invented story, the film is based on the real disability experiences of screenwriter Neal Jimenez.

REFERENCES

1. *Americans with Disabilities Act of 1990.* As Amended. Retrieved from http://www.ada.gov/pubs/ada.htm
2. The United Nations Programme on Disabilities. *The United Nations Convention on the Rights of Persons with Disabilities.* Retrieved from http://www.un.org/disabilities/default.asp?navid=12&pid=150
3. Davis, Lennard, Ed. 2006. *The disability studies reader*, 2nd ed. London: Routledge.
4. Milligan, M.S., and Neufeldt, A.H. 2001. The myth of asexuality: A survey of social and empirical evidence. *Sexuality & Disability* 19(2): 91–109.
5. Jimenez, N. 1992. 'Waterdance' isn't a "crippled formula film. *Los Angeles Times* June 8, 1992. Retrieved from http://articles.latimes.com/1992–06-08/entertainment/ca-56_1_formula-film
6. Canby, Vincent May 13, 1992 May 13, 1992. Heroism and humor as paraplegics learn. *The New York Times.* Retrieved from http://www.nytimes.com/1992/05/13/movies/review-film-heroism-and-humor-as-paraplegics-learn.html

7

institutional power: *one flew over the cuckoo's nest*

bruce jennings

One Flew Over the Cuckoo's Nest (1975). Jack Nicholson, Louise Fletcher, William Redfield, Will Sampson. Directed by Milos Forman. Duration: 138 minutes.

DVD Scene 28 (Questioning Billy) 01:53.28–1:59.17

O NE FLEW OVER THE CUCKOO'S NEST, adapted from Ken Kesey's classic novel (1962) explores the themes of normalcy, mental illness, freedom, therapy, and *power* in the broadest sense of the term, particularly as they reflect the cultural transformation of America in the 1960s and 1970s. During this turbulent era, all forms of authority (including medical authority) and all forms of institutional structure were called into question in the name of individuality, liberation, and authenticity.[1] The film tells the story of Randle P. McMurphy (Jack Nicholson), who finds rules, schedules, and social structures of all kinds overly confining. When committed to a state mental hospital locked ward, he enters a "total institution"[2] unlike any he has encountered before. Gradually, he becomes entangled by and literally silenced by the bureaucratic coils that rule this institution. Interestingly, a male physician-psychiatrist does not dominate the power structure of the ward but rather Nurse Ratched (Louise Fletcher), an exceedingly controlling woman who fosters the dependency of the men on her and exercises total autocratic control of the ward.

The power struggle between McMurphy and Nurse Ratched reaches a climax in this scene. In events leading up to this encounter, McMurphy has attempted to foment some resistance among the other inmates, most of whom he believes have their psychological problems and symptoms not because they are really ill, but because they are being cowed and repressed by Nurse Ratched. In this sense, she personifies authority and power. In the case of Billy Bibbit (Brad Dourif), a deeply troubled man with enormous guilt, McMurphy's prompting of disobedience and rebellion tragically misfires. As part of his subversive campaign, McMurphy contrives to throw an after-hours party on the ward, complete with liquor and two women prostitutes. One of these women and Billy have sexual relations during the evening. The following morning Nurse Ratched finds the ward in disarray and Billy in flagrante. She proceeds to shame and threaten Billy so severely (including saying that she will disclose his behavior to his mother, Billy's Achilles' heel) that he later commits suicide. Seeing this, McMurphy becomes enraged, loses his self-control, and assaults Nurse Ratched, nearly strangling her.

Bioethics, designed to deal with complex decisions in complex situations, most often focuses on individual agency and the rights and consequences at stake in actions taken, mainly by medical professionals, on patients, families, and society. *One Flew Over the Cuckoo's Nest* provides ample food for thought at the level of individual agency within the context of psychiatry and mental health nursing. Nurse's Ratched's ward is not a "snake pit" or an overtly abusive setting. The staff remains outwardly respectful and professional. With the possible exception of McMurphy, all the patients are either there voluntarily or because they need therapy and care. Throughout most of the film, one is hard pressed to judge Nurse Ratched as behaving unethically or to accuse her of professional misconduct. In the current scene, she does lose her composure and deals with Billy in an unprofessional and dangerous fashion, with tragic results. Is it ethically proper conduct for a health care professional to reveal information about a patient's behavior to his parent? After all, Billy is an adult, although he may be incompetent in the eyes of the law. Is it ever ethically proper for a health professional even to threaten to disclose confidential information? Such coercive threats, especially among patients who are vulnerable to them, like Billy, can be used effectively to bring a patient in crisis under control.

Where do we draw the line between ethically grounded therapy, on the one hand, and domination or the exercise of power, on the other? If we remain within the therapeutic frame, the perspective that has predominated in medical ethics and bioethics, psychiatry has been one area of medicine in which the bioethical balance between respect for autonomy and beneficence has been especially problematic and difficult to strike.[3,4] Involuntary commitment negates much of the moral space of autonomy. But, not all of it: The patient does not lose all rights, and many forms of treatment and experimentation, once accepted and widely used, are now forbidden. Respecting autonomy means taking seriously and, at least in large domains of conduct not harmful to others, deferring to the *reasons* that a person gives for what he wants to do or to have done to/for him. But, according to a mainstream view in psychiatry, mental illness is a condition in which reasons are not to be trusted or taken at face value; in a psychotherapeutic encounter, reasons are interpreted as rationalizations or symptoms of something more real that stands behind them.[5] The therapeutic task is to discover and to reveal—slowly, carefully, delicately, and usually against great resistance—what lies beneath. To refuse to accept reasons at face value is the path to restore reason.[6,7]

If bioethical analysis often focuses on the ethics of agency and foregrounds the individuals making decisions and those for whom decisions are made, it is also necessary to attend to the background conditions that constrain and shape decisions and actions. Most importantly, *One Flew Over the Cuckoo's Nest* leads bioethicists to consider alternatives to that therapeutic framework and the way it defines and identifies ethical issues. The alternative framework underscores the ethics of the use of power and social control.

To be sure, the therapeutic framework conceptualizes power in its own way. But the power it renders visible is mainly within the dyadic and interpersonal connections at work in the relationship between physician and patient, one quite evident in the case of Nurse Ratched and McMurphy. Each is a complex and flawed character; neither is a hero or a villain. But how much of what they did and who they were came from within, so to speak, and how much was a function of the circumstances they were in and of the social, cultural, and economic forces at work on them? When bioethics neglects this question, it ignores crucial aspects of "institutional or structural power." This power, operative in the background of interpersonal transactions and decision making, grows from how bodies of knowledge are codified and made accessible (Foucault's work emphasizes this aspect)[7] and the ways in which social rules, roles, and relationships over time are organized into institutions (Goffman emphasizes this aspect).[2] In this sense, then, power is not something extrinsic that expert knowledge or institutionalized authority simply uses; instead, power is inherent and constitutive of scientific knowledge and social institutions as such. The structuring of power also forms the necessary background and context within which individual acts of exercising power, such as those of physician vis-à-vis patient, occur.

During the past half century, the therapeutic framework has been challenged by the power framework (the so-called "antipsychiatry movement"),[5,8] which offers a critique and a moral delegitimation of psychiatric medicine. This challenge has come partially from within the discipline of psychiatry itself, but largely from sociology, history, and other fields that focus on the functions that certain categories and institutions play in the social control of deviant behavior. This alternative framework rejects the positivistic account of psychiatry as a descriptive and explanatory science and sees it instead from a social constructionist point of view, less as a service to individuals and more as a device of the state or society to label and control individuals. This view gained momentum in the United States through controversies such as the decision to remove homosexuality as a category of disorder in the *Diagnostic and Statistical Manual* of the American Psychiatric Association in 1973.[9] Moreover, the revelations in the West of the political uses of psychiatry in the Soviet Union contributed to the blurring of lines between political repression and mental health care.[10]

Does Nurse Ratched anticipate or intend that Billy be driven to suicide? This is ambiguous, as is the Nurse's passive-aggression. Clearly, however, she reacts to a personal and institutional imperative to maintain control, at whatever cost. This imperative should not be confused with the ethical commitment of a health care professional to protect and promote the well-being and healing of his or her patient. Billy and his misdemeanors pose no threat to institutional power and control. The real threat to her control, authority, and power is the sheer life force of McMurphy—an anarchistic element that neither the daily indignities of the ward routines, nor the violence (portrayed as tantamount to extreme physical punishment or torture) of electroshock treatments can suppress. If she did not intend Billy's extreme reaction, she surely did mean to provoke McMurphy into physical resistance, for she knew that such primal opposition would be his downfall. Although it is his undoing, this assault may ironically be a sign of McMurphy's moral growth. At the beginning of the film, it is hard to imagine him caring so much about the death of Billy, or any other inmate. In the confusion when Billy's body is discovered, McMurphy could have gone through an open window and made good his escape. He decides to stay. In the end, he has developed a capacity to feel a sense of responsibility and a righteous demand for justice that takes the form of violence. The struggle against institutional power is not a game.

The confrontation between Randall McMurphy and Nurse Ratched in *Cuckoo's Nest* is an allegory of the controversies that continue to swirl around contemporary psychiatry. The fact that, in recent years, the practice of psychiatry has become increasingly pharmacological does little to quell this controversy. Success in altering certain overt behaviors and subjective feelings doesn't settle the issue of whether we should alter them therapeutically or instead accommodate and mitigate them socially. Surely, a decent and just society would find some constructive outlet for McMurphy's *élan vital*. Moreover, McMurphy and Ratched, each with a skewed and incomplete understanding of the human condition, pose but do not resolve the question of wherein madness resides. Like Ratched and McMurphy, psychiatry and sociology—the therapy of illness and the deconstruction of power—see a part of madness, but not the whole.

REFERENCES

1. Fox, R.C., and Swazey, J. 2008. *Observing Bioethics*. New York: Oxford University Press.
2. Goffman, E. 1961. *Asylums: Essays on the social situation of mental patients and other inmates*. Garden City, NY: Anchor Books.
3. Beauchamp, T.L. 2009. The philosophical basis of psychiatric ethics. In S. Bloch, and S. Green (Eds.), *Psychiatric Ethics*, 4th ed., pp. 25–48. New York: Oxford University Press.
4. Culver, C.M., and Gert, B. 1982. *Philosophy and medicine: Conceptual and ethical issues in medicine and psychiatry*. New York: Oxford University Press.
5. Boyers, R. 1971. *R.D. Laing and anti-psychiatry*. New York: Harper and Row.
6. Rosenhan, D.L. 1975. On being sane in insane places. In T.J. Scheff (Ed.), *Labeling madness*, pp. 54–74. Englewood Cliffs, NJ: Prentice Hall.
7. Foucault, M. 2009. *History of madness* (trans. J. Murphy). New York: Rutledge.
8. Kotowicz, Z. 1997. *R.D. Laing and the paths of anti-psychiatry*. London: Routledge.
9. Bayer, R. 1987. *Homosexuality and American psychiatry*. Princeton, NJ: Princeton University Press.
10. Bloch, S., and Reddaway, P. 1977. *Psychiatric terror*. New York: Basic Books.

8

ethical conflicts of a complex humanitarian emergency: *the last king of scotland*

alan roth

The Last King of Scotland (2006). Forest Whitaker, James McAvoy,
Kerry Washington. Directed by Kevin MacDonald. Duration: 123 minutes.

DVD Chapter 2 scene 00:5:30 to 00:09:26

THE LAST KING OF SCOTLAND tells the story of Nicholas Garrigan (James McAvoy), an idealistic young physician fresh out of medical school, who comes to 1970s Uganda to join a medical humanitarian mission. In this scene, Dr. Garrigan has arrived in the jungle camp of Dr. David Merrit, who, with his wife Sarah, is caring for numerous Ugandan natives. Garrigan hopes to be of service, but is also attracted to the wife of the doctor whose hospitality he entertains. He seems bewildered, if not somewhat overwhelmed by the general surroundings in the Ugandan jungle. It quickly becomes clear that he is not morally, psychologically, or physically prepared to deal with the disease, people, or conditions he sees upon his arrival. Therefore, he decides to abandon his mission as a humanitarian. The film goes on to display many of the ethical dilemmas that result from that decision, as well as the frequent inability of Western medical professionals to handle their role as humanitarian professionals in a complex humanitarian emergency.

According to Beauchamp[1] (2009), medical ethics revolves around four broad principles: autonomy (respecting the decision-making capacity of individual patients through informed consent), beneficence (balancing risks and benefits of a given action), nonmaleficence (avoiding the causation of harm), and justice (distributing risks and benefits fairly). In the context of a complex humanitarian emergency, decisions made on an ethical basis may have significant and lasting impacts on the communities served.

One such example is the dichotomy of respecting local traditions and values when it comes in direct conflict with one's own training and belief system. A second example is the medical dilemma of choosing between providing basic care (for many) and maximizing care (for a few) with limited resources—a situation often present in a complex humanitarian emergency (CHE).[2] In fact, "certain ethical dilemmas may involve choices between equally undesirable alternatives or conflicting with moral codes"[3] (United Nations Disaster Management Ethics, p. 8).

The methodology needed for ethical decision-making must reflect the complexity of human and international relationships, technological developments, environmental vulnerability, and interdependency. Tensions and shifts in fundamental concepts of reason, truth, and goodness challenge longstanding decision-making procedures. The traditional tools of "objective" logic, rationality, and consistency may not be adequate. Ethics are standards of conduct and moral judgment, systems or codes of morals (concepts of right and wrong). Professional ethics involves the application of accepted principles or a moral code to the practice of a particular profession. Ethical behavior and actions of individuals, groups, or professions conform to values, morals, and standards of conduct. One example is the "Code of Conduct for the International Red Cross and Red Crescent Movement and Non-Governmental Organizations (NGOs) in Disaster Relief"[4] (Appendix A).

One tenet of a complex humanitarian emergency is that health needs overwhelm available human and material resources. In making the difficult ethical decisions, medical knowledge alone will not sufficiently render decisions in this environment. In a leadership position among medical professionals, how individuals deal with the ethical issues has not been clearly established. More specifically, how ethical decision-making relates to an environment of conflict and political violence has not been sufficiently addressed.

Complex humanitarian emergencies are still rare events, and yet individuals must plan to be ready to deal with the consequences of these events. Medical professionals must learn to prepare, cope, and survive these events. Medical humanitarian professionals must use their knowledge and extraordinary sense of "doing the right thing" as the catalyst to train for the next event. Leaders must identify gaps in their education, training, sensitivity, and cultural diversity to enable humanitarian professionals to prepare for CHE. Medical education does not have as part of the curriculum how professionals articulate a sense of fairness, accountability, and value judgment to manage life-and-death situations. In a CHE, the ethical conflict arises when resources are scarce and capacity has been overwhelmed, rather than the loss due to the limits of medical science. Moreover, an inherent cultural bias related to the concept of health and sickness exists between the humanitarian professional and the particular geographic area in which he or she is working.

Professional codes of conduct must reflect our obligation to our patients, under conditions tempered by severe environments. Those medical professionals on the "front lines" will need to examine how they make ethical choices in this particular environment. Humanitarian programs need to access the impact of CHE on not only the individuals but also on humanitarian professionals, organizations, and geography. The question to be determined is how medical responders cope with end-of-life decisions during a CHE in an ethical way that is different from the way they handle this procedure in a hospital or hospice situation. What leadership skills will be necessary to facilitate this change in behavior? What training may be necessary to handle the mental health aspects of this effort? The need to examine the ethical issues that arise from a CHE or pandemic not only affects those who are the victims of the disaster but also the persons intimately involved in the care of those individuals.[5]

To address the ethical questions, one needs to understand (a) who will be prioritized for scarce resources such as medications, hydration, ventilators; (b) how the decision is made to give less or no care to some when one is trained to give optimal care to all, (c) what is the human toll by which an individual or group can do this, and (d) what planning or guidance can our teams learn to facilitate during events which, by their very nature, are overwhelming?

Basically, there are three types of ethical dilemmas. The first involves choices between options with conflicting merits. This type of dilemma is addressed through professional training. The second dilemma centers on moral subjectivity, reflecting how to act when values of an intended beneficiary clash with those of humanitarian professionals. Such conflicts are addressed through mechanisms of participation and empowerment. The third type of dilemma is moral conflicts perceived within a hierarchy of moral obligations (i.e., the sanctity of life as the ultimate value).[6,7]

The decision to keep or withdraw staff from an emergency operation due to the insecurity of and threat to the lives of its humanitarian workers is probably one of the most difficult to make for any humanitarian agency. In choosing to become a medical professional in a CHE, the person understands that such a profession entails risk. It follows that these workers should expect to be among the last persons evacuated when the humanitarian mission can no longer be performed (UNDP, p. 33).

Medical professionals engaged in CHE response need to recognize that they must assume responsibility for the long-term impacts of their efforts. These humanitarian professionals are moved by compassion to work, often under extreme duress and danger, to alleviate the suffering they witness.[8] In particular, humanitarian professionals want to do well, and they are willing to make personal sacrifices to do it. The divergence of good works producing untoward negative effects is distressing. Humanitarian professionals want to find clear and unambiguous ways to express their humanity (UNDP, 38). A United Nations Development Program (UNDP) Report reflected on the experiences of an aid worker:

> You arrive and there are people dying right in front of you. You know you must do something to save them. Every night you are absolutely exhausted, but you know you've done good. Your efforts have saved the lives of children and adults who would not have survived without your food, your medicines, and your help. It is gratifying to be able to do this work. (UNDP, p. 38).

The goal of an organized and coordinated response to a CHE should be to maximize the number of lives saved. Changes in the usual standards of health and medical care in the affected locality or region will be required to achieve the goal of saving the most lives in a CHE. Rather than doing everything possible to save every life, it will be necessary to allocate scarce resources in a different manner to save as many lives as possible[9] (AHRQ, 2005). The basis for allocating health and medical resources in a CHE must be fair and clinically sound. The process for making these decisions should be transparent and judged to be fair by those one serves. The elements of trust and distrust may change a particular outcome, particularly when related to the non-Western view of sickness and health.

Protocols for triage (i.e., the sorting of victims into groups according to their need and the resources available) need to be flexible enough to change as the size of a CHE grows and will depend on both the nature of the event and the speed with which it occurs. Triage efforts need to focus on maximizing the number of lives saved. For example, instead of treating the sickest or the most injured first, triage would focus on identifying and reserving immediate treatment for individuals who have a critical need for treatment and are likely to survive. The goal is to maximize the number of lives saved. Complicating conditions may have an impact on an individual's ability to survive (AHRQ, 2005), and providers may need to make treatment decisions based on clinical judgment. If resources for medical testing are exhausted, treatment based on physical exam, history, and clinical judgment will occur.

This movie reveals many ethical dilemmas faced unsuccessfully by the main characters. Seduced by Uganda's new leader, Idi Amin, Dr. Garrigan chooses to participate in the dictator's government and becomes his personal physician and close advisor. He witnesses murder, torture, and Amin's gradually increasing use of violence to maintain power. His personal crisis rapidly escalates as, rather than speak truth to power, Garrigan accepts gifts (such as a Mercedes-Benz), has an illicit affair with one of the dictator's wives, and becomes responsible for many deaths before he is able to escape the country thanks to the personal sacrifice of a colleague. In this way, the film exemplifies what humanitarian assistance is not, particularly in regards to understanding local health care practices; comprehending differences in values in sickness and health, cultural, and political bias; and the ethical dilemmas resulting from breaches of trust, the cruelty of war, and the crimes of genocide.

APPENDIX A:

Code of Conduct for the International Red Cross and Red Crescent Movement and NGOs in Disaster Relief Principle Commitments:

1. The Humanitarian imperative comes first.
2. Aid is given regardless of the race, creed, or nationality of the recipients and without adverse distinction of any kind. Aid priorities are calculated on the basis of need alone.
3. Aid will not be used to further a particular political or religious standpoint.
4. We shall endeavor not to act as instruments of government foreign policy.
5. We shall respect culture and custom.
6. We shall attempt to build disaster response on local capacities.
7. Ways shall be found to involve program beneficiaries in the management of relief aid.

8. Relief aid must strive to reduce future vulnerabilities to disaster as well as meeting basic needs.
9. We hold ourselves accountable for both those we seek to assist and those from whom we accept resources.
10. In our information, publicity, and advertising activities, we shall recognize disaster victims as dignified human beings, not hopeless objects.

REFERENCES

1. Beauchamp, T., and Childress, J. 2009. *Principles of biomedical ethics*, 6th ed. New York: Oxford University Press.
2. Toole, M., Waldman, R., and Zwi, A. 2006. Complex humanitarian emergencies. In M.E. Merson, R.E. Black, and A.J. Mills (Eds.), *International public health: Diseases, programs, systems, and politics*, 2nd ed. pp. 445–512. Sudbury, MA: Jones and Bartlett Publishers.
3. United Nations General Secretariat Department of Humanitarian Affairs. 1997. *Disaster management ethics: The Disaster Management Training Program* (DMTP). Retrieved from http://www.undp.org
4. *Code of Conduct for The International Red Cross and Red Crescent Movement and NGOs in Disaster Relief*. 1994. Retrieved from http://www.ifrc.org/publicat/conduct/code.asp.
5. Hunt, M. 2008. Ethics beyond borders: How health professionals experience ethics in humanitarian assistance and development work. *Developing World Bioethics* 8(2): 59–69. doi: 10.1111/j. 1471–8847.2006.00153. x.
6. Boyle, P., DuBose, E., Ellingson, S., Guinn, D., and McCurdy, D. 2001. *Organizational ethics in health care: Principles, cases, and practical solutions*. San Francisco, CA: Jossey-Bass.
7. Hogan, D., and Burstein, J. (Eds.). 2007. *Disaster medicine,* 2nd ed. Philadelphia, PA: Lippincott.
8. Bortolotti, D. 2006. *Hope in hell: Inside the world of Doctors Without Borders*. Buffalo, NY: Firefly Books.
9. United Nations General Secretariat Department of Humanitarian Affairs. 1997. *Disaster management ethics The Disaster Management Training Program* (DMTP). Retrieved from: http://www.undp.org

9

the physician's obligation to speak out against oppression: *the lives of others*

mohsen davoudi

The Lives of Others (2006). Martina Gedeck, Hauptmann Gred Wiesler, Sebastian Koch, Ulrich Tukur, Thomas Thieme. Directed by Florian Henckel von Donnersmarck. Duration: 137 minutes.

DVD Chapter 17 scene 1:23:42 to 1:24:36

S ET IN THE FORMER (EAST) German Democratic Republic, *The Lives of Others* occurs in 1984, five years before *die Wende*, German reunification and the end of Eastern European Communism. The lives of citizens are tightly controlled by the brutal state security apparatus or Stasi. At the time of its fall, the Stasi employed more than 90,000 full-time employees, along with an estimated 500,000 informants (3%–4% of the population), paid to spy on fellow citizens, co-workers, friends, and family. Captain Wiesler (Ulrich Muhe), a devoted and proud Stasi agent, has been assigned to execute a 24-hour surveillance operation targeting the nation's beloved playwright, Georg Dreyman (Sebastian Koch) and his actress girlfriend Christa-Maria Sieland (Martina Gedeck). As time goes on, he finds his own austere life dull and monotonous, compared to the colorful and vibrant intellectual and creative lives of his charges. Hence, despite discovering clear evidence pointing to their betrayal of his Communist ideals, Wiesler develops a certain respect and envy for Dreyman, Sieland, and their circle of artist friends. In the end, notwithstanding a senior Communist Party minister's persistent demands (for personal reasons) that Dreyman must go down, Wiesler, who has now clearly come to doubt his own loyalties, chooses to cover up the "treason" of his subjects, thus grievously putting himself and his career at jeopardy.

In this scene, Wiesler uses a taped interrogation session of an "enemy of Socialism" to train students aspiring to become Stasi agents. The prisoner, interrogated for helping a friend cross the Iron Curtain, is subjected to inhumane treatment, humiliation, and sleep deprivation that culminates in his tearful confession. When a student questions the inhumane interrogation techniques, Wiesler flags his name, presumably for future consequences, while justifying his behavior as defense of Socialism.

the principle

There is no human society that does not suffer from a degree of societal oppression or at least some neglect of human rights. Although this statement is not meant to equate the suffering of citizens living under authoritarian regimes or brutal military occupation with those living in nominally democratic conditions, when judged based on the civil, political, economic, social, and cultural rights envisioned in the United Nations Universal Declaration of Human Rights, we are hard-pressed to find a society that does not suffer from oppression. In the bigger picture, as citizens of the third-millennial global village, it truly hurts to think how many instances of human rights violation we are each aware of. This begs the question: As physicians, do we have a distinct social and moral obligation to speak out against societal oppression and the violation of human rights? It is a question that has had frequent and eloquent responses, but none that is widely accepted or adhered to. Rudolph Virchow called the physician "the natural attorney for the poor"[1,2] more than 100 years ago, whereas René Dubos recently submitted that "A physician worth his salt should be more than a 'body patcher'—to use Martin Luther's expression—and should be capable of dealing with all problems which affect the quality of life."[3] One would think that oppression and abrogation of human rights would certainly qualify as definitive effectors of quality of life.

So, why should we heed Paul Lowinger's call to be "healers of social as well as individual pathology?"[4] Responsibility for societal and political ills is obviously incumbent on each and every citizen. Hence, as stated in the original 1846 version of the American Medical Association (AMA) Code of Ethics, "As good citizens, it is the duty of physicians to be ever vigilant for the welfare of the community,"[5] the physician's social responsibility is basically an augmented extension of the duty of every vigilant citizen. Why augmented? Many rationales have been proposed for this. As a profession whose primary concern is the alleviation of suffering, the practitioner of medicine from ancient times was expected to heal: The inscription at the Athenian temple to Asklepios reads "These are the duties of a physician... he would be like god, savior equally of slaves, of paupers, of rich men, of princes, and to all a brother."[6] Even seen from the closed vantage point of delivery of care to patients, it can hardly be denied that an environment of oppression and injustice is a cause of disease and frustrates its cure. Patients, of course, are not isolated organisms, but people living in societies and families, and impacted by them. Additionally, physicians must empower patients as part of their therapeutic relationship, and it is not possible to fulfill this duty without opposing social and political circumstances that denigrate human rights and dignity. Hence, as Jonsen and Jameton have submitted, physicians' responsibility compels them to move beyond issues directly impacting patient care to those that are the "setting and context for society at large. It is not so much their medical knowledge, but their dedication to human good which it represents, which imposes the responsibility upon them."[1]

obstacles

In the decades since World War II, groups of physicians have bravely mobilized against war and genocide, nuclear proliferation and the spread of land mines, social and economic injustice, torture, racial discrimination and apartheid, inadequate access to health care and public sanitation, systematic and institutionalized health disparity, environmental degradation, poverty and endemic starvation, and many other forms of human rights violation. Investigators who have studied these activist movements have identified several obstacles that have diminished their efficacy and prevented their widespread acceptance. Many (if not most) physicians are politically conservative and consider activist movements as naïve, utopian, even impetuous, and irrelevant to their daily practice of medicine. This is more common in the United States; quoting Lowinger, American medicine has had a "conservative or passive attitude... toward social change."[4] To quote but one such view, Ingelfinger says that "The physician, of course, should be aware of the multiple influences that bear on health—the economic, marital, political, environmental,... but the doctor's basic responsibility is cure... his primary concern, in spite of all the utopian claims to the contrary, is sickness, not overall health."[7][i]

Many physicians have a medically focused scope of attention and are willfully ignorant of social, political, and environmental issues. As a group, they have little or no knowledge of, or experience with, activism or grassroots organizing. They have limited training in epidemiology, occupational medicine, public health, or the social sciences. And, especially in the United States, with its market-driven model of health care, they are predominantly preoccupied with their own financial circumstances.[8] Even when they do wish to speak up, society may not always be receptive, as many deplore the economic, cultural, and class differences that separate physicians from the majority of those in need of medical care.

These conditions may be slowly changing: as McCally foresees, "The health professions are in a moment of critical reflection, including renewed attention to the meaning of professionalism; debates about current systems of care; calls for response to the uninsured; inquiry into the socioeconomic determinants of health; efforts to address poverty, injustice, inequality; and a growing discussion of ecological and environmental health."[8] Recent hopeful evidence suggests that current U.S. medical students are considerably more likely to be liberal, which may bring about a change in attitudes toward social responsibility in future U.S. physicians.[9] Many, such as Rosemary Stevens (a "new public service ethos"[10]) are are advocating for a return to the paradigms of social responsibility championed by the likes of Virchow and Chadwick. Michael McCally quotes TA Brennan, heeding that "a 'civic' medical professionalism be understood as an ideology of social reform in which physicians advocate for patients as a class."[8] To reclaim their professionalism, it is argued, physicians must engage in activism and advocacy for the good of society.

what should be done?

The first question is how? The obvious response is: However one can. In the same way that physicians choose different specialties that suit their varied temperaments, the type and intensity of the activism and advocacy that each physician engages in should only be dictated by that physician's priorities and modus operandi. Each of us is a bit more or less political, emotive, analytical, energetic, brave, adventurous; the activism we choose will more likely succeed if it is in tune with these personal characteristics. The second principle, applying to all social movements, is to organize and act in a unified, organized fashion. Many nongovernmental organizations (NGOs) are primarily avenues for physicians' activism and relief efforts: to name but a few, Physicians for Human Rights (and its many chapters), International Physicians for the Prevention of Nuclear War, Médecins Sans Frontières,[ii] Physicians for Social Responsibility, Physicians for a National Health Program, and the Medical Foundation for the Care of Victims of Torture have each done immense good, with relatively limited resources. Physicians have also been important actors in organizations such as Human Rights Watch and Amnesty International. Alternately, physicians may not wish to join the existing formations, preferring to organize de novo. This, too, can be a perfectly feasible project, so long as efforts and energy are not wasted on opposing the work of others.

In the question of what to advocate for, the avenues are indeed boundless. But, for whichever cause, the physician's single most noble and prominent role must be *to bear witness*. In bearing witness, physicians identify transgressions and become the voice of the voiceless, using their platform and power to open the eyes of public consciousness.[11] This bearing witness can be directed against any and all actions, whether by governments, groups, or individuals that violate human rights and dignity. It can include revealing the atrocities of genocide, military occupation, and social exploitation, while protecting the safety and health of vulnerable populations unable to escape violent conflict; opposing war and the militarization of societies, in favor of peaceful conflict resolution and nuclear disarmament; advocacy for empowering, bottom-up aid programs to fight poverty in underdeveloped and developed nations, including working toward solutions to resolve systematic and institutionalized disparities in the distribution of wealth, health care, nutrition, and sanitation; fighting child labor and other exploitative labor practices; looking for, detecting, documenting, and prosecuting the egregious crime of torture, while categorically rejecting all excuses for torture and inhumane treatment of prisoners, whether with Landauesque pseudo-justifications or the use of jingoistic patriotism and national security excuses; educating the public about environmental destruction and its role in perpetuating repeated "natural" disasters and endemic poverty; incorporation of social responsibility and human rights protection in the curricula of medical schools worldwide; advocating for the fundamental "universal right to the highest attainable standard of health"; and taking leadership against all forms of discrimination, whether by race, ethnicity, caste, gender, religion, sexual orientation, or disease state.

While advocating against social depredations and abrogation of human rights, it is obviously incumbent upon physicians to keep their house in order. This has two components: unanimous and unflinching commitment to the worldwide protection of physicians who stand up for these ideals and are themselves subjected to intimidation and punitive actions,[12] and the prevention of medicine and medical personnel from themselves becoming instruments of oppression. Thus, physicians must not allow medical justifications to be used to protect deposed tyrants from justice for their heinous crimes, in what has been aptly called "Pinochet syndrome"; they should vehemently oppose the use of "missionary medicine" for religious and ideological coercion and proselytization; they must forcefully act against the medicalization of human rights violations (such as the use of psychiatric diagnoses to confine, drug, and torture political dissidents and other suspects) or any other usage of medicine or the medical sciences as instruments of social control; they must staunchly resist all violations of medical neutrality in conflicts. Physicians must condemn the participation or even presence of medical personnel during the administration of capital punishment. And, most importantly, physicians and medical organizations should act forcefully and with a unified voice against any physician or health care provider who participates, however tangentially, in what Sussman has rightfully called the most profoundly barbaric and inhumane act, torture.[13]

The most cardinal Nuremberg ethic, that individuals, whether physicians or not, cannot refrain from personal accountability for crimes against humanity by claiming to have just followed orders, laws, or any other form of state authority, even under the guise of national security or military necessity, must not be forgotten. "The standing of the entire profession suffers when physicians act as agents of the state to destroy life and health."[14] Regrettably, the World Medical Association (WMA), despite its many "lofty 'ethical' statements," has refused to exercise "any authority to identify, monitor, or punish either physicians or medical societies who violate its ethical principles."[14] This has been evident in the affair of notorious Nazi physician Sewering, as well as in the WMA's refusal to take a stand against apartheid in South Africa or respond effectively to evidence of physician participation in torture and gross human rights violations across the globe, from China, to the United States, the USSR, Israel, India, Latin America, and the Middle East.[15] It is in this setting that Grodin and others have suggested the creation of an "International Medical Tribunal," to act as a form of "Permanent Nuremberg Court." The author concurs with their conclusion that this "can be both a symbolic and practical act that can help prevent governmental subversion of medical skills and authority, and thus help foster human rights."[14]

Going back to Germany, where the movie takes place, Martin Neimoller's famous poem of regret comes to mind, in which he subtly accepts his guilt for the crime of apathy to the suffering of communists, trade-unionists, Jews, and many others subjected to the Nazis' genocidal atrocities. It drives home the principle that injustice and oppression refuse to be confined to one group or locale, making it not only a moral imperative to fight it, but a matter of self-preservation, of ensuring one's own survival. Or else we may find ourselves wistfully lamenting that "then they came for me—and there was no one left to speak out for me."

NOTES

i. This view, in the author's opinion, ignores the profound impact of seemingly symbolic acts that bear witness to the immense social injustices that surround us. This brings to mind "dramatic gestures of protest such as Jack Geiger writing prescriptions of food for his undernourished welfare patients."[1]

ii. The first three organizations are Nobel Peace Prize laureates.

REFERENCES

1. Jonsen, A.R., and Jameton, A.L. 1977. Social and political responsibilities of physicians. *Journal of Medical Philosophy* 2(4): 376–400.
2. Geiger, J. 1971. Hidden professional roles: The physician as reactionary, reformer, revolutionary. *Social Policy* 1: 24–33.
3. Dubos, R. 1976-1977. The despairing optimist. *American Scholar* 46: 11–17.
4. Lowinger, P. 1968. The doctor as political activist. *American Journal of Psychotherapy* 22: 616–625.
5. Jecker, N.S. 2001. Dividing loyalties: Caring for individuals and populations. *Yale Journal of Health Policy, Law, and Ethics* 1: 177–186.
6. Bailey, J.E. 1996. Asklepios: Ancient hero of medical caring. *Annals of Internal Medicine* 124: 257–263.
7. Ingelfinger, J. 1976. The physician's contribution to the health system. *New England Journal of Medicine* 295(10): 565–566.
8. McCally, M. 2002. Medical activism and environmental health. *Annals of the American Academy of Political and Social Science* 584: 145–158.
9. Frank, E., Carrerra, J., and Dharamsi, S. 2007. Political self-characterization of U.S. medical students. *Journal of General Internal Medicine* 22: 514–517.
10. Stevens, R.A. 2001. Public roles for the medical profession in the United States: Beyond theories of decline and fall. *Millbank Quarterly* 79(3). Retrieved February 24, 2010 from http://www.milbank.org/quarterly/7903feat.html
11. Orbinski, J., Beyrer, C., and Singh, S. 2007. Violations of human rights: Health practitioners as witnesses. *Lancet* 370: 698–704.
12. Corillon, C. 1989. The role of science and scientists in human rights. *Annals of the American Academy of Political and Social Sciences* 506: 129–140.
13. Sussman, D. 2005. What's wrong with torture? *Philosophy and Public Affairs* 33(1): 1–33.
14. Grodin, M.A., Annas, G.J., and Glantz, L.H. 1993. Medicine and human rights: A proposal for international action. *Hastings Center Report* 23(4): 8–12.
15. Yudkin, J.S. 2009. The Israeli Medical Association and doctors' complicity in torture. *British Medical Journal* 339: b4078.

conflicts of consultation: *red beard*

karma lekshe tsomo

Red Beard (1965). Toshimo Nifune, Yuzo Kayama. Directed by
Akira Kurasawa. Duration: 185 minutes.

Scene: chapter 21 Scene 01:41:14 to 01:42:12

IN *RED BEARD*, DIRECTOR AKIRA KUROSAWA turns his signature existential lens on a dilapidated clinic for the destitute in Tokugawa-era Japan. Focusing on the tragedies that befall the patients and staff, his camera unflinchingly observes the flawed nobility of human character. The stark portraits of the clinic's patients and medical staff wordlessly reveal the political and economic roots of social injustice. As the taciturn director of the clinic stalwartly devotes himself to caring for the indigent, he models kindness and dedication to his often ambivalent staff. His work is framed and frustrated by the interconnections between politics and patient care: poverty, illiteracy, government indifference, and a desperate lack of tools for his trade. Far more than a political statement, however, the film exposes the hearts of human beings at their most vulnerable moments: illness and death.

The film opens with the arrival of Noboru Yasumoto (Yuzo Kayama) at Koishikawa Public Clinic in Edo. A green and cheeky young medical graduate, he has just completed his medical training in Nagasaki, then Japan's port of entry for the latest in Western technology. Appalled by the desperate poverty of the clinic and its patients, he initially refuses to comply with the clinic's regulations or to share his potentially life-saving knowledge. The clinic's gruff, intrepid, and compassionate director, Dr. Kyojo Niide (Toshiro Mifune), addressed publicly as *Sensei* (teacher) and covertly as Red Beard, trains him through a series of trials. As he gains insight into the tragic lives of his patients, Yasumoto is gradually transformed from haughty courtier to humble, caring clinician. His arrogance gradually crumbles as he begins to recognize his own inexperience, ignorance, and vulnerability, and develops empathy for the sufferings of the poor.

In the course of Yasumoto's training, a series of human dramas unfolds. First, he barely escapes becoming the latest victim of the "Mantis," a beautiful psychopath who seduces and then devours her prey. This close brush with death betrays Yasumoto's impudence in imagining that he can cure her when others have failed and teaches him the compelling and potentially destructive power of desire, as he is magnetically drawn in by her allure and helplessness. Next, Yasumoto's weakness and naivete are unmasked as he reels under the torment of a woman having her intestines sewn back into her body. As the arrogance of power and privilege are shattered by repeated encounters with unimaginable suffering, a noble new character dawns.

Like much of Kurosawa's work, *Red Beard* is replete with Buddhist allusions and values. The first noble truth of suffering and dissatisfaction is vividly portrayed, both in the patient's physical maladies and in the wretchedness of their tragic lives. The immutable law of cause and effect is illustrated through the consequences of ignorance, attachment, and aversion in the lives of the film's rich cast of characters. The preciousness of human life and the potential for awakening are poignantly expressed in the story of the young physician, who, through a series of humiliations, gains insight into his own weakness and shallowness of character and develops the wisdom to see things "as they are," rather than distorted by self-interest. The film reminds us that pain and ignorance are not just something from a by-gone era, but salient characteristics of the human condition.

The ethical dilemmas represented throughout the film point to the interplay between circumstances and ethical agency. To what extent are human beings individually responsible for their lives, and to what extent are they buffeted by social and political circumstances? What happens when moral obligations collide? How are the concepts of right and wrong affected by human emotion and overshadowed by the inevitability of death?

In the film, Red Beard instructs Yasumoto to examine Rokusake, a skilled gold-lacquer craftsman who lies dying a solitary and agonizing death. As Yasumoto warily observes the man's last gasps, he is forced to confront the stark reality of death. The mystery of Rokusake's lonely life unfolds when his long-estranged daughter arrives at the clinic with her three hungry children. Distraught and too late to make amends, she divulges a horror story of ruthless betrayal by her mother and also her husband. Tortured by remorse at her own callous rejection of her father's love, she plaintively asks, "Was he in pain when he died?" Instead of recounting her father's agony, Red Beard assures her, "No, he died peacefully." Satisfied with the lie that startles Yasumoto, the distraught woman at last breathes a relieved sigh.

The scene raises questions of right speech and right intention in relationships between care providers and patients. To say that the woman's father died a peaceful death was patently untrue, yet the deceit allowed the woman to cast off the burden of guilt that she carried along with her three starving children. The psychological burden she carries from years of abuse, shame, and deception are momentarily lifted.

Is Red Beard's misrepresentation justified? In Japan, as in most societies influenced by Buddhism, truthful speech is a core ethical principle. Physicians and medical staff especially, being charged with life-and-death decision making, are expected to be honest and trustworthy. How can we feel confident about the safety of ourselves and our loved ones if those responsible for our welfare cannot be trusted? Honesty is fundamental even for ordinary decent folk. Naturally, medical professionals, being held to a higher standard, are expected to be straightforward and truthful. What if every physician misrepresented the circumstances of his patients' deaths?

Compassion is another core ethical principal in societies influenced by Buddhism. Conceived as the wish to free all beings from suffering, compassion becomes an overarching value in Mahayana Buddhist tradition. In accordance with the great compassion of the *bodhisattva* ideal, one is urged to sacrifice one's own welfare to relieve the sufferings of others. According to legend, in a past life as a *bodhisattva*, the Buddha sacrificed his own flesh to nourish a starving tigress and her cubs. A *bodhisattva* might even go as far as to sacrifice his or her own life for the benefit of humanity.

Honesty and compassion are regarded as compatible values, since speaking and acting with honesty and kindness generally ensure positive human relationships. However, there are times when truthfulness and compassion may collide. In the example above, sacrificing one's life for the benefit of another is certainly a compassionate act, but the act of sacrificing one's life is also the taking of a life, which transgresses the Buddhist principle of non-harm. In everyday life, and particularly in patient care, moral dilemmas like these are not easily resolved. They must be mediated by the wisdom to discern what is ultimately beneficial and harmful, and the skillful means to implement that wisdom.

Gradually, Yasumoto becomes aware that Red Beard not only examines and treats the physical bodies of his patients, but intuits the complex of emotions they are grappling with as well. Subtler than thoughts, emotions reveal life lessons that have been learned and ignored. Discerning the hopelessness and sense of failure that torture Rokusake's daughter, Red Beard respects her sincere grief and desire for atonement. He listens to her pathos with his heart and reflects back the honesty of her heart. Dispelling his authoritarian image, he emanates the spirit of Kwannon, *bodhisattva* of compassion, who graces countless Japanese Buddhist shrines and brings hope to so many. His compassion is not sentimental or heroic, but humble, even bumbling, and direct: "We can only try to alleviate pain and ignorance and cover up what we do not know." He knows that blackmailing the magistrate is perfidy, but he consciously perjures himself to spare the woman and her children: "From today on, if I'm arrogant, remind me."

When is it allowable to transgress one ethical principle for another? Is it humanly possible to maintain absolute ethical purity? By what standard can ethical values be judged, and who determines which standard applies in varying cultural contexts? Even if certain ethical norms are regarded as universal, what recourse is there when others do not honor these norms?

Ultimately, say the Buddhists, each of us must weigh our own actions and take responsibility for them. To act with honesty and compassion in the world is in our own best interests. If, in our own best assessment of a situation, compassion trumps honesty, that is our judgment to make. The law of cause and effect continues to operate as a natural working principle of the universe, however; it is not blithely overruled by our good intentions. If human kindness compels us to sacrifice one moral value for another, we must take responsibility for our decision and be bold enough to accept the consequences. Even taken at face value, as the episode of Rokusake's daughter demonstrates, standard moralistic judgments may prove utterly inadequate, in that they ignore entire chapters of a human being's experience. When simplistic moral prescriptions fail us, we must act nonetheless and be honest in assessing whether our motivation is purely to benefit others or contaminated by deceit and self-interest.

In the larger social and political schema, configurations of action and responsibility are not simple and straightforward. Especially given the complexities and disparities of contemporary global society, we uncritically presume the moral values of others at our own peril. No unitary moral code is adequate today; life has become too complex and human beings are too uniquely varied. Between the complex new technologies and diverse cultures present in our hospital wards, the terms for negotiating mortally important medical decisions have become endlessly complicated and multivalent. Some general moral guidelines are needed, but derived from where, incumbent upon whom, and enforced by what authority?

As *Red Beard* reveals, death is human beings' common denominator—the opportunity of a lifetime that none can refuse. Death is the moment of truth of each person's life, not simply in a metaphorical sense, but literally, as the measure of all our actions. It is the subtext in the relationship between physicians and patients, nurses and families, mentors and trainees. Death is the specter that unites the admirers of Shahachi, the selfless character who labors to expiate his imagined sins, to exclaim: "He's a man from the Buddha. He cannot die." But, in the end, he does. Through the lens of death, our wholesome and unwholesome thoughts, words, and deeds come into focus. Indeed, life is cruel enough as it is. Perhaps listening to the dying is humanity's most effective moral compass.

REFERENCES

1. Cleary, T. 2009. *Samurai wisdom: Lessons from Japan's warrior culture*. North Clarendon, VT: Tuttle Publishing.
2. Coberly, M. 2003. *Sacred passage: How to provide fearless, compassionate care for the dying*. Boston: Shambhala.
3. Cowie, P. 2010. *Akira Kurosawa: Master of cinema*. New York: Rizzoli.
4. Harvey, P. 2000. *An introduction to Buddhist ethics: Foundations, values and issues*. Cambridge: Cambridge University Press.
5. Kurosawa, Akira. 1983. *Something like an autobiography*. New York, NY: Vintage.
6. Dali Lama. 2001. *Ethics for the new millennium*. New York: Riverhead Books.
7. Lief, J.L. 2001. *Making friends with death: A Buddhist guide to encountering mortality*. Boston: Shambhala.
8. Richie, D. 1999. *The films of Akira Kurosawa*. Berkeley: University of California Press.
9. Suzuki, S. 2006. *Zen mind, beginner's mind*. Boston: Shambhala.
10. Tsomo, K.L. 2006. *Into the jaws of Yama, lord of death: Buddhism, bioethics, and death*. Albany, NY: State University of New York Press.

part six

rights, responsibilities, and research

rights to access health care: *article 99*

lawrence mohr

Article 99 (1999). Ray Liotta, Kiefer Sutherland, Forest Whitaker, Lea Thompson, John Mahoney, Troy Evans, Keith David. Directed by Howard Deutch. Duration: 100 minutes.

DVD Chapter 1, Scene 00:04:17 to 00:05:16

ARTICLE 99 TELLS THE STORY of veterans at a fictitious government veteran's hospital unable to receive needed medical care because of funding cutbacks and an arcane, bureaucratic regulation known as "Article 99." This made-for-the-movies regulation states that, even though a veteran is eligible for "full medical benefits," treatment for certain medical problems cannot be provided "as the diagnosed condition cannot be specifically related to military service." The contradictory illogic of this regulation creates confusion, frustration, and anger among the veterans seeking care, as well as the dedicated medical staff who violate hospital policy to ensure that the veterans receive the care. Dr. Henry Dreyfoos' (John Mahoney) nefarious actions heighten their anger. Dr. Dreyfoos, an ambitious and ruthless hospital administrator, uses "Article 99" as the rationale for prohibiting costly medical procedures in a self-serving effort to cast the hospital's "bottom line" in a favorable light to his superiors in Washington.

The movie begins with a Korean War veteran, Pat Travis (Troy Evans), leaving his farm and traveling to the veteran's hospital for triple-bypass open-heart surgery. As he bids farewell to his wife, with military discharge papers in hand, he confidently tells her "don't worry about anything, Uncle Sam's gonna take care of me just fine." However, upon arriving at the hospital, he finds a chaotic scene in the admitting area, with long lines of frustrated, boisterous veterans attempting to receive medical care. He witnesses one veteran, whose records were lost by the hospital eight months before, being told by a clerk that "without certification we have no actual proof that you are disabled." The veteran explodes with rage, removes his prosthetic leg and repeatedly slams it on the desk while shouting, "You want proof, here's the god-damned proof right here." Travis is jostled in the ensuing chaos and staggers into the presence of Luther Jerome (Keith David), a wheelchair-bound Vietnam veteran, who is the hospital's chief "rabble-rouser" and "hustler." The stunned Travis asks Jerome, "What the hell is going on here Luther?" Jerome tells Travis that "this is the VA, soldier," and informs him that "whatever you need you ain't gonna get." Travis exclaims that "I need a triple bypass." Jerome laughs and responds by saying, "Forget it unless you got a Congressman in your pocket; otherwise the only thing gonna be bypassed around here is you."

These opening scenes set the stage for the rest of the movie, in which veterans and a group of committed doctors take matters into their own hands, break the illogical and oppressive rules established by Dr. Dreyfoos, and do all they can with limited resources. Dr. Richard Sturgess (Ray Liotta), an accomplished, irreverent, and savvy surgeon, leads the rebellious doctors in this effort. We are first introduced to Dr. Sturgess and his team when they perform life-saving open-heart surgery on a patient only authorized to receive prostate surgery. When questioned about the propriety of this unauthorized procedure by an intern, Dr. Sturgess tells his team "Look, we're here, he's here; why don't we make the most of this?" They then proceed with the unauthorized open-heart operation and save the patient's life. When Dr. Dreyfoos becomes aware of the fact that unofficial open-heart operations are being performed, he goes on a personal crusade to clamp down on these procedures and punish the doctors involved. The situation becomes dire as a result of the Dreyfoos vendetta. The doctors respond by stealing valuable medical supplies from a well-funded animal research laboratory in order to continue the unauthorized procedures.

The plot of *Article 99* illustrates the conflict that physicians and other health care providers experience when bureaucratic obstacles prevent them from providing the care that patients need. It is widely believed by physicians and bioethicists that such obstacles are intrinsically unethical: Physicians have a responsibility to advocate for their patients and provide the best care that they can in spite of obstacles. The roots of this ethical construct can be found in the ancient writings of Hippocrates. In *Aphorisms*, Hippocrates states that "the physician must not only do what is right himself, but also to make the patient, the attendants, and externals cooperate."[1] That is, physicians have the responsibility to advocate for patients and remove obstacles to care by making others cooperate. This implies that the physician should take whatever actions are necessary to make sure that their patients receive the care they need. This fundamental ethical principle has withstood the test of time for more than twenty-four centuries. At present, it is clearly embodied in the American Medical Association's Council on Ethical and Judicial Affairs statement, which declares that physicians "must remain primarily dedicated to the health care needs of their patients" and that "regardless of any allocation guidelines or gatekeeper directives, physicians must advocate for any care they believe will materially benefit their patients."[2] Support for this position can be found in the writings of two prominent medical ethicists, Norman Levinsky and Edmund Pellegrino. Levinsky writes that physicians have a responsibility to assertively advocate for their patients "without regard to costs or other social obligations."[3] Pellegrino writes, "When conflicts or doubts arise, the physician's first responsibility is to the genuine needs and welfare of his or her patients—not the system, the plan, or its other members."[4]

The responsibility of physicians to advocate for their patients and take whatever actions are necessary to provide the care they need is dramatically illustrated as *Article 99* continues. The doctors must "turf" patients from one service to another to prevent them from being discharged before they receive the medical care they need. In the process, strong personal bonds develop between patients and the doctors who care for them. Dr. Peter Morgan (Kiefer Sutherland), a new intern, befriends a plain-spoken, World War II veteran named Sam Abrams (Eli Wallach), who instructs him in the finer points of "turfing" tactics. The intern is visibly moved when he incidentally discovers the Silver Star medal that this frail, elderly patient was awarded for heroism on D-Day. This poignant personal relationship strengthens Dr. Morgan's resolve to do all that he can to provide necessary medical procedures to the veterans under their care, in spite of the obstacles created by Dreyfoos. Shortly thereafter, Dr. Sturgess is identified as the ringleader of the group of surgeons who have been stealing surgical supplies in order to operate on their patients. A gloating Dreyfoos demands that Sturgess place himself on "voluntary suspension" pending a hearing of the medical review board. Dr. Morgan is appalled by Dreyfoos' decision and breaks into his office to obtain the surveillance camera video tape used to identify Sturgess. Dreyfoos finds Dr. Morgan in his office; the intern is also suspended after he confronts Dreyfoos with his disgust and walks out his office with the video tape that was used to identify Sturgess. As Morgan leaves the office, Dreyfoos threatens that he will never do anything significant in medicine. Morgan replies by saying, "There's always your job, sir."

In *Article 99*, Drs. Sturgess and Morgan demonstrate extraordinary courage in risking their medical careers to overcome the obstacles created by Dreyfoos. However, even though physicians have an ethical responsibility to do what they can to provide medical care to their patients, this does not necessarily imply that all individuals have a *right* to receive the medical care that they need. These are, indeed, two different, and often conflicting, ethical propositions. This ethical conflict is illustrated in the plot of *Article 99*. Throughout recorded history, the question of whether or not individuals have a right to receive health care has been addressed and debated through a complex mixture of religious doctrine, political thought, government laws, economic considerations, social theory, and ethical philosophy. There is no single unifying principle or definitive document that provides a generalized, universally accepted answer to this question. To this day, it is largely a matter of individual opinion based upon a conglomeration of individual beliefs. This has led to disparate views of varying intensity among individuals of different religions, political views, legal opinions, socioeconomic status, and ethical perspectives. Thus, the issue of whether access to health care is a right or a privilege is a complex proposition, with fervent arguments on each side of the issue. These arguments are summarized in the paragraphs that follow, since I think that a basic understanding of these arguments is necessary to appreciate their relevance to the plot of *Article 99*.

In my experience, most physicians and many nonphysicians would assert that access to health care is a fundamental human right, simply because it is the "right thing" to do. In Western civilizations, this common moral judgment has its roots in the Judeo-Christian religious beliefs that every human life is a sacred gift from God and human beings should "love thy neighbor as thyself." These beliefs are the foundation of the landmark *Pastoral Letter on Health and Health Care* published by the Roman Catholic bishops of the United States. This pastoral letter states: "Every person has a basic right to health care. This right flows from the sanctity of human life and the dignity that belongs to all human persons, who are made in the image of God."[5] Similar beliefs have been incorporated into secular thought through the philosophic writings of Immanuel Kant and Thomas Hobbes. Kant argued that all human beings have absolute worth simply because they exist and that one should "act in such a way that you always treat humanity whether in your own person or in the person of any other, never simply as a means, but at the same time as an end."[6] Hobbes thought that there are "Laws of Nature" that allow human beings to ascertain their obligations to each other through reason, including the obligation to preserve life.[7] Over the years, the widespread teaching of these religious and philosophical beliefs has led to a commonly held altruistic view that one person's need for health care requires others in society to help, and that the moral obligation to help overrides individual self-interest. As stated by Dr. Edmund Pellegrino, "A medical need in itself constitutes a moral claim on those equipped to help."[8]

On the other hand, arguments exist for the proposition that access to health care is a privilege and not a fundamental right. Such arguments are largely based upon the premise that the need for health care is no different from the need for other goods and services that are necessary to sustain human life.[9] Robert Sade clearly illustrates the practical dimensions of this premise: "No one can have a positive right, that is, an entitlement, to the efforts of those who provide health care services any more than they have an entitlement to the products and services of farmers and grocers to satisfy their need for food or of architects and builders to satisfy their need for shelter."[10] Leonard Peikoff states that "you have no right to the actions or products of others except on terms to which they voluntarily agree… nobody has the right to the services of any professional individual or group simply because he wants them and desperately needs them."[11] According to this line of thought, access to heath care requires an agreement or contract between a provider of health care and an individual who wishes to receive it. From an ethical perspective, proponents of this viewpoint believe that the only right to access health care is the right of an individual to enter into such an agreement and receive the promised services without the interference of other individuals or the government. They believe that there is no inherent ethical responsibility for a physician to provide health care to individuals with whom they have not established a doctor–patient relationship.

This is the Libertarian principle of *autonomy*. Its proponents believe that individuals are responsible for their own lives and should have the freedom to meet their own needs in accordance with their resources and their own judgment. In advancing this argument Peikoff states: "Observe that all legitimate rights have one thing in common: they are rights to action, not to rewards from other people."[11] In this worldview, the role of government should be restricted to protecting the freedom of individuals to take legally sanctioned actions that are necessary to meet their needs, to providing a legal framework for enforcing contracts and to establishing procedures for the resolution of disputes among parties who have entered into contracts.[10] This implies that government also has a responsibility to protect the freedom of an individual physician to satisfy his or her personal need to provide medical care to the poor and destitute as an act of charity. However, Libertarians argue that "voluntary charity, not government-enforced charity must answer to the moral claims of the needy."[12]

As *Article 99* continues, Drs. Sturgess and Morgan decide to return to the hospital and resume the unauthorized operations in spite of the fact that they have been suspended. Upon their return, they find that the hospitalized veterans have become increasingly angry about the actions and policies of Dr. Dreyfoos. The anger eventually reaches the "boiling point" and, under the leadership of Luther Jerome, the veterans go on a rampage and take over the hospital in order to allow the suspended surgeons to continue the unauthorized operations. The hospital siege also attracts the attention of the media, which gives extensive coverage to the plight of the hospitalized veterans. Although the veterans appear to act impulsively, the ethical basis for taking over the hospital is clear. The action they take is an expression of their strong belief that, as a result of their military service and wartime injuries, a contract exists between the government and the veterans for the Department of Veterans Affairs to provide the health care that the veterans need. Indeed, the storyline of *Article 99* is based upon the premise that the hospitalized veterans have *earned the privilege* to receive government-provided health care and that the self-serving policies of Dreyfoos have created an unethical obstacle to receiving the health care that the government has promised to provide. Thus, in taking over the hospital, the veterans are exercising their right to take action in accordance with the Libertarian principle of autonomy.

As the movie concludes, Dr. Sturgess convinces Luther Jerome to call off the siege while Dr. Morgan performs an emergency triple-bypass surgery on Pat Travis in a desperate attempt to save his life. With the siege ended, an experienced and empathetic Inspector General enters the hospital and quickly becomes aware of the abhorrent situation that Dreyfoos has created at the hospital. Dreyfoos is fired on the spot, Drs. Sturgess and Morgan are reinstated, Luther Jerome is cheered as a hero by fellow veterans, and Pat Travis survives as a result of the triple-bypass operation he received during the siege. Travis did not survive because Uncle Sam took care of him, as he expected when he first travelled to the hospital. He survived because his doctors acted courageously in providing him with the care he needed in spite of the obstacles created by Dreyfoos and because his fellow veterans exercised their right of autonomy in taking action to ensure that he received the health care he had the privilege to receive as a result of his military service. These are the ethical lessons of *Article 99*.

REFERENCES

1. Hippocrates. 1956. Aphorisms, Section I. In M.J. Adler, and W. Brockway (Eds.), *Hippocratic Writings*, p. 131. In R.M. Hutchins (Editor-in-chief), *Great books of the western world*, Volume 10. Chicago: University of Chicago Press.

2. American Medical Association, Council on Ethical and Judicial Affairs. 1995. Ethical issues in managed care. *Journal of the American Medical Association* 273: 330–335.

3. Levinsky, N. 1984. The doctor's master. *New England Journal of Medicine* 311: 1573–1575.

4. Pellegrino, E.D. 1995. Interests, obligations, and justice: Some notes toward an ethic of managed care. *Journal of Clinical Ethics* 6: 312–317.

5. Pastoral letter on health and healthcare. 1981. *Origins* XI: 396–402.

6. Arrington, R.L. 1998. Kant. In R.L. Arrington (Ed.), *Western ethics*, pp. 261–294. Malden, MA: Blackwell Publishers.

7. Hobbes, T. 1996. In R. Tuck (Ed.) *Leviathan*, Chapter XIV, pp. 91–100. Cambridge: Cambridge University Press.

8. Pellegrino, E.D. 1987. Altruism, self-interest, and medical ethics. *Journal of the American Medical Association* 258: 1939–1940.

9. Kelly, D. 1998. *A life of one's own: Individual rights and the welfare state*, pp. 83-90. Washington, DC: Cato Institute.

10. Sade, R.M. 2007. Ethical foundations of health care system reform. *Annals of Thoracic Surgery* 84: 1429–1431.

11. Peikoff, L. December 11, 1993. *Health care is not a right*. Manuscript of a speech delivered at a Town Hall Meeting on the Clinton Health Plan, Costa Mesa, California. Retrieved October 6, 2009 from http://www.bdt.com/pages/Peikoff.html

12. Friesen, T. 2001. The right to health care. *Health Law Journal* 9: 205–222.

2

rights to health care information:
and the band played on

jennifer s. bard

And the Band Played On (1993). Matthew Modine, Alan Alda, Patrick Bauchau, Nathalie Baye, Phil Collins, Richard Gere, Glenne Headly, Anjelica Huston, Saul Rubinek, Steve Martin. Directed by Roger Spottiswoode. Duration: 141 minutes.

DVD chapter 18 Scene 00.51.47 to chapter 19 scene 00:54:53

A ND THE BAND PLAYED ON[1] is a 1993 made-for-television movie based on the 1987 book, *And the Band Played On: Politics, People, and the AIDS Epidemic* by Randy Shilts.[2] Not only does the story of the early days of AIDS in the United States serve as a warning about how easily values of justice and compassion can be put aside in the face of fear, but it is also important to understand how infectious disease in general "got left out of bioethics" because, until the coming of AIDS, it was seen as no longer a threat.[3] In chronicling the start of the last great epidemic, this movie presents an opportunity to reshape bioethics, so that we are better both medically and ethically to address the emerging, and reemerging, infectious threats that are sure to come.

The movie, like the book, represents itself as a nonfictional account of the history of the AIDS epidemic in the United States, from the first awareness of clusters of cases of inexplicable immunodeficiency in young homosexual men in 1981 until the early 1990s when HIV/AIDS[4] had become a terrifying fact of life in the United States. It does so by telling the story from the perspective of Don Francis, an epidemiologist of the Centers for Disease Control (CDC), who was in fact one of the first people assigned to track down the source of the new epidemic. The movie is structured around the experiences of Francis, his colleagues at the CDC, and the public health officials in cities such as San Francisco and New York, with whom he joined to first identify and then try to contain the epidemic.

Watching events unfold, the scenes demonstrate that, despite rising death tolls, societal, and by extension political, prejudice against homosexuals made it impossible to marshal the resources needed to study and fund the disease until it started affecting "innocent victims," such as babies born with HIV and hemophiliacs infected through use of clotting factor made from the blood of hundreds of donors. It starkly presents the concept of the "innocent" versus "noninnocent" victim that so often marks the outbreak of any new disease and which, in the case of AIDS, still lingers. As the epidemic spreads throughout the country, so does the story as Francis and his team become active participants in private meetings and public hearings to combat the disease. With the benefit of hindsight, it is frustrating to see resistance to taking steps that might have slowed its spread. Residents of the Castro in San Francisco, still remembering the assassination of activist Harvey Milk, believed that the infection was being used as an excuse to close the bathhouses where men often had sex with multiple partners. It is almost impossible for those who did not live through those times to understand the secrecy and shame with which most homosexuals outside of the Castro in San Francisco, California, led their lives and therefore how valuable that neighborhood was as a refuge.

Even more horrifying than frustrating, the blood industry refused to use the first tests that could detect the virus. Concerned both that the test had too great a false-positive rate, which would require them to discard substantial amounts of donated blood, and that any publicity about possible infection through the blood supply would result in lowered demand, the industry decided to do nothing and let the virus spread freely. The movie demonstrates the fear and discrimination that accompanied an AIDS diagnosis. As the CDC investigators conduct interviews in San Francisco, the movie documents the horror of a wealthy young couple who must learn from them that the wasting disease suffered by the wife is actually AIDS acquired in a blood transfusion. The husband collapses as he hears what is effectively a death sentence. In another scene, the brother of a recently deceased wealthy San Francisco bachelor resists the efforts of CDC doctors who want to trace his contacts, a reminder that in the late 1980s the stigma of being a homosexual was far greater than that of being sick. Yet, as the disease spread with little understanding of how it was transmitted and no effective means of combating it, those diagnosed began to face severe discrimination if not ostracism. People with AIDS were literally untouchable. The power of the actual news footage of celebrities such as Prince Diana or Michael Jackson hugging people diagnosed with AIDS is lost without an understanding of the depth of that fear and discrimination.

It is because of this discrimination against those diagnosed with AIDS that people became aware of a need for stronger laws to protect patient privacy. Writing in 1995, Dr. Molly Cook reminds us of the realities of that time, noting that it was understandable when patients did not want their HIV status noted in their charts;

> It is true that individuals can lose both their employment and their insurance if their HIV status becomes known. In addition, some insurers specifically exclude HIV from coverage, or severely cap benefits for HIV infection, functionally depriving individuals of coverage to which they are entitled by virtue of having paid premiums, and to which other individuals with diseases of similar prognosis continues to have access.[5]

These AIDS-specific laws are a thing of the past, but the concern about medical privacy remains. The Health Insurance Portability and Accountability Act of 1996 (HIPAA)[6] was a direct outcome of a new awareness of the need to keep health information private. Heralding the implementation of the law, then Secretary of

Health and Human Services (HHS) Tommy Thompson stated, "Today, I am pleased to announce that the President is taking a bold and definitive step to protect the rights of citizens to keep their medical records confidential."[7] Today, while the seemingly endless paperwork and often petty rule-making of HIPAA have permeated the health care industry, its message that patients own their own health information has not. Although the law is clear that, on request, patients must receive "a copy of your health records" and "to have corrections added to your health information"[8] recent reports indicate that patients in the hospital still find it very difficult to see their own charts. Ironically, health care workers often justify this by reference to HIPAA's confidentiality requirements. Reports of patients told that they must file a written request and wait to receive copies of a chart hanging at their own bedside seem a deliberate violation of the law's letter and spirit.

Yet, the government's refusal to acknowledge or address the epidemic overshadowed both public response and the obstinacy of the blood industry. The movie raises issues of political ethics and historical revisionism that challenges what has become an increasingly hagiographic memory of Ronald Reagan as not just universally beloved but an example of compassion combined with fiscal conservatism. In a 2004 interview, Don Francis confirms that many of the dramatic events portrayed are quite true and that he did indeed "pound the table" and shout in frustration at the complete lack of interest the Reagan administration had in recognizing, let alone providing the funds to combat, the disease.[9] Looking back, Francis says, "I despise Ronald Reagan and the people around him for what they did to public health in the United States and the rest of the world.... I don't know what was going on in their minds to obstruct our efforts to protect the public's health, but they did, and have been hardly held accountable for that.... In the end, their more than impassive inaction and their active obstruction of actions that were necessary, allowed HIV to get a firmer hold around the world and had to be the result of millions of deaths in the long run."[10]

The movie, inevitably, reflects only what was known at the time. But its presentation of theories that have now been discredited, such as that AIDS was brought to the United States by a French-Canadian flight attendant, the so-called "Patient Zero,"[11] are instructive lessons in the dangers of jumping to early conclusions. Both in recreating the history of an epidemic and in challenging what has become conventional wisdom, the movie functions as an essential teaching tool now that there are at least two generations of Americans with absolutely no memory of a time without AIDS. Today, when we understand exactly how to prevent the transmission of AIDS, including how to treat these patients without personal risk to health care professionals, and when, even more significantly, we have drugs that can often convert it into a manageable chronic condition rather than a death sentence, it is easy to forget the initial shock and the instinct to lash out against and disassociate ourselves from the victims of a disease that came out of nowhere and killed everyone who contracted it.

Despite their powerlessness against the virus, the movie portrays medical doctors as caring healers who express deep compassion for the suffering of their patients. Since clinical care is not, however, at the core of the movie's interest, very little details the realities of those times, including the extent to which care of those patients challenged the paradigms of medicine in an era which believed it had conquered infectious disease. Perhaps the best supplement to this movie in teaching about those days is Dr. Kate Scannell's *Death of the Good Doctor*, a collection of her beautifully written essays about how, as a young doctor, she was put in the completely unfamiliar situation of presiding over young men dying of a disease that defied any available medical intervention.[12]

The movie ends on what we now know is an unduly positive note. By 1993, many of the battles to prevent the spread of AIDS in the United States seemed to have been won. The gay community itself organized around the crises and became very effective in educating people about prevention, causing a significant drop in new diagnoses. The AIDS crisis also if not created then perfected the phenomena of grassroots lobbying for medical research, which has now been widely adopted. Moreover, although treatment was still in its early stages, the success in identifying the virus, the scenes showing the less than heroic in-fighting between the Pasteur Institute and Dr. Robert Gallo in claiming credit for the discovery are very good, and led to optimism that a vaccine would soon follow.

Watching the movie 15 years later, we know that this optimism was cruelly unwarranted. Continued refusal by the United States and the World Health Organization (WHO) to take aggressive measures in preventing AIDS in India, Africa, and Asia resulted in the disease spreading through those countries unchecked.[13] Moreover, the complexity of the virus and its ability to mutate rapidly means that there is no vaccine and no particular hope of one in the foreseeable future. This reality raises issues of global public health ethics and shows how the failure of the United States to advocate and fund international prevention campaigns, indeed its refusal to do so—based on political pressures not to promote contraception—have destroyed the hopes expressed in 1993 that once identified, the virus could be contained.

The movie ends with a photomontage of real victims, as well as the AIDS Quilt, which, when last displayed, covered almost the entire distance from the Capital to the Washington Monument in Washington, D.C. While one theme is that AIDS had spread far beyond any one community and killed babies, young mothers, and old people who acquired it innocently through blood transfusions, another is that the coming of AIDS forced Americans to recognize that people they already loved, whether celebrities like Rock Hudson or members of their own family, were homosexuals. AIDS made homosexuals visible, in that it manifested itself with marks such as Kaposi's sarcoma, a skin lesion that characterizes an impaired immune system, and what became a familiar and horrible progression from perfect health to wasting death. The discrimination faced by AIDS patients has led to federal protection of health information. While this has brought more protection than before, the battle to give patients full access to information about their own health is still being fought. *And the Band Played On* brings bioethics outside of the hospital and laboratory to show how easily values such as justice, privacy, and compassion can become compromised in the face of fear.

REFERENCES

1. *And the Band Played On.* Directed by Roger Spottiswoode (1993) (First Broadcast HBO September 11, 1993).
2. Shilts, R. 1987. *And the band played on: Politics, people and the AIDS epidemic.* New York: St. Martins' Press.
3. Battin, M.P., Francis, L.P., Jacobson, J.A., and Smith, C.B. 2009. *The patient as victim and vector: Ethics and infectious disease,* p. 42. Oxford: Oxford University Press.
4. Although this essay follows the contemporary practice of describing anyone infected with the virus as having either "HIV" or "AIDS," distinctions were made when it was still thought likely for someone to be infected with the HIV virus and not develop AIDS symptoms.
5. Cooke, M. 1995. Patient rights and physician responsibility: Four problems in AIDS care. *Seminars in Dermatology* 14(3): 252–258.
6. 45 C.F.R. §§ 160–164.
7. Retrieved November 23, 2009 from http://www.hhs.gov/news/press/2001pres/20010412.html
8. Retrieved November 23, 2009 from http://www.hhs.gov/ocr/privacy/hipaa/understanding/consumers/index.html (accessed November 23, 2009).
9. Retrieved August 15, 2009 from http://www.pbs.org/wgbh/pages/frontline/aids/interviews/francis.html
10. Id.
11. Henry, W.A. III. June 24, 2001. The appalling saga of patient zero. *Time Magazine.* Retrieved from http://www.time.com/time/magazine/article/0,9171,965791,00.html
12. Scannell, K. 1999. *Death of the good doctor: Lessons from the heart of the AIDS epidemic.* San Francisco, CA: Cleis Press.
13. McFarlane, D.R. 2006. Reproductive health policies in President Bush's second term: Old battles and new fronts in the United States and internationally. *Journal of Public Health Policy* 27(4): 405–426.

3

gender discrimination in medicine: *to kill a mockingbird*

nicholas m. lampros and kristen r. monroe

To Kill a Mockingbird (1962). Gregory Peck, John Megna, Frank Overton, Rosemary Murphy, Robert Duvall. Directed by Robert Mulligan. Duration: 129 minutes.

DVD Chapter 39 scene 2:06:54 to 2:07:54

Like the pulitzer prize-winning book on which it is based, the film *To Kill a Mockingbird* focuses on a family in fictional Maycomb, Alabama: Atticus Finch (Gregory Peck), a small-town lawyer and single father, and his children, ten-year-old Jem (Phillip Alford) and six-year-old Scout (Mary Badham). The film, set during the Great Depression, centers on a series of summers during which Jem and Scout attempt to lure their reclusive neighbor, Boo Radley (Robert Duvall), out of his house. Their idyllic childhood pastimes are interrupted, however, when a local black man, Tom Robinson (Brock Peters), is accused of raping a white woman. While much of the town assumes Tom's guilt, Atticus agrees to defend Tom in court. Over the course of the trial, Atticus proves that Mayella and her alcoholic father have fabricated the "rape" allegation, but the all-white jury convicts Tom anyway.

This scene occurs at the end of the film, in the aftermath of the trial and Tom's subsequent lynching. Scout and Jem are returning home from a Halloween pageant when Bob Ewell, drunk and angry with the Finch family for the embarrassment Atticus caused him during the trial, attacks the two children, breaking Jem's arm. Fortunately, a mysterious stranger intervenes, fighting Bob off and carrying Jem back to the Finch home. The film's closing scene reveals that the children's rescuer is none other than Boo Radley, who had been secretly watching over them and leaving them small presents for some time. As the film ends, Scout walks Boo home and reflects on something her father taught her about empathy, saying in voice over, "Atticus was right. One time he said you never really know a man until you stand in his shoes and walk around in them. Just standing on the Radley porch was enough." It is this idea of empathic understanding—putting yourself in the place of another—which individuals, doctors included, can take from *To Kill a Mockingbird*.

Like most good films, *To Kill a Mockingbird* raises a number of issues to contemplate, but one of the most important concerns discrimination. The question raised as we watch *To Kill a Mockingbird* and think about the medical profession is why gender discrimination remains so endemic in medicine. Too often, in medicine as in contemporary society, behavior that would be recognized as clearly racist or anti-Semitic if exhibited toward a black or a Jew, is ignored when directed toward women.

Much aggregate data demonstrates this, and we cite only a few statistics to buttress our argument. According to the United States Census Bureau, women earn roughly 25% less than their male counterparts. This disturbing aggregate statistic, however, actually reflects progress from 1970, when women earned 41% less than men. The gender gap found in all occupations is especially acute in medicine and health management. In these categories, women earn only 63% of their male counterparts' salaries. Consider nursing, which remains a predominantly female field, with nine out of ten registered nurses (RNs) women; female nurses earn only 88% of what male nurses make. Even when levels of education and experience are comparable, female nurses earn less than their male equivalents. While both men's and women's salaries in nursing have increased annually, males still exceed the average salary for females by over $3,000. For nurse practitioners, the gap is even larger, with a discrepancy of $8,650 in annual salary.[i] Part of the differential arises from the fact that male nurses tend to work in the intensive care unit (ICU), coronary care unit (CCU), emergency room, or psychiatric ward, all areas viewed as valuing "male" characteristics such as physical strength. These areas of nursing also offer the highest pay, the annual average being at least $60,000 versus $49,634 for all nursing fields. Some justify this differential because men perform hard labor (e.g., lifting patients, etc.) that women do not, and should therefore be compensated for it. However, prior to World War II, many schools would not accept men in their nursing field, thereby leading to an almost all-female nurse force. During these times, women still did not receive equivalent pay.

This brief discussion suggests the need for more nuanced data to detect discrimination. We conducted a study of attitudes toward gender equality among both female and male faculty, including medical professionals at UCI School of Medicine. (See Monroe et al., 2008 for a fuller description of these data and findings.) In-depth interviews were conducted with full-time members of the academic Senate, including both male and female faculty, over a five-year period beginning in 2002. The attitudes of male faculty, both in the medical school and in the broader campus, toward women were intriguing, especially since they diverged dramatically from the views expressed by female faculty.

Most male faculty said they saw no outright discrimination and were not aware of anything wrong. Many described themselves as close to their mothers, sisters, and female friends, but they never saw much discrimination against these women. They described their wives as being "independent" women, yet many also related that their wives had stopped their career and/or education because of various family issues. Most cited having children as the main reason for stopping career/education, but an equally frequent cause was moving because of the husband's profession. When male faculty were asked if family issues would create difficulties for women—perhaps *the* major obstacle to equality in the eyes of the female faculty we interviewed—male faculty noted that they could see that being a problem but that they had not really seen that happen too often. Those who did acknowledge that women often struggle with the balance between career and family could give no real solution to the issue. This finding stands in stark contrast to interviews with female faculty, for whom the challenge of juggling career and family remains especially acute in the bench sciences and clinical sciences. These women specified medicine as an especially difficult field for women in which to combine career and family.

Most male faculty, especially the older faculty, emphasized that change had occurred over the generations and emphasized how much equality has been given over time. We heard frequent comments about how many women are currently studying in various academic fields, such as medicine. These comments expressed no regret at this change but did contain negative views about the institutionalized mechanisms to achieve gender equality, with male faculty noting that they felt reverse discrimination was a problem. Interestingly, many male faculty said, in effect, that "maybe there is discrimination in other departments, but not in the one I work in. I'm certainly not prejudiced and I treat all women equally." Each male faculty member we interviewed expressed some variant on this statement. One doctor added, as proof that things were improving for women, that women now could vote.

These interviews come from only a handful (less than 100) of male faculty at only one university. Further, not all the faculty was in medicine, so they are hardly dispositive. But the level of insensitivity to the situation for women in medicine, as in academia more generally, was striking. Our interviews suggest that Harper Lee's movie against racial discrimination awaits a contemporary counterpart highlighting the ongoing problem of gender equality among the professoriate and among the medical profession. Walking around the equivalent of Boo Radley's porch might increase sensitivity to this issue.

NOTE

i. According to the 2005 National Survey of Nurse Practitioners, male nurse practitioners make an average annual salary of $82,647 compared to women's salary of $73,986. That is an 11.7% difference, 7% higher than the difference of 10% in 2003.

4

the use of experimental therapies: *awakenings*

rebecca e. wolitz and christine grady

Awakenings (1990). Robert De Niro, Robin Williams, John Heard, Julie Kavner, Penelope Ann Miller, Max Von Sydow. Directed by Penny Marshall. Duration: 121 minutes.

Scene: DVD chapter 53 scene 1:42:57 to 1:43:53

PATIENTS AT BAINBRIDGE HOSPITAL SUFFER from several severe chronic psychiatric and neurological disorders. Among them is a postencephalitis population of patients who have been unable to move or speak for decades. Despite little clinical experience, Dr. Sayer (Robin Williams) believes that these catatonics may possess active minds. Aware of L-DOPA as a treatment for Parkinson's disease, Sayer asks for permission to administer it to one of his patients, Leonard (Robert De Niro). Although Leonard "awakens" from his long sleep, this miracle is short-lived. The health of the catatonic patients Sayer treats rapidly deteriorates due to side effects and tolerance to L-DOPA.

In this scene, Leonard proudly shows Dr. Sayer the wood models he has been working on: "It feels good while I'm working. It feels good here." Being able to work, to communicate—these are the humble yet profound benefits Leonard experiences on L-DOPA. L-DOPA, however, has a darker side. Shortly after these assertions of contentment, Leonard suffers violent side effects. Convulsing, he implores Dr. Sayer to "Learn! Learn! Learn from me!" *Awakenings* raises important issues about how to characterize the use of experimental therapies and whether this use, particularly in vulnerable patient populations like Dr. Sayer's, is ethical.

What differentiates clinical practice from clinical research? The purpose of clinical practice is to promote the well-being of individual patients through "diagnosis, preventive treatment, or therapy."[1] Clinicians are charged solely with caring for and making medical decisions in their patients' best interests. By contrast, physician researchers are responsible for conducting good science while protecting the rights and welfare of patients. Clinical research is designed to test scientific hypotheses and create generalizable medical knowledge.[2]

Given this distinction, is Dr. Sayer's experimental use of L-DOPA properly considered clinical research or clinical practice? Although Sayer has extensive nonhuman research experience, he is employed as a clinician and must attend to his patients' best interests and well-being. Indeed, these motivations drive Dr. Sayer toward finding a treatment, as nothing else has helped these "locked-in" patients. His assumption, although challenged throughout the film, is that if a treatment could restore normal functioning, it should be pursued because it is in these patients' best interests.

Still, part of Dr. Sayer's motivation in giving L-DOPA to Leonard is to see whether it is a successful therapy generalizable to his other catatonic patients. Leonard's initial favorable response to L-DOPA is compelling evidence to give others the drug. Moreover, as made explicit in his conversation with Leonard's mother, Dr. Sayer had no idea what effect L-DOPA might have on catatonics. It is unclear whether Dr. Sayer conceives of his experimental activities as research, but if held to these standards, several problems arise in light of well-established standards for ethical research involving humans.[3]

For research to be ethical, it must be scientifically valid. Without validity, research is a waste of time that "cannot justify exposing subjects to burdens or risks."[3] Although a research protocol's details are uninteresting to movie-goers, *Awakenings* provides scant evidence that Dr. Sayer has a scientifically sound plan capable of generating reliable data. To the contrary, his use of L-DOPA seems somewhat haphazard. Moreover, if a study design exists, Sayer deviates from it by secretly doubling Leonard's dose. These actions cast additional doubt on the scientific validity of Dr. Sayer's project.

Ethical clinical research must also have a favorable risk–benefit ratio.[3] Clinical research is justifiable when the risks are minimized and outweighed by the overall potential benefits. Although determining a risk–benefit ratio is inherently speculative, neither Dr. Sayer nor his supervisors appear to engage in this analysis. Moreover, he does not mention any potential risks of L-DOPA to Leonard's mother. It is unclear whether he gives any significant thought to these issues even after Leonard experiences severe side effects; Dr. Sayer reacts not by reassessing use of the drug, but by increasing Leonard's dosage.

Additionally, consideration of emotional risks appears to be eclipsed by the hoped-for benefits of L-DOPA. Dr. Sayer does not wrestle with reservations about whether bringing this population "back to life" is, all things considered, the right course of action. Nor does he appear to reflect on what it means to suffer, or whether some forms of suffering are worse than others. Several patients, for example, experience intense emotional anguish after "awakening." Realizing that decades of life have evaporated, or that exercising newfound autonomy will be thwarted, can be deeply distressing. Add to that the trauma of discovering that L-DOPA eventually fails to maintain normal functioning lives. How should these risks have been accounted for? And by whom? Dr. Sayer appears convinced that such suffering, emotional or otherwise, is not worse than a life suspended. But do others share this conviction? Whose views should count the most? Weighing the potential risks and benefits of research is a difficult endeavor. Some attempt, however, at this calculus is necessary.

Given potential risks, the decision to enroll in research is significant. Consequently, informed consent is an important ethical requirement.[3] Research participation should be informed, voluntary, and consistent with the interests, values, and preferences of the prospective subject.[3] Mentally incapacitated individuals, like those in *Awakenings*, are unable to consent for themselves and therefore require additional protections. At many institutions, including the National Institutes of Health, for example, incapacitated adults are allowed to participate in limited categories of research calibrated by risk–benefit ratios with the consent of an authorized surrogate decision maker.[4] Because Dr. Sayer's patients are mentally incapacitated and the risk–benefit ratio of L-DOPA is so unclear, this case demands careful consideration of whose permission is sufficient for procuring consent. Although it seems a safe assumption that Leonard's mother is his legal guardian, *Awakenings* does not provide any details about who is consenting for the other catatonic patients.

Surrogate decision makers are charged with ensuring that research participation is consistent with the interests, values, and preferences of the inca- pacitated individual. These evaluations can be extremely difficult, especially for patients like Sayer's who may have lost capacity as children and/or lack a surro- gate with knowledge of this intimate information. *Awakenings* does not address the issue of whether those without an appropriate surrogate should receive L-DOPA or the complex consent issues that arise from this drug temporarily reinstating capacity. At the time of revival, the patients are all adults and appear to function normally, raising the question of who ought to be making medical decisions—surrogates or patients? Even if these awakened patients possess some capacity for decision-making, the Bainbridge physicians do not appear to treat them as such.

Appropriate oversight remains an important component of ensuring that research is ethical.[3] Independent review by, among others, institutional review boards and ethics committees, allows for an unbiased assessment of whether a proposed study satisfactorily meets criteria necessary for conducting ethical research. Dr. Sayer's L-DOPA experiments, however, are subject to only minimal and, arguably, inadequate oversight. Although he does seek his superior's permission, this is the extent of his "independent review." It does not appear that his precise plans are scrutinized. When considered as clinical research, Dr. Sayer's use of L-DOPA has several ethical transgressions. But is it appropriate to hold his activities accountable to these standards?

It is generally accepted that not all experimentation is research.[1,5,6] The line between practice and research can be difficult to draw.[2] Some propose that a middle ground exists, sharing features of each. Referred to as "informal research," "innovative" or "nonvalidated" therapy, such activities are often, but not always, "offered to a patient, generally as a last resort, in the hope that it might save the patient's life or improve a serious illness."[7] Innovative therapies are like research in that their efficacy is not vetted, yet like clinical practice in that their use is intended for individual patient benefit.

It is uncertain, however, what ethical standards ought to apply to this in-between category. Clear criteria articulating when a technique or therapy counts as genuinely "innovative" remain largely undefined. How much deviation from standard practice constitutes innovation? Given that some clinical practice is supported by very little evidence, what levels of evidence are appropriate for making useful distinctions? Exploring these questions may help guide which ethical standards are most applicable to an experimental therapy. Holding smaller deviations, for example, to ethical standards set for clinical research may be excessive, yet clinical practice standards may be too permissive.

Off-label prescribing is a common practice, and generally accepted to be within the prerogative of a physician if he or she genuinely thinks it is in the patient's best interests. Unfortunately, off-label use can also result in serious unanticipated complications; one example is the serious pulmonary hypertension and heart valve damage caused by the off-label use of the popular combination fen-phen for weight loss.[8] New drugs, and new combinations, frequently lack sufficient evidence supporting their appropriateness for a particular off-label use and time to track what serious side effects might occur over time.[9] In 1969, when L-DOPA was administered off-label to these catatonic patients, it had only been on the market for two years.[10] Some have suggested that when there is very low certainty of net benefit, as seems the case with Dr. Sayer's patients, "investigational off-label use... generally should be limited to the context of research protocols."[9]

This analysis seems correct. The safety and interests of these vulnerable patients suffering from encephalitis-induced catatonia—both present and future— are likely to be best served by adhering to the ethical and scientific standards of clinical research. Given the uncertainty involved, the dramatic departure from standard practice, as well as the clearly defined population that could benefit from improvements in care, it seems most appropriate to experiment with L-DOPA in the context of research. This, however, does not necessarily indicate that Sayer's use is impermissible. Reasonable people—and reasonable review committees— may disagree about whether giving L-DOPA to Leonard and his fellow patients should have been held to the standards of clinical research or to the less rigid and less well-defined standards of innovative therapeutic use in clinical practice. Justifications for when an experimental therapy can be tested both within research and practice, as opposed to only one or the other, remain to be explored. Many issues merit further consideration.

NOTE

i. The opinions expressed are the view of the authors. They do not represent any position or policy of the U.S. National Institutes of Health, the Public Health Service, or the Department of Health and Human Services.

REFERENCES

1. Levine, R.J. 1986. *Ethics and regulation of clinical research* 2nd ed., p. 452. Baltimore: Urban & Schwarzenberg.
2. Miller, F.G., Rosenstein, D.L., and DeRenzo, E.G. 1998. Professional integrity in clinical research. *Journal of the American Medical Association* 280(16): 1449–1454.
3. Emanuel, E.J., Wendler, D., and Grady, C. 2000. What makes clinical research ethical? *Journal of the American Medical Association*, 2000. 283(20): p. 2701–2711.
4. NIH Intramural Program Medical Administrative Series, M87-4 Research Involving Adults Who Are or May Be Unable to Consent. 9 July 2008. Policy and Communications Bulletin.
5. Freedman, B.1989. Nonvalidated therapies and HIV disease. McGill/Boston Research Group. *Hastings Center Report* 19(3): 14–20.
6. Margo, C.E. 2001. When is surgery research? Towards an operational definition of human research. *Journal of Medical Ethics* 27(1): 40–43.
7. Mariner, W.K. 1992. AIDS research and the Nuremberg Code. In G.J. Annas, and M.A. Grodin (Eds.), *The Nazi doctors and the Nuremberg Code: Human rights in human experimentation*, pp. 286–303. New York: Oxford University Press.
8. Brody, H. 2008. *Ethics, the medical profession, and the pharmaceutical industry.* Lanham MD: Rowman and Littlefield.
9. Largent, E., Miller F., and Pearson, S. 2009. Going off-label without venturing off-course: Evidence and ethical off-label prescribing. *Archives of Internal Medicine* forthcoming.
10. Sacks, O.W. 1999. *Awakenings*. 1st ed., p. 408. New York: Vintage Books.

5

subject participation in research: *frankenstein*

edmund g. howe

Frankenstein (1931). Boris Karloff, Colin Clive, Mae Clarke, Dwight Frye.
Directed by James Whale. Duration: 76 minutes.

DVD chapter 7 scene 0:30:50 to 0:34:19

FRANKENSTEIN IS THE STORY OF a creature or, some might say a "monster," made by Dr. Frankenstein in an attempt to create "life." The creature initially seeks companionship, like all humans. Yet, from his very start, he is brutalized by Dr. Frankenstein and others. He escapes the castle in which he was created and imprisoned and meets a young girl named Maria, who wants to befriend him and play. She throws a flower into the water. He then throws her into the water, thinking this too is part of their game. She drowns. He becomes violent. The townspeople come after him and kill him.

I have had the rare fortune as a teacher of being able to present this story to medical students, annually, as a one-act play. This is because an actor, Jon Spelman, wrote a script from Mary Shelley's classic and now performs it. Teachers of ethics could, I believe, use this movie or its fragments as effectively.

This story captures the misery of this creature's isolation and depicts Dr. Frankenstein's abysmal treatment of him as solely a "subject" of his research.[i]

The creature's sense of isolation is, however, profound: "Everywhere I see bliss, from which I alone am irrevocably excluded" (Shelley, p. 97). Shelley writes here, for example, that the creature's "unearthly ugliness rendered it almost too horrible for human eyes" (Shelley, p. 95). Part of this may have been due to how the creature looked.

In response, presumably to this isolation and to the hurt the creature endured from others, he at the end contemplates carving up the face of a young woman, "blooming in the loveliness" of her youth, so that she could then be like him and he no longer so alone. He says to himself, chillingly, "My companion must be of the same species, and have the same defects. This being you must *create*" (Shelley, p. 139). He doesn't, but flees.

This story can be, then, a springboard for raising questions regarding research in general, and more particularly, how researchers should treat research participants.[1,2] The specific scene that best exemplifies this subject occurs when the creature (Boris Karloff) first becomes conscious and "emerges." Dr. Frankenstein (Colin Clive) shows his colleagues how the creature can obey simple commands.

He opens a skylight, and the creature is drawn to this light, innocently holding out his hands. As the skylight is closed, the creature again faces the dark. The doctor's assistant, Fritz (Dwight Frye), then taunts the creature with a burning torch. The creature retreats like a wounded animal in fear. Believing that the creature is dangerous, Dr. Frankenstein and his colleagues beat the creature and lock him back in his "prison cell."

This scene, by implication, raises the key ethical conflict in research ethics: Researchers want, on one hand, to obtain findings beneficial to others; yet, at the same time, they must respect and protect the rights of participants.[3] No participant who is competent, for example, should ever be forced to partake in a procedure without his or her consent. This consent should be free and not too strongly affected by the circumstances that the participant is in.[4] The risks they take on should not be too unequal to those taken on by others, and these risks, in any case, should also not be too great. Presently, institutional review boards, or IRBs, formally review research protocols and decide whether criteria designed to adequately protect research participants are met.[5] These boards consist of not only experts in medicine and the scientific method, on one hand, but nonscientists, representing the community at large, or people chosen to be on a jury, on the other.

The options differ for doctors treating patients versus those conducting research. Doctors in clinical contexts can generally place their patients' interests first, but doctors conducting research may have to draw certain lines between the needs of their research and the needs of those who participate in it. In many studies, for example, patients may want to participate because, although it is unknown whether an experimental drug will harm or help them, they still may benefit. They may not otherwise have access to a new and promising, but not fully tested, drug. Researchers may not be able to include these people, however, because they do not meet inclusion criteria that the research requires.

As a second example of researchers' different options, some research contexts demand that researchers can't give information as frequently as they would to individual patients in their clinical care. An example of this is research that needs extraordinarily large numbers of people to determine whether or not a new vaccine, such as one to protect people from acquiring HIV, is effective.[6] This type of research might pursue this question by dividing participants into two groups. One half of the group could be given the vaccine and the other half, a placebo. This study would show that the vaccine was effective if—but only if—enough people in both groups engaged in risky drug use or unprotected sex to show a significant difference. In a clinical setting, doctors might inform individual patients "constantly" about these risks, but in the research setting, they could not. They instead might inform participants only to the degree that this was required by the research, as the usual standard of clinical care. Doctors conducting this research, then, might be less able to tailor their clinical interventions to patients' individual and even idiosyncratic personal needs.

Participants who may become involved in research may have increased stress from the first moment that they consider this endeavor. They first must decide whether or not to enter a research protocol. They may do better in a protocol because the standard treatments haven't worked well. With experimental treatments, rather than standard treatments, they may at the same time do worse. In addition to being torn between entering a protocol or "just" receiving standard treatment, they could also be stressed because they could opt for a third choice— palliative treatment—instead of either.

Even when researchers can give participants as much information as they want, this itself may be ethically problematic. Some participants may, for instance, want extensive information regarding the research's potential benefits and risks. Others, however, may find this same amount of information overwhelming and unduly stressful. Therefore, researchers, and then IRBs, must determine how much is the "right" amount of information to give, best for all, in every protocol.

Although all research participants are vulnerable in these respects, some, like the creature, are especially vulnerable, and this is foreseeable.[ii] Consequently, present research regulations give special protections to these participants. Categories of people within this group are, for example, prisoners and children.[7] Prisoners are more vulnerable for many reasons. They could volunteer in the hope that this could result in their gaining earlier parole. They could also feel guilty for their crime and want to make up for this to society. Children are vulnerable primarily because they lack decision-making capacity. Thus, there are more strict requirements when research involves children. However, these greater restrictions pose another problem. They may result in less research being done with children. This, in turn, may result in doctors then having less evidence-based data to guide them in providing children with optimal treatments. Those establishing research requirements again must draw a line between allowing researchers to obtain findings that will help future patients on one hand, while simultaneously protecting these exceptionally vulnerable, potential participants on the other.

Frankenstein also highlights the importance of the relationship between participants and researchers. This relationship is important both at the beginning and throughout the research. Researchers can, for example, greatly help participants cope with their feelings of being isolated and alone. They may, for example, fear, unconsciously or consciously, that they are "guinea pigs." They may worry that researchers regard them in ethical terms, as Dr. Frankenstein regarded the creature, as primarily the means to others' ends. Researchers can reassure them that this isn't the case. Researchers can explain to participants, for example, that in other contexts, physicians commonly give their patients treatments that have not been fully tested and this is solely to benefit them. Doctors give patients drugs, for example, that are "off-label" or that haven't been "approved" for this purpose as evidence-based. Likewise, they may give patients treatments not yet fully tested for "compassionate" reasons when patients have a serious illness, and this alone may help. These participants' situations may be the same.

In rare instances, treatments not fully tested may be given to people to protect them. Then, although these treatments are untested, this is not research at all. In Iraq, during the first Gulf War, for instance, soldiers were required to take a vaccine to protect them from botulism, because it was feared that Saddam Hussein might use rockets containing botulism against them, although this vaccine hadn't been tested for this use.[10] This was solely done for their protection. It would, of course, have been "unethical" to expose soldiers or anyone to this biological weaponry in an effort to predetermine the extent to which this vaccine was effective against this biological weaponry.

NOTES

i. This movie is based upon Mary Shelley's classic novel, *Frankenstein* (Mary Shelley, *Frankenstein* (New York: Penguin Books, 1992), first published in 1818. (See, Richard Carter. 1999. Mary Shelley's nightmare (1797–1851): *Frankenstein*; Her life, literary legacy, and last illness. *World Journal of Surgery* 23: 1195–1201.

ii. Initially, the creature is open to others and shows tenderness in both the movie and book. In the book, for example, the creature comes to greatly admire humans. He says, for instance, "The gentle manners... of the cottagers greatly endeared them to me: when they were unhappy, I felt depressed; when they rejoiced, I sympathized in their joys." (Shelley, p. 109)

REFERENCES

1. Holm, R.P. 2006. Frankenstein, a story of scientific discovery turned to dread, with a lesson in ethics. *Pharos of Alpha Omega Alpha Honor Medical Society* 69: 30–34.
2. Davies, H. 2004. Can Mary Shelley's Frankenstein be read as an early research ethics text? *Medical Humanities* 30: 32–35.
3. Appelbaum, P.S., Lidz, C.W., and Klitzman, R. 2009. Voluntariness of consent to research: A conceptual model. *Hastings Center Report* 39: 30–39.
4. Emanuel, E.J., Wendler, D.W., and Grady, C. 2000. What makes clinical research ethical? *Journal of the American Medical Association* 283: 2701–2711.
5. Enfield, K.B., and Truwit, J.D. 2008. The purpose, composition, and function of an institutional review board: Balancing priorities. *Respiratory Care* 53: 1330–1336.
6. Fauci, A.S., Johnston, M.I., Dieffenbach, C.W., et al. 2008. HIV vaccine research: The way forward. *Science* 321: 530–532.
7. Schwenzer, K.J. 2008. Protecting vulnerable subjects in clinical research: Children, pregnant women, prisoners, and employees. *Respiratory Care* 53: 1342–1349.
8. Bayne, T., and Levy, N. 2005. Amputees by choice: Body integrity disorder and the ethics of amputation. *Journal of Applied Philosophy* 25: 75–86.
9. First, M.B. 2005. Desire for amputation of a limb: Paraphilia, psychosis, or a new type of identity disorder. *Psychological Medicine* 35; 919–928, at 26.
10. Howe, E.G., and Martin, E.G. 1991. Treating the troops. *Hastings Center Report* 21: 21–24.

power and patient/subject exploitation: *the elephant man*

lester d. friedman

The Elephant Man (1980). John Hurt, Anthony Hopkins, John Gielgud, Anne Bancroft, Wendy Hiller, Freddie Jones. Directed by David Lynch. Duration: 124 minutes.

DVD chapter 1 scene 00.21:04 to 00.23.38

IRECTED BY DAVID LYNCH, WHO later became famous for quirky films such as *Blue Velvet* (1986), *Wild At Heart* (1990), and the TV series *Twin Peaks* (1990–1991), recounts the compelling story of Joseph Merrick (called John in the movie) in *The Elephant Man*. Profound, unsightly changes rendered Merrick (John Hurt) odious to polite Victorian society, and his condition initially condemned him to life as a sideshow spectacle, displaying his misshapen body to curious gawkers.[1] Ultimately, his condition drew the attention of young Dr. Frederick Treves (Anthony Hopkins), an ambitious surgeon who rescued him from the hideous world of freak shows and brought the ailing man to the Royal London Hospital. Lynch's movie traces Merrick's evolution from circus oddity to London celebrity, slowly exposing the gentle man with artistic sensibilities buried beneath a hideous exterior that denied him normal human contact. Shot in striking, often shimmering, black-and-white cinematography, Lynch continually juxtaposes Merrick's personal story with evocative images of a rapidly industrializing London, showing the brutality that permeates both Merrick's struggle to have his humanity recognized and that of the changing world surrounding him.[2]

As the scene begins, a bright light emanating from a projector floods the screen, gradually dimming to reveal a lecture hall filled with well-dressed physicians awaiting a presentation by Dr. Treves. At his direction, two men wheel in a small, tent-like contraption and, upon his command, they part the curtains to reveal its human contents: the Elephant Man. Previously, Lynch always presented Merrick in oversized clothing and covered his face with a hood, so the audience just watched the reactions of others to him. Now, the director continues to tease and tantalize, not permitting us to peek beneath the tent or view this spectacle of human deformity directly. We see only the crooked, shadowy outline of Merrick's malformed body. As Treves delivers a dry, medical description of Merrick's manifold physical ailments, Lynch intercuts faces from the crowd of medical men, who sit stunned and staring at the figure before them. Their faces register shock, discomfort, and disgust at the sight revealed to them, which further piques our curiosity to see

Merrick. Treves begins his talk by stating that he has never "met with such a perverted or degraded version of a human being as this man"; he ends by noting that Merrick's genitals are intact and unaffected by his condition. As he concludes, the doctors applaud, the men wheel Merrick offstage, and the scene fades to the bright projector light with which it opened.

Throughout this scene, Lynch cleverly positions the viewer in relationship to Merrick. First, Treves stands behind a table at the front of the room with anatomical pictures behind him. As the scene progresses, he appears no better than Merrick's former "owner," Mr. Bytes (Freddie Jones), a barker who abused and exploited him as a freak. In fact, while Bytes physically mistreats Merrick, Treves inflicts deeper psychological wounds by offering a cruel introduction and concluding with taste-less comments about the state of his genitals (which we assume are uncovered). Lynch arranges the well-dressed assemblage of doctors like the gawkers who paid their guineas to stare at Merrick in the circus. No one protests Treves' callous presentation, his insensitively to Merrick's physical pain, or his lack of basic respect for another human being. Finally, Lynch incorporates the audience as an equally guilty participant in this dispassionate travesty, linking our curiosity to view Merrick's abnormalities with the numb response to human tragedy exhibited equally by the unruly circus goers and the austere doctors.

In class, I have actually watched medical students crane their necks, vainly trying to catch a glimpse of Merrick's veiled body behind that curtain.

Although set in the 1890s, *The Elephant Man* raises myriad issues relevant to 21st-century bioethics, including how to respond to a broad spectrum of difference (the "Other" in contemporary parlance) ranging from physical deformities to socioeconomic disparities to racial dissimilarities. It also confronts the subjects of how doctors deal with incurable diseases and the politics of hospital care. At its heart, however, the film delves equally into the education of Frederick Treves, who changes from callow professional to compassionate provider, and into the plight of John Merrick, who comes to value his own personhood through the caring of his physician: "I am not an elephant! I am not an animal! I am a human being! I am a man!" As such, the film spotlights the evolution of a doctor–patient relationship and raises contemporary questions about the boundaries between patient exploitation, professional exhibitionism, and appropriate medical treatment.

Even in our modern age of technological marvels and genomic medicine, the doctor–patient relationship remains the cornerstone of the entire medical system. This human connection underlies the fundamental moral concepts and forms the foundation for the bioethical principles commonly cited as essential: autonomy, confidentiality, beneficence, truth telling, nonmaleficence, and justice. Although scholars offer various descriptions of this bond between physician and patient, most follow the basic model outlined by Emanuel and Emanuel[3]: paternalistic/ priestly (the doctor as parent/priest provides selective information to encourage the patient to choose what the physician considers the best option), informative (the doctor as technical expert supplies factual information and offers no opinions), interpretive (the doctor as counselor tenders factual information and helps the patient reach a decision consistent with his or her values), and deliberative (the doctor as teacher/friend engages in a dialogue with the patient about what actions best suit the situation and his or her values). Treves actually progresses through each of these models; he begins the film by looking at Merrick simply as a study specimen and ends by embracing him as a friend, ultimately discovering the man inside the severely deformed patient.

Each of Emanuel and Emanuel's principally dyadic relationships contains at least one common element: a shifting power linkage between the patient and the physician that ranges from one-sided and slyly dictatorial to a partnership between consenting adults. As Dupuy[4] notes, controversies around the use and misuse of power in society, often within the medical arena, have fascinated a wide range of thinkers, prominent among them: Friedrich Nietzsche (*Twilight of the Idols*, 1889), Michel Foucault (*The History of Sexuality*, 1976–1984), Ivan Illich (*Medical Nemesis*,1975), and Howard Brody (*The Healer's Power*, 1992). William Carlos Williams' provocative short story, "The Use of Force" (1938), has attained canonical status in many medical humanities and bioethics programs for its dramatic presentation of the circumstances under which doctors may/should/might over-rule the wishes of patients for their own well-being. On a more theoretical level, Foucault claims that power inequities exist everywhere and play a significant role in every aspect of all human relationship, including, of course, between doctor and patient. Brody,[5] who sees power as the central ethical problem in medicine's moral discourse, identifies three intersecting levels of medical power: *Aesculapian*, the power a physician possess by virtue of his or her medical training; *charismatic*, the power a physician possess by virtue of his or her personality, independent of medical knowledge; and *social*, the power a physician possesses by virtue of his or her social status. To these three, others scholars have added *hierarchical*, denoting the power a particular physician has within the medical structure itself.

Every interaction with medical professionals incorporates power issues ranging from the trivial to the profound.[6] In what other circumstances would you find yourself nearly naked discussing the intimate details of your life with a person you met scant minutes before? A vast body of literary and cinematic works aptly demonstrates that even doctors who become patients suffer from these power inequities, as their illness transforms them from competent professionals into insecure, frightened, and vulnerable patients. Despite some extremely rare examples, such that as depicted in *Lorenzo's Oil* (1992), laymen cannot hope to match the physician's knowledge of medical matters, even with the vast resources of the Internet at their disposal. In the scene under discussion, Treves exhibits all of Brody's levels of power over Merrick, as well as his own professional ambitions.[7]

The history of Western medicine is replete with examples of the exploitation of patients—particularly the poor, the uneducated, the incarcerated, the mentally ill, and the racially different—yet as Brazier[8] argues, humankind has benefited from experiments that treat human beings merely as subjects rather than individuals. Although what one doctor considers exploitation another may characterize as necessary for the good of humanity, some historical events illustrate unmistakable miscarriages of ethical behavior in which vulnerable segments of the population have been dehumanized and exploited. No controversy, for example, exists about the brutal Nazi experiments performed upon unwilling concentration camp victims. Few people today know that the Nazi doctors defended themselves during the Nuremberg Trials by citing similar studies performed by physicians on prisoners and racial minorities in the Allied countries. As Pressel[9] points out, their lawyers specifically cited malaria experiments conducted at the Statesville Penitentiary in Illinois (1940s), as well as various mistreatments of blacks, as comparable to their clients' treatment of medical subjects. Similarly, the infamous Tuskegee longitudinal study of untreated syphilis (1932–1972) incorporated over 400 poor, illiterate, black men. To these blatant examples, we might add the feeding of radioactive oatmeal (sponsored by Quaker Oats and led by MIT researchers) to "mentally retarded" children at The Walter E. Fernald School for the Feebleminded (Massachusetts) in the 1950s, and the Willowbrook State School where, between 1963 and 1966, doctors inoculated healthy children with the virus that causes hepatitis to gauge the effects of gamma globulin in combating it.

Such past cases remain important to remember and vital to teach, but current students often sweep them aside as ancient history, claiming that such abuses no longer exist in the modern medical world. Such is not the case, despite the role of institutional review boards meant to eliminate subject exploitation. Research offers the most obvious opportunities for abuse, particularly when the goal of the project looms larger than the risks to the participants.[10] The pervasive infusion of funding from pharmaceutical companies increases the risk of mistreatment, since so much financial support, personal prestige, and institutional solvency hinges upon research efforts coinciding with corporate goals. With so much money and power at stake, the temptations to place positive outcomes over subject autonomy remains evident.

Although the field of medical research contains palpable minefields, the risks for patient exploitation exist in virtually every aspect of the medical system. Some that spring immediately to mind include the sexualization of the doctor–patient relationship[11]; the involuntary incarceration of those labeled mentally disturbed; the pressures of a changing fiscal and reimbursement system; the advancements in technology that prolong death rather than life; the (very human) prejudices and biases of physicians; the marginalization of patients from different racial and socioeconomic classes[12]; the stigmatization of patients with atypical lifestyles, disabilities, or sexual orientations; the effects of direct advertising upon patient care; the use of pharmaceutical choices based on drug company incentives; and the positive and negative effects of Internet sites. Direct financial incentives for recruitment of patients from a physician's practice, so-called "finder's fees," for participation in research protocols provide a current example of potential abuse of physician power. These fees can be as high as $5,000 for each patient enlisted in a study. Doctors who know that the enrollment of each patient will bring significant financial rewards may be tempted to find every possible way to convince their patients of the advantages of participation.

The power inequities intrinsic to the practice of medicine allow the potential for patient exploitation to remain possible in all medical encounters. Howard Brody speculates that within our "primitive depths" lies the desire "to victimize others less powerful and to enjoy it—to glory in the fact that they and not we are the victims."[i] Juxtaposed to such unsettling and chilling assumptions, however, are the words of warning uttered by two physicians separated by centuries: "If a doctor forgets his patient's fears, he's in danger himself—flirting with the seductions of tyranny" (William Carlos Williams); "May I never see in the patient anything else but a fellow creature in pain" (Moses Maimonides). In this scene, the doctor clearly exploits the patient. Yet, *The Elephant Man* allows the viewer to accompany Treves on this journey toward empathizing with, rather than utilizing, a "fellow creature in pain." We follow Treves as he finds the beauty beneath the beast, simultaneously becoming more aware of our own frailties and misconceptions, of the power inequities inherent within medical culture, and of how an egotistic sense of superiority make us prey to exploiting others.

NOTE

i. From Howard Brody, *The healer's power* (Yale University, 1992, p. 21). Brody speculates on how the use and misuse of power must be explicitly addressed in medical ethics.

REFERENCES

1. Born on August 5, 1862, Merrick was afflicted with proteus syndrome, an extremely rare disorder of mosaic growth dysregulation resulting in severe deformities, including marked asymmetric enlargement of the skull, overgrowth of the right side of the body, a nonfunctional flipper-like right hand, severe dysarthric speech, painful disabling arthritis, scoliosis of the spine, shortness of breath, and large distorting subcutaneous growths of the face and body. Sir Frederick Treves (1st Baronet) eventually attained prominence in British medical circles and finally became personal physician to King Edward VII, whose life he saved in 1901. Merrick, who spent his final four years in relative comfort at the Royal London Hospital, died in his sleep on April 11, 1890, at the age of 27, the large overgrowth of his head and surrounding tissues reportedly having suffocated him.

2. Lynch's film follows in the footsteps of others intrigued by Merrick's condition and his life, including a seven-paragraph pamphlet, *The Autobiography of Joseph Carey Merrick*, purportedly written by Merrick himself. Treves published his own account of their interaction, *The Elephant Man and other Reminiscences* (London: Cassell and Company, 1923); the eminent anthropologist Ashley Montague later came forth with *The Elephant Man: A Study in Human Dignity* (New York: E.P. Dutton, 1979), and

Bernard Pomerance's Tony award winning play, *The Elephant Man* (New York: Grove Press, 1979) debuted first in London and then on Broadway. Although the story that Michael Jackson offered half a million dollars for Merrick's skeleton seems more urban myth than fact, Graham and Oehlschlaeger (pp. 187–190) point out that the performer incorporated "Elephant Man" motifs in his famous *Moonwalking* music video (1988) and recalled his fascination with Merrick in his autobiography, *Moonwalk* (1988).

3. Emanuel, E.J., and Emanuel, L.L. 1992. Four models of the physician-patient relationship. *JAMA* 267: 2221–2226.

4. Dupuy, J.-P. April 26, 2004. Medicine and power: A tribute to Ivan Illich. *ComPlexUs* 1: 1:44; 157–163.

5. Brody, H. 1993. *The healer's power*. New Haven: Yale University Press.

6. Waitzkin, H. 1993. *The politics of medical encounters*.New Haven: Yale University Press.

7. Graham, P.W., and Oehlschlaeger, F. 1992. *Articulating the Elephant Man: Joseph Merrick and his interpreters*. Baltimore: Johns Hopkins University Press.

8. Brazier, M. 2008. Exploitation and enrichment: The paradox of medical experimentation. *Journal of Medical Ethics* 34: 180–183.

9. Pressel, D.M. (December 2003). Nuremberg and Tuskegee: Lessons for contemporary American medicine. *Journal of National Medical Association* 95(12): 1216–1225.

10. Resnik, D.B. 2002. Exploitation and the ethics of clinical trials. *The American Journal of Bioethics* 2(2): 28–29.

11. Rogers, N. (May 2007). Race and the politics of polio: Warm Springs, Tuskegee, and the March of Dimes. *American Journal of Public Health* 97(5): 784–795.

12. Hall, K.H. 2001. Sexualization of the doctor-patient relationship: Is it ever ethically possible? *Family Practice* 18: 511–515.

the ethics of international research:
the constant gardener

annette rid and seema k. shah

[1]*The Constant Gardener* (2005). Ralph Fiennes, Rachel Weisz, Hubert Kuondé.
Directed by Fernando Meirelles. Duration: 129 minutes.

DVD chapter 10, Scene 0:51:30 to 0:53:30

N A REMOTE AREA OF Northern Kenya, British lawyer and activist Tessa Quayle
is found brutally murdered. The evidence points to a crime of passion, but
Tessa's widower, Justin Quayle (Ralph Fiennes), starts his own investigation.
Reexamining his marriage to a woman he never really knew, Justin learns that Tessa
had uncovered the fraudulent research activities of a Swiss-Canadian pharmaceutical company and the Kenyan branch of a multinational firm. After British officials
failed to silence her, these companies arranged for Tessa's murder to prevent their
criminal undertakings from being publicized.

Although central to the plot, the film provides little information about the
drug trial conducted in the slums of Nairobi. The Swiss-Canadian company has
outsourced the clinical testing of, Dypraxa, an investigational agent against
multidrug-resistant tuberculosis, to a multinational firm that appears to have no
specific qualifications for conducting research. The trial reveals that Dypraxa has
serious side effects. However, both companies deliberately conceal these results—
including more than 60 deaths—in the interest of profit. Corporate intimidation
stifles public scrutiny. Although it is difficult to imagine a pharmaceutical
company risking its reputation with a drug that has blatant lethal side effects and
committing murder to promote such a product, *The Constant Gardener* raises
important questions about the ethics of research in developing countries. Given
the increasing internationalization of clinical trials,[1] this is a timely topic for
students to explore.

In the selected scene, Justin Quayle attempts to carry on his wife's work by
investigating the death of a young Kenyan woman named Wanza Kilulu. In a slum
of Nairobi, he finds Wanza's children waiting outside a portable medical clinic to
receive a dose of Dypraxa. Before they receive the medication, the children must
turn in a medical record card on which the box for informed consent has been
checked. While Justin is talking with Wanza's child about his mother's death, he
observes a woman being turned away from the clinic, sobbing. The woman has
been denied medication for her child after she stopped taking Dypraxa. Justin,
upset that she is being denied medical care unrelated to research because she

withdrew from the study, approaches a man in a white coat who appears to be connected to the research: "Not much of a choice, is it? I suppose they're not even informed that they're testing a new drug."

Indeed, in this scene, people appear to be signing informed consent documents without fully understanding them because they have few, if any, options to obtain health care outside of research. It may be helpful to begin the lesson by asking students what they think is ethically problematic about what Justin witnesses. One obvious problem is that Wanza's oldest son, who is still a minor, could not legally give consent for his younger sibling to be involved in research. Additionally, if the research participants were indeed not informed about their involvement in a clinical trial, the researchers failed to obtain informed consent. The scene also raises a more complex and interesting question about the voluntariness of the informed consent. When multinational clinical research is conducted by sponsors from developed countries in resource-limited settings, significant concern always exists about the voluntariness of consent because participants may be coerced or unduly influenced.

Ethicists have argued that research participants "in dire health or extreme poverty" are vulnerable to coercion when they are offered medical care through participation in research.[2] Coercion occurs when one person threatens to harm another if he or she does not perform a certain action. A paradigmatic example of coercion is when a thief holds a gun to someone and demands, "Your money or your life." At first glance, it may appear that the thief is offering a choice to the person. However, this is coercion disguised as a choice because the thief threatens to take something away from the person. The difference between a coercive threat and an offer is that an offer increases the number of options a person has, whereas a threat takes options away.[3]

As a result of widespread global injustice, many people in developing countries have no reasonable alternative but to enroll in research to obtain treatment they would otherwise not receive. Nevertheless, the fact that researchers are likely to encounter participants suffering from unfair background conditions does not turn an offer of research participation into a threat. The offer to participate in research and receive medical care provides an additional option for people; it does not take some of their options away.

A more critical concern is that research participants may be unduly influenced to participate in research in order to receive desperately needed medical care.[4] People may be unduly influenced when incentives to participate in research are "so attractive [that they] can blind prospective participants to potential risks or impair their ability to exercise proper judgment."[5] Giving someone a reason to do something he or she might not otherwise do, however, is not necessarily problematic. For instance, people are paid salaries to perform their work—and as long as we think the work they do is acceptable, the fact that people have monetary reasons to do their jobs does not concern us. If a night watchman is paid to work in a museum, but would not choose to spend his nights guarding the building for free, we would hardly be troubled that he has been unduly influenced by the money to make a bad decision.[5]

Similarly, when an independent ethics committee has determined the risks of a study are acceptable, then it is not clear that research participants are making a bad choice. In a situation in which people lack access to health care, and the research poses a favorable ratio of risks to benefits (unlike the Dypraxa trial), research participation might be a perfectly rational and sound decision. A valuable take-away lesson for students is to understand that we should be wary of unjustified paternalism in attempts to protect research participants, and that research in developing countries raises complicated questions beyond consent.

In addition to portraying how, in the Dypraxa trial, the participants' consent was not fully informed or voluntary, the movie also provides examples of several other international research ethics issues. For example, the research trial would have been unethical for several reasons even if consent had been valid.[6] The Dypraxa trial was scientifically flawed because research results were manipulated. This undermined the trial's social value, thus exposing participants to risks without the potential to benefit future patients. Moreover, the high number of drug-related deaths in the study suggests that the risks to participants were excessive. The trial apparently lacked common safeguards for minimizing risks to participants, such as independent scientific and ethical review and oversight. These mechanisms would have prevented continued enrollment once the drug's serious side effects had become apparent.

The Dypraxa trial also illustrates that research in resource-limited settings raises concerns about exploitation. One would think that such research would not be exploitative if it is responsive to local health needs and priorities. However, responsiveness to local needs does not safeguard against exploitation. For example, if an investigational drug proves to be safe and effective but is marketed at a high price worldwide, it would probably not be affordable in the country hosting the trial. In this case, hosting communities would assume the risks and burdens of testing the drug whereas its benefits would have accrued mostly to patients in more developed countries.

To avoid this scenario, international ethics guidelines often require that proven interventions are made reasonably available after the trial.[7] However, participants and communities could still receive an unfair level of benefits, or assume an unfair level of risks or burdens, if this requirement is fulfilled. For example, for drugs proven to be unsafe or ineffective, reasonable availability offers no benefits to the participants or the community. Responsiveness and reasonable availability are therefore not always effective in minimizing exploitation in international research.[8]

An alternative approach is to let research participants, communities, and researchers determine which level of benefits is fair, and what types of benefit should be provided.[9] Benefits are thus more broadly defined in order to avoid unwarranted paternalism and enable communities to focus on what matters most to them. This approach would minimize exploitation and help build a spirit of collaborative partnership. However, none of the above considerations regarding exploitation—responsiveness, reasonable availability, or collaborative partnership—seems to have played a role in the Dypraxa trial.

The Constant Gardener describes a clear example of scientific and ethical misconduct. However, it is important for students to recognize that even well-motivated researchers struggle with the complex ethical issues involved in international research. It may therefore be helpful to have students discuss other case studies of research in developing countries, such as the Malorone trial in Thailand, which provides a better illustration of issues related to exploitation in international research.[10] This approach should help students become aware of the challenging and nuanced nature of questions that arise more frequently in international research ethics.

ACKNOWLEDGMENTS

Annette Rid is grateful for financial support from the Swiss National Science Foundation.

NOTE

i. The opinions expressed are the authors' own. They do not represent any position or policy of the National Institutes of Health, Public Health Service, or Department of Health and Human Services.

REFERENCES

1. Thiers, F., Sinskey, A., and Berndt, E. 2008. Trends in the globalization of clinical trials. *Nature Reviews Drug Discovery* 7: 13–14.
2. Carr, D.M. 2003. Pfizer's epidemic: A need for international regulation of human experimentation in developing countries. *Case Western Reserve Journal of International Law* 35(1): 15–53.
3. Wertheimer, A., and Miller, F.G. 2008. Payment for research participation: A coercive offer? *Journal of Medical Ethics* 34(5): 389–392.
4. Emanuel, E.J., Currie, X.E., and Herman, A. 2005. Undue inducement in clinical research in developing countries: Is it a worry? *Lancet* 366(9482): 336–340.
5. Office for Human Research Protections (OHRP). *IRB guidebook*. Washington, DC: OHRP. Retrieved July 28, 2009 from http://www.hhs.gov/ohrp/irb/irb_guidebook.htm
6. Emanuel, E.J., Wendler, D., Killen, J., and Grady, C. 2004. What makes clinical research in developing countries ethical? The benchmarks of ethical research. *Journal of Infectious Disease* 189(5): 930–937.
7. Council for International Organizations of Medical Sciences (CIOMS). 2002. *International Ethical Guidelines for Biomedical Research Involving Human Subjects.*

Geneva: CIOMS. Retrieved July 28, 2009 from http://www.cioms.ch/frame_guidelines_nov_2002.htm

8. Wolitz, R., Emanuel, E.J., and Shah, S. Rethinking the responsiveness requirement for international research. *Lancet* (in press).

9. Participants in the 2001 Conference on Ethical Aspects of Research in Developing Countries. 2002. Fair benefits for research in developing countries. *Science* 298(5601): 2133–2134.

10. Lavery, J.V. 2007. *Ethical issues in international biomedical research: A casebook.* New York: Oxford University Press.

8

state intervention in parental decision making: *gone baby gone*

armand h. matheny antommaria

Gone Baby Gone (2007). Casey Affleck, Michelle Monaghan, Morgan Freeman, Ed Harris. Directed by Ben Affleck. Duration: 114 minutes.

DVD Chapter 18, Scene 1:32:41 to 1:42:36

GONE BABY GONE CENTERS ON the abduction of a young girl, Amanda McCready (Madeline O'Brien). Neighborhood private detectives Patrick Kenzie (Casey Affleck) and Angie Gennaro (Michelle Monaghan) search for Amanda under the false premise that she has been kidnapped by a drug dealer to force her mother, Helene (Amy Ryan), to return $130,000 she stole from him. In fact, she has been abducted by police officers, including Captain Jack Doyle (Morgan Freeman), the head of the Crimes Against Children Unit, at the behest of her uncle Lionel (Titus Welliver). Lionel fears for her welfare if her mother moves away with her. The police initially convince Patrick and Angie that Amanda is dead by staging a botched ransom exchange. Their cover-up begins to unravel after a lead in Patrick's investigation of Amanda's disappearance results in him finding another abducted child, who has been sexually abused and killed, and executing the perpetrator.

Not yet fully comprehending the situation, Patrick and Angie drive to Jack's country house. After Angie unsuccessfully tries to change his mind, Patrick confronts Jack alone. During their exchange, the viewer hears the screen door open and sees Amanda run off the porch into Jack's arms. Patrick finally understands what really happened. Both Jack and Angie attempt to dissuade Patrick from calling the state police. Jack emphasizes Amanda and her future children's welfare and his own greater experience. He states, "… and you ask yourself is she better off here or better off there? You know the answer…" Angie focuses on Amanda's happiness and Jack's love for her. She also asserts returning Amanda to her mother will irreparably damage Angie and Patrick's relationship. Patrick emphasizes the importance of family integrity, as well as the wrong of kidnapping and the right of keeping promises. The viewer sees the state police cars silently arrive with their lights flashing as the score swells. Jack passively goes into custody, but Amanda has to be extracted from his wife's arms.

One of the fundamental issues raised by Gone Baby Gone is the nature of the relationship between parents and children and when, if ever, others should intervene. The extreme ends of the spectrum are the views that the state should raise children and that parents should have absolute authority over their children. The dominant, contemporary view is that there is a rebuttable presumption in favor of parental autonomy and family privacy.[1] This view can be justified both in terms of the benefits of families and the harms of state intervention. Many authors emphasize the intimate nature of family relationships and the necessity of that intimacy for children's development and well-being.[1,2] Parents are also likely to know more about their children's needs and their family's values and priorities.[1,3] Conversely, expert knowledge of child development and proper parenting is limited.[3] Because families bear the burdens of decisions about their children, they should have control over them.[3] In addition to arguing that domestic privacy generally protects children's basic interests,[1] one can also justify a presumption against state intervention based on its limited efficacy.[2,3]

Although a presumption exists in favor of parental autonomy and family privacy, this presumption is rebuttable in cases of abuse or neglect. There are a variety of potential ways to define child abuse and neglect. One can focus primarily on the parent or perpetrator's intention or on the harm to the child. Excessive emphasis on the parent's intention can have several negative consequences. Children may be harmed in the absence of the intention to do so.[4] A focus on parental intent may also increase the likelihood of interventions that produce more harm than good.[3] While not excluding consideration of intention, most definitions of child abuse and neglect view harmful consequences as central. Lori Legano and colleagues define physical abuse as "any nonaccidental injury inflicted or allowed to be inflicted by a parent or caretaker."[5]

One of the central issues remains the relevant threshold for intervention. Medical ethics typically emphasizes that parents should act in their child's best interest. While this standard may be relevant in other domains, such as child custody, it imposes unreasonable demands on parents and disregards other competing interests or rights. One could focus instead on minimum needs or community standards. Focusing on community standards may be problematic because of the difficulty in establishing the standard and because of the variation among communities.[4] Standards are needed to address the magnitude of any intervention, but also to protect the child in the likelihood that something occurs. Thresholds may vary relative to the nature or degree of intervention.

Consider, for example, the boundary between corporal punishment and physical abuse. Parents may inadvertently harm children even if their intention is to correct them, so that their intention is not sufficient. What is the relevant degree of harm? In its "Guidance for Effective Discipline," the American Academy of Pediatrics provides examples of forms of physical punishment that are unacceptable, and identifiable as child abuse. It lists striking a child with an object, striking a child with such intensity that marks lasting more than a few minutes occur, and physical punishment delivered in anger with intent to cause pain as unacceptable, whereas beatings, scaldings, and burnings are examples of child abuse.[6] Setting the threshold too high inadequately protects children, while setting it too low violates family privacy and may also indirectly harm children.

Other considerations, whose detailed discussion are beyond the scope of this chapter, include due process protections.[3] Justice includes consideration not only of fair outcome but also fair process. Basic procedural safeguards may include the ability to present evidence and confront accusers, the guarantee of legal representation, and the specification of who bears the burden of proof and what level of evidence must be met.

Addressing child maltreatment requires the coordinated activities of many entities.[5] Potential abuse and neglect must be identified and reported. In most states, health care providers and others with regular contact with children, such as teachers, are mandated reporters. The threshold for reporting is typically reasonable suspicion.[5,7] Child protective service agencies evaluate reports and, if abuse or neglect is substantiated, intervene by seeking the least intrusive alternative. While lack of resources does not excuse maltreatment, intervention should address contributory factors such s drug abuse.[8] Home visitation is a proven prevention strategy.[5,9] Neglect often requires long-term intervention, support, and follow-up.[8] Removing a child from his or her home and placing the child in foster care may not produce the best outcome. The court functions as a check on state power. The public, in addition, must be willing to support this system for it to function properly.

While *Gone Baby Gone* does present a horrendous example of child sexual and physical abuse, Amanda is portrayed as neglected rather than abused. Neglect can be characterized as physical (including inadequate provision of food, clothing, hygiene, shelter, or supervision), medical, emotional, or educational.[5] Having inherited a unit in a multiplex, Helene and Amanda have stable housing. In spite of the depiction of a messy home with dirty dishes and open junk food on the counters, Amanda appears to have adequate food and clothing and appropriate hygiene. The nonmalevolent natures of Helene's intentions are illustrated by her concern that Amanda's kidnappers might not be feeding her. Although Helene is an alcoholic and drug abuser, it appears she uses drugs outside of the home, and Amanda may not be at substantial risk for inadvertently ingesting them. Emotional neglect is poignantly suggested by Helene's lack of knowledge of her daughter's favorite doll's name, which is revealed in a conversation between Amanda and Patrick at the film's close. While Helene does not necessarily act in her daughter's best interests, Amanda's basic needs appear to be met.

Supervisory neglect is central to the story—Helene leaves Amanda alone at home on the night she is abducted, forsakes her in a car on a sweltering day, and takes her to a bar and along on a drug deal. The American Academy of Pediatrics lists a number of factors to consider in deciding when lack of supervision is neglect, including the length of time and time of day, the child's knowledge of emergency telephone numbers and procedures, and the child's accessibility to his or her parent or to another, specific, informed caregiver.[10] Amanda, a four-year-old, is too young to care for herself. The concern is not only these prior events, but also the possibility that Helene will take Amanda away. Does the likelihood and severity of this risk justify intervention?

The film depicts an extreme, private intervention. Reporting Helene to child protective services is never seriously considered. Although they are police officers, Jack and his colleagues act outside of their official roles. They effectively terminate Helene's parental rights without any due process protections. Less-intrusive alternatives, such as drug treatment for Helene or placement of Amanda with her aunt and uncle, are not considered. The film vividly demonstrates the limitations of prediction and beneficent motives. Patrick and Angie's unanticipated involvement leads the officers to cover up their actions by killing two drug dealers and potentially even Amanda's uncle. Their actions are justified in their minds by a sharp dichotomy between child abusers and protectors. While Patrick's killing of the pedophile is viewed by some characters simply as just retribution, caring for neglected children is complex. The importance of graded and long-term intervention is captured by the final image of Patrick sitting on the couch with Amanda watching cartoons while her mother goes on a date.

REFERENCES

1. Miller, R.B. 2003. *Children, ethics & modern medicine.* Bloomington: Indiana University Press.
2. Goldstein, J., Freud, A., and Solnit, A.J. 1979. *Before the best interests of the child.* New York: The Free Press.
3. Wald, M. State intervention on behalf of 'neglected' children: A search for realistic standards. *Stanford Law Review* 27: 985–1040.
4. Abrams, N. 1979. Problems in defining child abuse and neglect. In O. O'Neill, and W. Ruddick (Eds.), *Having children: Philosophical and legal reflections on parenthood,* pp. 156–164. New York: Oxford University Press.
5. Legano, L., McHugh, M.T., and Palusci, V.J. 2009. Child abuse and neglect. *Current Problems in Pediatric and Adolescent Health Care* 39: 31.e1–26.
6. American Academy of Pediatrics. Committee on Psychosocial Aspects of Child and Family Health. 1998. Guidance for effective discipline. *Pediatrics* 101: 723–728.
7. Levi, B.H. 2008. Child abuse and neglect. In P.A. Singer, and A.M. Viens (Eds.), *Cambridge textbook of bioethics,* pp. 132–140. Cambridge: Cambridge University Press.
8. Dubowitz, H., Giardino, A., and Gustavson, E. 2000. Child neglect: Guidance for pediatricians. *Pediatric Review* 21:111–116.
9. Tenny-Soeiro, R., and Wilson, C. 2004. An update on child abuse and neglect. *Current Opinion in Pediatrics* 16: 233–237.
10. Hymel, K.P. and the Committee on Child Abuse and Neglect. 2006. When is lack of supervision neglect? *Pediatrics* 118: 1296–1298.

9

physician participation in torture and interrogation: *iron jawed angels*

irene martinez

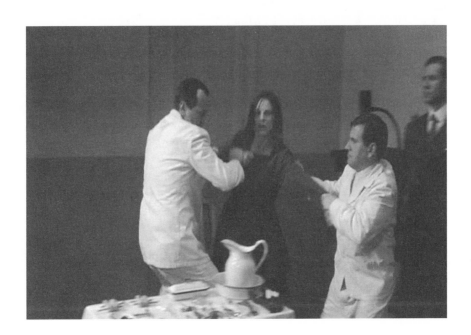

Iron Jawed Angels (2004). Hilary Swank, Frances O'Connor, Julia Ormond, Angelica Houston. Directed by Katja Von Garnier. Duration: 123 minutes.

Scene: DVD chapter 14 Scene 01:41:13 to 01:42:50

I RON JAWED ANGELS TELLS THE story of the struggles and persecution of World War I-era suffragettes led by Alice Paul and Lucy Burns, who advocated a Constitutional Amendment granting women the right to vote. Seen as an embarrassment by the Wilson administration, Paul and other suffragettes were unlawfully incarcerated for picketing in front of the White House. Subjected to mental and physical abuse during their incarceration, Paul brought attention to their unjustified detention and maltreatment by going on a hunger strike. Her fellow imprisoned suffragettes soon joined her.

To prevent the public scandal that would follow Paul's death, government officials ordered her to be force-fed. First, a prison physician interrogated her to determine her mental capacity and intent. To the dismay of the authorities, Paul gave sound and compelling reasons for her refusal to eat. While the film takes some liberties, combining the histories of Alice Paul and Lucy Burns, it effectively portrays the cruelty and horror of force-feeding. The scene to be discussed shows Alice Paul taken in a straightjacket to the jail infirmary by medical personnel. There, she is tied to a chair, her nostrils blocked to compel her to open her mouth, a speculum forced into her oral cavity, and a rubber tube inserted through her esophagus into her stomach as food is poured into her body. This treatment is depicted several times during the film, sometimes with the rubber tube inserted through her nose. Alice Paul suffered from vomiting throughout these procedures and from local injury including bleeding from the gums, mouth, and nostrils. In addition, the treatment was demeaning and humiliating. Suffragettes thus rightly categorized force-feeding as a form of torture, as it would subsequently be defined by the United Nations Convention Against Torture as "cruel, inhuman, or degrading treatment."[1]

Historically, hunger strikes have been associated with some form of protest. Such fasts were undertaken primarily to recover debts, or to obtain justice for perceived wrongs. The primary goal was to "shame" the authority into granting the protestor's demands. In India, such practices date back to as early as 750 BC. In pre-Christian Ireland, where fasting was known as *Troscadh*, contemporary civic codes specifically regulated its use. Allowing a person to die famished at one's doorstep for a wrong of which one was accused was considered a great dishonor. In the past century, prisoners have engaged in hunger strikes and occasionally endured force-feeding, most notably in Ireland and Turkey and, most recently, at Guantanamo Bay. In early 20th-century Great Britain, when suffragettes were incarcerated and routinely subjected to force-feeding, several deaths resulted and the Prisoners' Temporary Discharge of Ill Health Act (1913) responded by provid-ing for the release of fasting suffragettes who became dangerously weak.

The ethical issue of physician participation in force-feeding has been addressed in two separate declarations of the World Medical Association (WMA). The first, promulgated in Tokyo in 1975, is aimed primarily at forbidding physician participa-tion in torture, but contained a proviso on hunger strikes, specifically prohibiting artificial feeding (Article 5, 1975; Article 6, 2006).[2] These provisions were meant to provide support for doctors confronted with prisoners who were victims of torture if these prisoners undertook hunger strikes. Doctors would not be compelled to force-feed or resuscitate detainees in order to make them fit enough to return to torture. The second, the WMA's 1991 Declaration of Malta on hunger strikes (updated in 2006), explicitly forbids force-feeding by physicians, judging the principle of respect for patient autonomy to overrule the principle of beneficence in such cases.[3]

Force-feeding, involving physical restraint, of being held down forcibly while pain- and injury-causing instruments invade the body is cruel, inhumane, and degrading treatment; and thus meets the criteria of torture as defined under the 1975 WMA Tokyo Declaration, which prohibits "the deliberate, systematic, or wanton infliction of physical or mental suffering by one or more persons acting alone or on the orders of any authority, to force another person to yield informa-tion, to make a confession, or for any other reason."[4] The Declaration explicitly prohibits medical doctors from any participation in torture whether actively, passively, or through medical knowledge.

The ethical prohibition against physician participation in torture adopted by the WMA grows out of the experience of World War II and resonates within a broader framework of human rights and the non-derogable prohibition of torture. The most notorious incidents of medical torture were the often-deadly experiments carried out by Dr. Josef Mengele. But other countries, including Japan and the Soviet Union, employed physicians to assist in torture during World War II. In the wake of these revelations, the WMA was created after World War II to ensure the independence of all physicians and to promote and achieve the highest possible standards of ethical behavior and care. While the WMA dec-larations are not enforceable treaties, they internationally recognize guidelines on ethical principles and serve as a template for the medical associations of more than 80 countries, including the American Medical Association (AMA). Using the Declaration of Tokyo as a model, other professional societies passed their own codes condemning medical complicity with torture. The International Council of Nurses, the World Psychiatric Association, the American College of Physicians, and the American Psychiatrics Association are all examples.

Passed in 1976, the UN's International Covenant on Civil and Political Rights stipulated that "no one should be subjected to torture, or cruel, inhuman, or degrading treatment or punishment."[5] While the treaty has been signed by 174 states, it has not yet been ratified (and thus rendered legally binding) by eight of those states, and even when ratified, may contain significant reservations, be poorly enforced, or be effectively nullified by states' legal maneuvering. This treaty was thus followed, in 1987, by the UN Convention Against Torture and Other Cruel, Inhumane or Degrading Treatment or Punishment that specified any act of torture as potentially subject to prosecution by the International Criminal Court at The Hague (a body to which the United States does not currently belong). In 2006, the Optional Protocol to the Convention Against Torture (OPCAT) obligated participating states to submit regular reports and provided for the establishment of a system of "regular visits undertaken by independent international and national bodies to places where people are deprived of their liberty, in order to prevent torture."[6] As of December 2008, 40 countries have become parties to OPCAT, and another 29 countries have signed but not ratified the protocol.

Numerous nongovernmental organizations (NGOs) have attempted to enforce applications of these treaties at the local level. For example, The Los Angeles Offices of the American Friends Service Committee, the Physicians for Social Responsibility, and Program for Torture Victims have coordinated a campaign supporting passage of a California bill outlining physician responsibility in cases of torture. At the international level, the WMA, International Rehabilitation Council for Torture Victims, Human Rights Foundation of Turkey, and Physician Human Rights USA collaborated on the Istanbul Protocol, the first set of international guidelines for identifying evidence of torture, adopted by the UN in 1999.[7]

Despite these international, national, and professional prohibitions, medical complicity with torture and abuse of prisoners remains common in nearly 100 countries, and a third to half of survivors report physicians overseeing torture. Physicians, psychologists, and other medical personnel collude with torture by devising techniques to minimize physical scars and certify prisoners "fit" for abuse, transfer, or rendition; by monitoring vital signs during mistreatment and providing approval for intensified abuse; or by concealing evidence of abuse in medical documents or death certificates.[8]

Addressing the key conflict faced by health professionals called upon both to serve state or military officials by assisting in torture and to abide by the Hippocratic oath, the International Dual Loyalties Working Group in 2003 refined principles laid out by the Nuremberg and Tokyo Declarations and reiterated that it is not permissible for health professionals to perform medical interventions for "security purposes."[9] The "torture memos" released by President Obama in early 2009 document how medical personnel at American detention centers supervised a litany of abuses, notably "multiple water-boardings."[10] Following the release of these memos, the AMA reaffirmed its condemnation of any member's participation in medically assisted torture.

While some physicians have assumed great personal risks to assist prisoners and have become victims themselves, far more physicians remain complicit with abusing prisoners than work in programs to treat torture survivors. The Tokyo Declaration was a landmark event in medical ethics, but Steven Miles and Alfred Freedman recommend that it should go farther, ensuring that physicians complicit in torture are held professionally and criminally accountable and that the declaration should be more readily understandable.[8]

How can local and international associations protect physicians and their families who refuse to take part in torture and interrogations? Article 7 of the Tokyo Declaration states, "The World Medical Association will support, and should encourage the international community, the National Medical Associations, and fellow physicians to support the physician and his or her family in the face of threats or reprisals resulting from a refusal to condone the use of torture."[4] How this recommendation is implemented merits serious discussion and further solutions.

As we have seen, the prohibition against physicians' participation in torture is not only institutionalized by international human rights protocols, but rooted in the time-honored ethics of the Hippocratic Oath to respect doctor–patient relationships, practice beneficence, and do no harm. To fully abide by these commitments, physicians should not only refuse to participate in torture, but become an active voice against torture, in a manner that would make individuals aware of the influence of human rights principles in their daily lives, including the ways in which their own comfort and privilege may rest, directly or indirectly, on acts of torture. Human rights should be taught and discussed at all levels of education and play a key role in medical training.

Considering the ill-treatment of suffragettes such as Alice Paul and Lucy Burns is both a way of recognizing the cruel and degrading nature of force-feeding and of better understanding international struggles for human rights and the prohibition of torture. Above all, their story illustrates the crucial role physicians must play in these struggles by refusing to facilitate torture and honoring their professional commitment to protect their patients from harm and injustice.

REFERENCES

1. United Nations Convention Against Torture or other Cruel Inhumane or Degrading Treatment or Punishment (UNCUT). Retrieved November 15, 2009 from www.hrweb.org/legal/cat.html

2. World Medical Association. 1975. *Declaration of Tokyo* Retrieved August 4 2009 from http://www.wma.net/e/policy/c18.htm. The declaration was revised in 2006, and Article 5 is now Article 6.

3. World Medical Association. 1991. *Declaration on Hunger Strikers* [Declaration of Malta]. Retrieved August 4, 2009 from http://www.wma.net/e/policy/h31.htm. The declaration was revised in 2006.

4. World Medical Association. 1975. *Declaration of Tokyo*. Retrieved August 4, 2009 from http://www.wma.net/e/policy/c18.htm

5. International Covenant on Civil and Political Rights, G.A. res 2200A (XXI), 21 U.N. GAOR Supp. (No.16) at 52, U.N. Doc. A/6316(1966), 999 U.N.T.S. 171; entered in to force March 23, 1976.

6. Optional Protocol to the Convention against Torture (OPCAT). Retrieved November 15, 2009 from http://www2.ohchr.org/english/bodies/cat/opcat/index.htm

7. The Istanbul protocol: International standards for the effective investigation and documentation of torture and ill treatment. 1999. *The Lancet*, 354: 1117.

8. Miles, S., and Freedman, A. 2009. Medical ethics and torture: Revising the Declaration of Tokyo. *The Lancet*, 373(9660): 344–348.

9. Physicians for Human Rights and University of Cape Town Health Sciences Faculty. 2003. *Dual Loyalty and Human Rights in health professionals practice (DLHR)*. Retrieved November 15, 2009 from http://physiciansforhumanrights.org/library/2003-03-06.htm

10. Hopkings, W. 2009. Willing accomplices: Medical complicity and torture. *Medical Foundation for the Care of Victims of Torture* June 16, 2009. Retrieved August 8, 2009 from http://www.torturecare.org/uk/newsfeatures/2544

rights of prisoners: *the lives of others*

silvia quadrelli[i]

The Lives of Others (2006). Martina Gedeck, Hauptmann Gred Wiesler, Sebastian Koch, Ulrich Tukur, Thomas Thieme. Directed by Florian Henckel von Donnersmarck. Duration: 137 minutes.

DVD Chapter 2 scene 00:01:20 to 00:05:56

THE LIVES OF OTHERS IS about the former East Germany, five years before the fall of the Berlin Wall, while it was still controlled by the secret police, the Stasi. The Stasi had about 90,000 employees, but recruited a network of thousands of unofficial employees to report on co-workers, friends, and even family. Stasi Captain Wiesler (Ulrich Muhe) follows orders strictly; his newest assignment is to wiretap a famous author Georg Dreyman (Sebastian Koch) and his girlfriend, actress Christina-Maria (Martina Gedeck). As Wiesler starts to listen, he begins to like the couple, gets caught up in their lives, and sees the emptiness of his own life. As time passes, Wiesler comes increasingly under pressure. A Central Committee official has made it clear to Wiesler and his supervisor Lieutenant Colonel Grubitz (Ulrich Tukur) that Dreyman has to go down. Finally, he finds himself so enchanted by the couple's love and spirit that he decides to remain silent rather than work in the interests of the organization he had so proudly served.

In this scene, Wiesler interrogates a prisoner suspected of helping a friend from the West. The director moves to a scene of a classroom where Wiesler lectures on "enemies of socialism." He is playing an audio tape that demonstrates methods of interrogation, and states how methods such as sleep deprivation can break a liar and provide information. When one of the students says "but this method is so inhumane," Wiesler replies that it is necessary, and identifies the student as one whose judgment is unreliable.

This scene is a good trigger to discuss rights of prisoners and the response that noninvolved witnesses are morally obliged to exert. First of all, it exemplifies a timely concept, namely that of "torture lite," a phrase used to describe a range of techniques that do not obviously injure the victim's body, but may include sleep deprivation, forced stays in stress positions, isolation, noise bombardment, or mock execution, among others.[1] This term has been coined in an attempt by some liberal democracies to justify the use of torture, as if "torture lite" is not "formal torture." This play on words is necessary because torture is considered legally and morally abhorrent.

In the past decades, several international treaties and declarations have condemned the practice of torture by public officials. Promulgated international agreements include the International Covenant on Civil and Political Rights (ICCPR) (prohibiting cruel, inhuman, or degrading punishment), the Geneva Convention (including provisions governing prisoners of war and Common Article 3, which prohibits torture and "outrages on personal dignity"), and the UN Convention Against Torture and Other Cruel, Inhuman, or Degrading Treatment or Punishment (CAT) (prohibiting both torture and cruel, inhuman or degrading treatment in all circumstances). The United Nations charter also prohibits torture, calling upon UN member countries to promote "universal respect for, and observance of, human rights and fundamental freedoms for all… ."); the Universal Declaration on Human Rights states in Article 5 (1948) that "no one shall be subjected to torture or to cruel, inhuman, or degrading treatment or punishment." The CAT, which furthermore requires parties to prohibit the use of torture and mandates the punishment or extradition of torturers found within their territorial jurisdiction, has been signed by over 140 states, including the United States. Torture is also prohibited in the Genocide Convention (1948), the Supplementary Convention on the Abolition of Slavery (1956), the International Convention on the Elimination of All Forms of Racial Discrimination (1965), International Covenant on Civil and Political Rights (1966, entered into force 1976), and the International Convention on the Suppression and Punishment of the Crime of Apartheid (1973).

CAT defines torture as "any act by which severe pain or suffering, whether physical or mental, is intentionally inflicted on a person… by or at the instigation of or with the consent or acquiescence of a public official or other person acting in an official capacity." This definition does not include "pain or suffering arising only from, inherent in, or incidental to lawful sanctions." Importantly, both the European and American Conventions on Human Rights prohibit derogation even in times of war and public emergency, even when those emergencies threaten the survival of the state (common article 15). In a similar way, the International Committee of the Red Cross stressed in the 1949 convention that: "no possible loophole is left; there can be no excuse, no attenuating circumstances" in which torture may be permitted. The World Medical Association's defines torture in the Tokyo Declaration of 1975[2] as "the deliberate, systematic, or wanton infliction of physical or mental suffering by one or more persons acting alone or on the orders of any authority, to force another person to yield information, to make a confession, or for any other reason."

Methods of torture may include various interrogation and detention practices such as isolation, use of extreme temperatures, sensory bombardment, sleep deprivation, forced nakedness, severe humiliation and degradation, or sensory deprivation. Some may be officially authorized by military and civilian officials during certain periods of incarceration. Additional practices include beatings and other forms of severe physical and sexual assault as a part of a regime of brutality during interrogation or detention.[3]

It has been well demonstrated that torture has devastating health consequences on an individual's physical, psychological, and social well-being with a permanent combination of physical and psychological impacts.[4] Sequelar pain from beatings can produce recurrent, intrusive memories of prior torture. Depression resulting from trauma may produce headaches, vertigo, and stomach aches. Torture often results in individuals becoming withdrawn and socially isolated, and impacts a whole community by promoting a culture of fear and general mistrust. Torture and other cruel, inhuman, and degrading treatments of detainees in any of the forms that violate human dignity carry a high risk of psychological damage. Many torture survivors suffer, therefore, from debilitating psychological damage that comes from intense and prolonged fear, shame, humiliation, horror, guilt, and grief, as well as mental and physical exhaustion.[4]

Not only is torture considered legally wrong, but there is a broad consensus (although not unanimous) that it is morally wrong. As Sussman says: "Since the Enlightenment at least there has been a broad and confident consensus that torture is uniquely 'barbaric' and 'inhuman': the most profound violation possible of the dignity of a human being. In fact, during philosophical and ethical discussions, torture is commonly used as one of the few unproblematic examples of a type of act that is morally impermissible without exception or qualification.[5]

Yet the question remains: If no decent person has problems subscribing to the prohibition of torture because it is abhorrent, violates the physical and mental integrity of the person subjected to it, negates autonomy, and deprives one of human dignity by coercing a person to act in a manner that may be contrary to one's most fundamental beliefs and values, why is it now coming under increasing discussion? Some contemporary writers submit that, given the threat terrorists pose to innocent lives, society should consider whether it is better to inflict pain on one guilty person than to place at risk hundreds or even thousands of innocent people, all potential victims of a terrorist atrocity. These writers, as well as many politicians, consider torture as the "lesser evil," accepting the idea of an ethics that, during emergencies, allows leaders to choose between different evils.

It is not the first time that democracies have justified torture. In the 1950s, France believed that it was confronting an entirely new form of warfare in Algeria, and the French police and army believed that "unconventional methods," such as torture, were required. In 1971, the Compton Committee was established to investigate claims that British authorities in Northern Ireland had tortured and abused suspected Irish Republican Army (IRA) terrorists. Currently, the U.S. Defense Department argued that the administration of drugs to detainees would violate the prohibition on torture only if it was calculated to produce "an extreme effect." The Department of Justice insisted that, to count as torture, a prisoner's treatment must inflict more than just moderate or fleeting pain and that, "torture must be equivalent in intensity to the pain accompanying serious physical injury, such as organ failure, impairment of bodily function, or even death."

The defense of licensing torture is associated mainly with Allen Dershowitz because he has strongly defended the argument in several publications, but similar ideas are widely held in both popular and political discourse in the United States. Dershowitz[6] assumes, with absolutely no doubt, that if American law enforcement officers had a captured terrorist who knew about an imminent attack but refused to provide the information, they would try to torture the terrorist into providing the information. His position is that the real question is not whether torture would be used—because it would—but whether it would be used outside of the law or within the law. And so he proposes that torture should be permitted through a "torture warrant" being issued by a judge, based on the absolute need to obtain immediate information in order to save lives. This warrant would limit the torture to nonlethal means, such as sterile needles being inserted beneath the nails to cause excruciating pain without endangering life. Dershowitz's case draws directly from Bentham's utilitarian defense of torture. His proposal for judicially approved "torture licenses" draws upon the findings of the Landau Commission in Israel (1987), whose justification of torture was based on the hypothetical "ticking-bomb" terrorist. In this scenario, a bomb has been planted that is likely to kill large numbers of civilians, and the security services have apprehended a suspect who they believe knows the whereabouts of the bomb but is refusing to talk.

In a similar way Mirko Bagaric and Julie Clarke[7] argue that, when we have a choice between saving the life of an innocent person and not harming a terrorist or other offender, it is indecent to prefer the interests of the offender and that even as brutal an act as torture may be permissible if it has the potential to save innocent lives. They claim that the "main benefit of torture is that it is an excellent means of gathering information." The slippery slope argument can be easily dismissed with the assertion that capital punishment is limited to a relatively small number of crimes and that, as torture is widespread, it is better to adopt a "realistic" rather than moral approach and regulate the practice, thereby making it more responsible. Sanford Levinson[8] notes that the debate over the moral and legal nature of the prohibition on torture is, for the most part, a debate between deontologists and consequentialists. It is one example of the deep difference between accepting that certain actions may be inherently morally wrong, regardless of the consequences of such actions, and that the value of such actions is dependent on their consequences. Deontologists will support an absolute prohibition on torture even in times of catastrophe. Consequentialists will accept that the duty not to torture may be canceled by rival values in certain exceptional circumstances. Bentham clearly believed that in some cases the greater public good required that the prisoner be tortured because the torture of one guilty person for the purpose of saving more than one innocent person satisfies the cost–benefit ratio and is therefore justifiable. On the other hand, others will object that human rights are absolute and categorically without exception.

Many moral theorists have argued against the fallacy of those arguments. Anne O'Rourke, et al.[9] and also Mary Strauss[10] have clearly stated that most of historical, medical, legal, and military evidence refute the efficacy of torture as an information-gathering method. There are many studies showing that false confessions under violent conditions are not only ineffective at getting to the truth, but can actually serve to encourage rather than undermine terrorist groups by strengthening hatred of the torturers.

Beyond the potential ineffectiveness of torture, another moral argument is that tormenting a prisoner violates the key principle of noncombatant immunity that any "just war" requires. By its very nature, torture involves deliberately inflicting harm upon noncombatants. Once a potential terrorist is taken prisoner, he ceases being a combatant, mainly because he is no longer a threat. A person under interrogational torture is completely powerless before his torturers and, no doubt, there is something deeply immoral about damaging someone when he is down, attacking him when there is nothing he can do to defend himself. Terrorism is claimed to be morally and politically abhorrent mainly because it involves harming noncombatants. Therefore, torture is wrong for precisely the same reasons. The prohibition of torture is a peremptory rule.

Concerning the utilitarian concept that the "ends justify the means," Professor Strauss reminds us that such a rationale has never been viewed as the basis of the justice system and that many rules have been developed to precisely guard against such a philosophy.[10] But, additionally, using such an argument to justify the torture of terrorists will cause any nation to lose the moral high-ground in the war against terrorism, lowering them to the same level as the terrorists. As Professor Kremnitzer observed, "the license to employ physical pressure in interrogations constitutes a victory for terror, which has succeeded in causing the State to stoop to quasi-terrorist methods."[10] Torture is evil, not only because of what it does to those tortured, but also because of the great cost to the torturer and society. When the state itself beats and extorts, it can no longer sustain that it rests on foundations of morality and justice, but rather on force. By employing torture, a state reduces the moral distance between a government act and a criminal act.[10] Much research that has been undertaken in the fields of law, medicine, psychiatry, and politics demonstrates that when societies legitimize violent practices, all concepts of morality become distorted and produce practical consequences such as higher arrest rates;. In the words of Anne O'Rourke[11], "these actions become not merely corrosive but implosive, as the atrocity environment turns against itself." In countries where torture has been permitted, a degrading process makes the practice proliferate in the police apparatus, as has been documented in democratic countries (such as with France, in Algeria) and in nations with limited democracy.

Even if torture were morally justified as self-defense in narrow circumstances, and even possibly effective, a strong argument against permitting it is the impossibility of defining when, how, and which circumstances are exceptional enough to permit implementing it. It simply shows that the ticking-bomb scenario is quite useless as a moral reasoning and that by invoking fear through the use of an extreme, yet unrealistic, construction of facts constitutes what David Luban describes as "intellectual fraud."[11] The ticking-bomb scenario is absolutely unrealistic—the reality is that captors typically do not know whether there is a ticking bomb at all or whether their captive has any useful information about it.[12] Certainly none of the instances of torture in the U.S. war on terror have come close to the ticking-bomb scenario, and a great problem with creating an exception for those exceptional circumstances is slippage.[13] If the practice becomes normalized, the justification to use it drops from the extreme need to save lives to the wish to extract rapid information. No matter how much one tries to confine the use of torture to extreme circumstances, the temptation to broaden those circumstances is inevitable.[13] There is also some evidence that slippage and normalization are occurring in the war on terror, and evidence from Israel, the United States, the United Kingdom, and elsewhere suggests that, in normative contexts wherein the judiciary is prepared to tolerate torture, its use becomes easily extended. Once the absolute moral prohibition has vanished, its authorization turns into only a bureaucratic procedure.

A difference exists between completely ignoring truly catastrophic cases and focusing our attention mainly on those cases when designing general rules and policies.[14] Ignoring the consequences of catastrophic cases may result in turning the legal system unrealistic and inadequate, and legal rigidity in the face of severe crises may be hypocritical or even detrimental.[13] Advocates of absolute prohibition of torture face the dilemma of what to do in catastrophic cases, but most absolutists seem to resolve the dilemma by conceding that catastrophic cases call for exceptional treatment, but not for general policies. Therefore, it can be said that, in spite of controversial voices, the prohibition of torture is a peremptory rule of international law. It is also contrary to the ethics of war because it violates the principle of noncombatant immunity, as all prisoners are noncombatants and must not be harmed. Morally, it violates the essential principle of human dignity.

Those considerations are extended to any kind of torture. There is enough experience showing that "torture lite" victims suffer long-term consequences such as persistent amnesia, serious physical complications, and temporary psychosis with permanent damage. In addition, "torture lite" methods have contributed to death, as in the case of the Afghani prisoner who froze to death after being stripped naked and left in an interrogation cell without blankets.[1]

The Lives of Others does not raise the issue of a doctor's participation in torture, but discussing the permissibility of torture in a medical ethics group will necessarily call attention to that subject. In that field, ethical scenarios are much less controversial. No doubt, safeguarding the health, integrity, and dignity of all detainees (whether they are guilty or not) is a duty for the medical profession.[15] Preventing torture is everyone's business—but three professions seem to be especially well suited to prevent torture: medicine, law, and the military.[16] Physicians have the obligations that come from their universally recognized and respected role as healers. As Sagan and Jonsen[17] observed, the medical skills used for healing can be maliciously perverted "with devastating effects on the spirit and the body"; therefore, it is "incumbent upon the medical profession and upon all of its practitioners to protest in effective ways against torture as an instrument of political control." As Kotow[18] states "an ethical crossroad lies between accepting that warlike conditions may temporarily obliterate medical rights, duties, and the moral convictions of medicine on the one hand, and witnessing how bioethics distorts and adjusts its normative language to the needs and whims of strategists on the other. Moral justification of medical participation in bellicose acts is an unfortunate distortion of professional ethics."

In 1975, the World Medical Association adopted the Declaration of Tokyo,[2] which is very clear about the subject: "The doctor's fundamental role is to alleviate the distress of his or her fellow men, and no motive whether personal, collective, or political shall prevail against this higher purpose. The doctor shall not countenance, condone, or participate in the practice of torture or other forms of cruel, inhuman, or degrading procedures, whatever the offence of which the victim of such procedure is suspected, accused or guilty, and whatever the victim's belief or motives, and in all situations, including armed conflict and civil strife." And it goes on to state that "the doctor shall not be present during any procedure during which torture or other forms of cruel, inhuman, or degrading treatment are used or threatened."

The British Medical Association in its Torture Report[19] states the duty of doctors to inform on activities breaching the Declaration of Tokyo and specifies that this duty transcends any question of national security: If a doctor knows of some activity breaching the Declaration of Tokyo, then the doctor has a duty to speak out, thus making clear the difference between the doctors and the state. In the same vein, the American Medical Association supports calls for a new investigation into whether doctors were complicit in the torture of prisoners held by U.S. military forces in Iraq and Afghanistan, with the intention of censuring, suspending, or expelling any member found to have violated its principles of medical ethics.

Politicians, philosophers, and society itself may manage to find reasons to accept torture of any kind, but the involvement of health care professionals should not be ethically accepted in any way. The physician–society relationship is mainly based on trust, and both the medical professions and society need the reassurance that, while taking part in any sort of war, the participation in torture by those engaged in caring and helping will never receive ethical approval. The first principle is still "do not harm."

NOTE

i. The editors intentionally choose to devote two essays to this movie (see M. Davoudi, *Speaking out against oppression*) in order to illustrate how various scenes from the same film can be used to initiate discussion on related topics: in this case, a society's responsibility to speak out against oppression, in conjunction with one's moral obligation to protect individual rights.

REFERENCES

1. Wolfendale, J. 2009. The myth of "torture lite." *Ethics & International Affairs* 23: 47–61.

2. World Medical Association. 1975. Guidelines for medical doctors concerning torture and other cruel, inhuman or degrading treatment or punishment in relation to detention and imprisonment. In the *Declaration of Tokyo*. Retrieved January 2, 2010 from http://web.amnesty.org/pages/health-ethicswmatokyo-eng

3. Physicians for Human Rights. *Report: Broken laws, broken lives: Medical evidence of torture by US personnel and its impact*. Retrieved February 2, 2010 from http://brokenlives.info/?page_id=69

4. Physicians for Human Rights. 2005. *Break them down: The systematic use of psychological torture by US forces*. Retrieved February 2, 2010 from http://physiciansforhumanrights.org/library/report-2005-may.html [hereinafter PHR Break Them Down].

5. Sussman, D. 2005. What's wrong with torture? *Philosophy and Public Affairs* 33(1): 2.

6. Dershowitz, A. January 22, 2002. Want to torture? Get a warrant. *San Francisco Chronicle*.

7. Bagaric, M., and Clarke, J. 2005. Not enough official torture in the world? The circumstances in which torture is morally justifiable. *University of San Francisco Law Review* 39: 581.

8. Levinson, S. 2005. In quest of a 'common conscience': Reflections on the current debate about torture. *1 Journal of National Security Law and Policy* 231, 232.

9. O'Rourke, A., Chaudhri, V., and Nyland, C. Torture, slippery slopes, intellectual apologists, and ticking bombs: An Australian response to Bagaric and Clarke. *University of San Francisco Law Review* 40: 85–108.

10. Strauss, M. 2004. Torture. *48 New York Law School Review* 201, 261–262.

11. Luban, D. 2005. Liberalism, torture, and the ticking bomb. *Virginia Law School Review* 91, 1425–1454.

12. Colb, S.F. 2008. Why is torture 'different' and how 'different' is it? *Columbia Public Law & Legal Theory Working Papers*. Paper 08148. Retrieved from http://lsr.nellco.org/columbia_pllt/08148

13. Bellamy, A. 2006. No pain, no gain? Torture and ethics in the war on terror. *International Affairs* 82:121–148.

14. Gross, O. 2007. Torture and an ethics of responsibility. *Law, Culture and the Humanities* 3: 35–54.

15. Chariot, P., Martel, P., Penneau, M., and Debout, M. 2008. Guidelines for doctors attending detainees in police custody: A consensus conference in France. *International Journal of Legal Medicine* 122:73–76.

16. Annas, G.J. 2005. Unspeakably cruel—torture, medical ethics, and the law. *The New England Journal of Medicine* 352(20): 2127–2132.

17. Sagan, L.A., and Jonsen, A. 1976. Medical ethics and torture. *New England Journal of Medicine* 294: 1427.

18. Kottow, M.H. 2006. Should medical ethics justify violence? *Journal of Medical Ethics* 32: 464–467.

19. Working party of the British Medical Association investigating the involvement of doctors in torture. 1986. *The torture report*. London: British Medical Association.

part seven

reproduction, genetics, and sexuality

artificial insemination:
and then came love

patricia digilio and nazanin z. rohani

And Then Came Love (2007). Vanessa Williams, Michael Boatman, Jeremy Gumbs. Directed by Richard Schenkma. Duration: 90 minutes.

DVD chapter 3 scene 00:11:30 to 00:15:00

JULIE DAVIDSON (VANESSA WILLIAMS) IS a confident, autonomous, successful woman who, several years earlier, had decided to become a single mother by resorting to artificial insemination by an anonymous donor. When her son Jack begins inquiring about his father and social pressures from school begin to mount, Julie begins a quest for the original donor, one which will ultimately lead her to change her life.

In this scene, Julie is called for a meeting at her son's school. Apparently, behavioral problems are negatively interfering with Jack's learning. Teachers suggest this might be the result of his peculiar family situation. Upset by the situation, Julie tells a family friend that she had paid special attention to the donor's physical and intellectual qualities, finally deciding upon one with high grades from a prestigious university. Julie wonders whether Jack's problems at school might not be due to hereditary factors, and she becomes suspicious of the truth about her anonymous donor. To clear up any doubts, she embarks on her quest, breaking the rules of confidentiality and anonymity that govern the practice of artificial insemination.

Separating procreation from sexuality prompts questions about many assumptions of our culture in regard to life's origins, transmission of biological and cultural inheritance, kinship bonds, maternity, and paternity. Nowadays, many extraordinary operations are possible; cells are extracted, donated, and used as the exchange products of social relationships. This has caused deep alterations in our way of thinking about procreation. The analysis of ethical issues derived from these new conditions must take into account that insemination fulfills the needs of couples or persons wishing to have children, and elicits a new series of material and discursive practices in the biomedical sciences that drastically alter many basic assumptions of our culture.

The technical complexity of artificial insemination is not directly proportional to the ethical, legal, and social problems arising from its implementation. One question is whether the difference between a natural form of reproduction and an artificial or technological one implies a values hierarchy: granting privilege to one person over another. Either a "natural" and immutable family cell exists, or the way in which families can be constructed is the result of science and social phenomena, and thus liable to transformation. If this is the case, these new forms of parent–child bonding constitute family forms with specific problems that demand consideration from new perspectives.

The leading character in *And Then Came Love* resorts to artificial insemination from an anonymous donor in order to procreate. Artificial insemination consists of placing sperm into the female reproductive tract without intercourse. The inseminated sperm may belong to the male partner in a couple or may come from an anonymous donor. This last method is usually suggested in cases of sterility, when there is low or zero sperm mobility in the couple's male partner, or when the male is carrying a serious hereditary disease. Nevertheless, as shown in the movie, its implementation has been extended to other cases, such as when a woman desires a child but does not want or have a male partner.

The decision to resort to a donor is followed by the difficult decision of donor selection. Accordingly, three general conditions must be observed. First, donor sperm, which must not contain harmful germs or a genetic profile liable to endanger the child, must be able to fertilize the female's eggs. Second, the donor must have physical characteristics that are not discordant with the couple or the recipient nucleus. Measures are also taken to prevent matching a donor and a recipient who may present with equal risks for child pathology. When the donor is anonymous, there is an additional ethical and contractual requirement of preserving anonymity.

Anonymity is presented as an ethical rule that allows for the circulation of procreative substances while safeguarding the confidentiality and privacy of all parties involved in the transaction. This results in a direct contradiction and confrontation between two value systems. The first, mandating unconditionally the anonymity of the donor protects the private life of the couples and/or individuals participating in this process. The second, by affirming the right of all children to know their biological origins, protects a person's right to biological identity and rejects establishing anonymity as an absolute rule. The family created by artificial insemination is thus founded on a secret that cannot be revealed (the identity of the donor) but that is always present and whose consequences on the life of the child (and parent) cannot be predicted. The consequentialist interest in protecting the donors' market and avoiding the concern of potential donors about future paternity claims provides additional arguments in support of anonymity.

In recent years, however, an increase in gamete donation has been followed by a trend advocating nonanonymity in donor programs and disclosure to offspring of donor gamete conception.[1] Legislation in some countries allows offspring access to information about the donor.[2] Internationally, most countries endorse anonymous gamete donation. Some countries (France, Denmark and Norway) do not allow donor offspring any information about their conception. Others, such as Sweden, Austria, and Switzerland allow identifying information. In the United States, no legislation at either the federal or state level prohibits or enforces anonymous gamete donation.[3] In the United Kingdom, anonymity is preferred but not compulsory. Some investigators and mental health professionals have noted, however, donors' increasing willingness to be made known to recipient parents and offspring.[4,5]

Anonymity is designed to protect prospective parents, donors,[6] and intermediaries, including medical practitioners.[7] There is no doubt that, where a choice must be made between the interests of birth parents and donors and the interests of donor offspring, the presumption should be in favor of the children. When interests are in conflict with those of offspring, resolution has usually been in favor of the former.

This philosophy is changing, in part because of the increased consideration of the vulnerable nature of children, as recognized by family law and the United Nations Convention on the Rights of the Child.[8] Many ethicists feel that policies of anonymous gamete donation contravene Article Seven of the Convention on the Rights of the Child, which includes the right to know one's parents, and Article Eight of the European Convention on Human Rights (respect for family life). Taking into account that those conventions were not focused on this newly available technology, the Council of Europe stated, "it is not possible—at the present moment—to draw decisive arguments from the Convention for the Protection of Human Rights and Fundamental Freedoms either in favor of or against the anonymity of donors."[9]

Evidence suggests that parents are unwilling to tell their children that they were conceived with donated gametes. Several studies found that 70%–90% of parents had not informed their donor offspring of the circumstances of their conception.[3] It is evident that couples are not comfortable with secrecy, however, and many are in fact reluctant to use the word "secrecy" to describe their behavior.[10] The best interests of donor offspring will be sustained against those arguments for anonymity, stating that infertile individuals or couples and gamete donors are voluntary participants of a process, but that donor offspring have no control over the secrecy regarding mode of conception or the identity of their gamete donor.[11] This means that children are at the mercy of their birth parents, their gamete donors, and the legal system. They are the only ones who cannot provide an opinion about their desire to know their genetic heritage.[12] Trust within the family could be irreparably damaged if donor offspring do one day learn, perhaps from someone other than their birth parents, the truth of their conception. Additionally, extrapolating from what we have learned from adoption, a concrete concern is the development of "genealogical bewilderment"; that not knowing one's origins could have a bewildering effect on children, induce a great state of confusion, and have a negative effect on the adoptee's personal growth.

In conclusion, the exaggerated power that today's culture attributes to genes in the physical and psychic formation of an individual is illustrated in *And Then Came Love* by Julie's precautions and demands when considering donor selection. Some argue that children should be told whether one (or both) of their birth parents is not their genetic relative, and that gamete donor(s) should be disclosed because lack of knowledge of one's genetic origins has potentially adverse psychosocial implications, and because our genetic heritage is part of our identity. Others claim that focusing so strongly on anonymity versus disclosure is just another example of genetic essentialism, whereby providing knowledge of one's genetic parents is given special importance beyond that given to nongenetic ones.

In one sense, we might question whether Julie's desire for a son might not also have included a desire for other guarantees relating to "product" quality. Artificial insemination thus risks becoming a means to an end, as if requesting a child of a particular sex might also include the request that the child carry specific physical or intellectual attributes. We can only contemplate the ethical and social consequences of granting privilege to a deterministic vision in which the innate prevails over the acquired in characterizing the human condition: Individual destinies would be naturally fixed "in the genes." How then, would freedom and autonomy be affected? What will become of genetic patrimonies, and what new modes of discrimination might our society encounter as new social categories are thus constructed?

REFERENCES

1. Sheib, J.E., and Cushing, R.A. 2007. Open-identity donor insemination in the United States: Is it on the rise? *Fertility and Sterility* 88: 231–232.
2. Ethics Committee of the American Society for Reproductive Medicine. Informing offspring of their conception by gamete donation. *Fertility and Sterility* 81: 527–531.
3. Frith, L. 2001. Beneath the rhetoric: The role of rights in the practice of non-anonymous gamete donation. *Bioethics* 15(5-6): 473–484.
4. Crawshaw, M., Blyth, E.D., Daniels, K.D. 2007. Past semen donors' views about the use of a voluntary contact register. *Reproductive Biomedicine Online* 14: 411–417.
5. Shehab, D., Duff, J., Pasch, L.A., et al. 2007. How parents whose children have been conceived with donor gametes make their disclosure decision: Contexts, influences, and couple dynamics. *Fertility and Sterility* 89:179–187.
6. Daniels, K.R., and Taylor, K. 1993. Secrecy and openness in donor insemination. *Politics and Life Sciences* 12: 200–203.
7. Haimes, E.V. (1993). Do clinicians benefit from gamete donor anonymity? *Human Reproduction* 9: 1518–1520.
8. United Nations General Assembly. 1989. *The Convention on the Rights of the Child*, Articles 3, 8.
9. Council of Europe. 1998. *Medically assisted procreation and the protection of the human embryo comparative study on the situation in 39 States*, p. 27. Strasbourg.
10. Landau, R. 1998. Secrecy, anonymity, and deception in donor insemination. *Social Work in Health Care* 28(1): 75–89.
11. Johnston, J. 2002. Mum's the word: Donor anonymity in assisted reproduction. *Health Law Review* 11(1): 51–55.
12. Triseliotis, J. 1988. Identity and genealogy. In N. Bruce, A. Mitchell, and K. Priestley (Eds.), *Truth and the child: A contribution to the debate on the Warnock report*. Edinburgh, UK: Family Care.

abortion: *if these walls could talk*

lawrence j. nelson

If These Walls Could Talk (1996). Demi Moore, Sissy Spacek, Anne Heche, Cher, Xander Berkeley, Jada Pinkett Smith. Directed by Nancy Savoca and Cher. Duration: 97 minutes.

DVD chapter 5 Scene 00:23:25 to 00:26:17

IF THESE WALLS COULD TALK, a made-for-television movie originally broadcast on HBO, portrays three women's personal conflict over abortion, all of whom happened to live in the same house over the course of five decades. The first story, set in 1952, deals with Claire Donnelly (Demi Moore), a nurse whose husband recently died during the Korean War. Claire discovers she is pregnant after having an emotional, late-night encounter with her brother-in-law, who had confronted her about her excessive drinking while grieving. Desperate to end her pregnancy, maintain her own reputation and life, and protect her late husband's family from the shame of her having an illegitimate child by one of their own, Claire tries unsuccessfully to self-abort with an overdose of prescription medication and a knitting needle. As a medical abortion is illegal, she then turns to a cash-up-front, back-alley abortionist who ends her pregnancy while she is stretched out on her kitchen table… and she shortly thereafter loses her life due to a massive hemorrhage.

Barbara Barrows (Sissy Spacek), a supermom of four children and wife to a police officer working nights, wrongly thought she was done with having and raising babies. Her life is so crowded with domestic chores (she does the shopping, washes the dishes, cleans her children's rooms for them, irons, cooks, etc.) and college that it takes her the better part of a day to tell her husband the surprising and troubling news. While at school, she borrows the first edition of *Our Bodies, Ourselves* from the library and reads about abortion. Her deep desire to stay in school and conversations with her best friend who has had an abortion ("Do you regret it?" "No, I really don't," she responds. Her friends told her she'd be depressed and feel guilty, but "Honestly, I was so relieved. But not everyone's the same"), her high school senior daughter ("You know, Mom, you can get one at any health clinic. It's your legal right"), and her husband ("I don't know what the hell else you want to do. I don't know what you have in mind. What do you think the alternative is?") don't make her struggle any easier. Ultimately, she decides not to have an abortion: "I'm going to have the baby. I don't know if it's the right decision. It's just the only one I can live with."

The third story, set in 1996, concerns Christine Cullen (Anne Heche), a college student having an affair with her married architecture professor and who unintentionally becomes pregnant by him. He gives her some money, presumably to have an abortion, and leaves her on her own to deal with the pregnancy. Her roommate and best friend describes her as someone who "doesn't believe in abortion," but Christine thinks she can't go through with the pregnancy and visits a reproductive health clinic. There, she meets some antiabortion protestors who urge her to reconsider, offer her help with lodging and baby supplies, and suggest the fetus will feel pain during the abortion. Christine leaves the clinic still pregnant and tells the protestors that she couldn't go through with it. The protestors rejoice and pray in gratitude for a life saved. That night, she gets drunk at a party and tearfully begs her best friend (who has previously told her that if she has an abortion, she is "on her own") to help her ("Patti, I made a mistake. I made one hell of a big mistake. Could you forgive me for making a mistake, friend?"). They both return to the clinic on the following day while a large and loud protest ensues outside. Christine is determined to go through with the abortion, and escorts scramble to get her past the demonstrators (on both sides of the controversy) and into the clinic. Right after the procedure is finished, one of the protestors bursts into the room and proceeds to shoot the physician (Cher) to death in a shower of blood. The story ends with Christine holding the physician's head in her lap and futilely shouting for help.

Abortion can be considered a third-level moral issue, reached only after considering the ethics of engaging in potentially reproductive sexual activity and the use of contraception. Many feminists claim that, as women's choices in these areas are often constrained, their access to abortion should not be.[1,2] The three stories don't directly address these issues, but they show how they happened to play out for these particular women. Claire—probably drunk, surely lonely and angry over the loss of her husband—has sex with her brother-in-law after he confronts her over her heavy drinking and initiates intimate contact. She considers it a mistake, and when he apologizes for what happens, she tells him "it never happened" and conceals her pregnancy from him. Contraception isn't mentioned, but then, in the 1950s and in such circumstances, there's not much to say. Barbara conceived after fully consensual sex with her husband, but we're told nothing about their use of contraception. Barbara says, "I just thought I was done [having kids], that's all. I thought I was finished." Due to what? Menopause? Wishful thinking? Christine has an affair with her professor ("I'm screwed for screwing the nutty professor") and gets pregnant. Again, we're not told if they used contraception or if it failed. And we're left wondering if, in the last analysis, it really matters.

The film doesn't take us very far, if at all, into the conceptual moral questions at the heart of the abortion controversy: What is the moral status of the fetus? Does it change over the period of gestation? Does its moral status depend entirely upon the will of the pregnant woman? If it's wrong to claim that fetal life is morally unimportant, isn't it equally wrong to claim that the woman's life—with her varied relationships, hopes, plans, and values—is unimportant? Should early abortion be legal and readily available to women, while late abortion should be restricted to cases in which the women's life or health are at serious risk? This well-acted and produced film allows us to experience some small part of what comes to bear upon the minds and hearts of women—and those related to them—when an unexpected and unwanted pregnancy presents itself. After all, abortion is not just a meta-ethical problem about who has what rights and interests, the nature of moral and legal personhood, and who should ultimately decide when someone becomes a mother and father, with the heavy responsibilities of raising a child in today's uncertain world.

I have shown this film to many of my undergraduate ethics classes, and the clear majority of my students do not find it to be a heavy-handed piece of pro-choice propaganda. To be fair, the movie is clearly sympathetic to women truly having choice—the choice to bear a child even in the face of personal and family adversity (Barbara), as well as the choice to end a pregnancy for reasons the woman finds compelling (Christine), without her being impelled by circumstances and the legal system to do so in a dangerous manner (Claire). All three stories, although compact and incomplete, are believable and rightly make the point that there is no such thing as a generic pregnancy: Every prenatal human exists inside an individual woman with her own story. The film does, however, contain several graphic and potentially disturbing images: Claire sticking a knitting needle into her womb; blood on the floor as she bleeds to death following the illegal abortion she so desperately sought; the clash (both physical and moral) between the pro-life and pro-choice demonstrators at the clinic where Christine seeks to end her pregnancy; and the bloody, terrible violence of the shooting death of the physician.

This film has significant educational value in several ways. First, the overwhelming majority of today's students were not alive when abortion was illegal in the United States. Claire's story takes them back to that time and can help them experience and understand the desperation of a woman with an unwanted and unintended pregnancy, the disclosure of which would devastate her and her family. Second, all three stories show how gender affects abortion. Claire faces her situation alone and takes the burden of dealing with it entirely upon herself. After using the knitting needle, Claire tearfully discloses her pregnancy to her sister-in-law who responds "How could you do this?…If my mother ever finds out about this, it'll kill her. So, I don't give a damn what you do. How dare you shame us like this?" Barbara, the 40-something, old-fashioned, stay-at-home, do-it-all mom, finally gets to go back to college after some 20 years of taking care of her four children and husband… and is surprised with a pregnancy. Her husband can't seem to appreciate how she hates the prospect of losing the part of her life that she has regained or even mention abortion as an option. Christine receives no support or help from the man who, along with her, is responsible for the pregnancy—other than an envelope with money he expects her to use to pay for the abortion. She tells the clinic counselor, "It's so not fair. It just doesn't seem fair at all. He goes about his life and I'm here, making this decision. And I'm having a hard time thinking about the baby being ripped out of me." Christine wants to, but doesn't, tell her Irish Catholic mother about her pregnancy because she is the "good girl" in the family, and her parents are dealing with her brother who is only recently out of drug rehab.

No one film can possibly delve very deeply into the moral, human, and social tangle of abortion. Some more recent popular films address pregnancy, but don't even allude to abortion (*Knocked Up*, *Waitress*). The pregnant teen in *Juno* actually goes to an abortion clinic and meets a single, likewise teenaged antiabortion protestor, but both encounters are, rightly or wrongly, treated with the writer's tongue more than firmly planted in her cheek. *If These Walls Could Talk* gives us a more serious look at the personal struggle that an unwanted pregnancy can throw a woman into, a look that may lead us to better appreciate what that struggle, that bit of hell, is like now—and what it was like in the past.

REFERENCES

1. Sherwin, S. 1992. *No longer patient: Feminist ethics & health care*, pp. 99–116. Philadelphia, PA: Temple University Press.
2. Tooley, M., Wolf-Devine, C., Devine, P.E., Jaggar, A.M. 2009. *Abortion: Three perspectives*, pp. 120–175. New York: Oxford University Press.

3

enhancement technologies:
the incredibles

michael j. green

The Incredibles (2004). Craig T. Nelson, Holly Hunter, Samuel L. Jackson, and Jason Lee. Directed by Brad Bird. Duration: 115 minutes.

DVD Chapter 4: Scene 00:14:48 to 00:15:38[i]

DVD Chapter 24: Scene 01:29:30 to 01:30:25[ii]

THE INCREDIBLES IS AN ANIMATED film about the midlife crises of former superheroes no longer appreciated by the public who once adored them. At their peak, Mr. Incredible and Elastigirl were popular crime fighters, until a series of lawsuits forced "supers" like them underground, to be relocated into a witness protection program so they could live "normal" (and anonymous) lives. Fifteen years pass, and Mr. Incredible and Elastigirl marry, have children, and are now known exclusively by their new identities, Bob and Helen Parr.

Bob works in the insurance industry and is frustrated by his job and his insufferable boss; he yearns for more excitement and meaning in his mundane, suburban life. When Bob is contacted by a mysterious woman and offered the chance to once again play the role of Mr. Incredible, he eagerly pursues the opportunity. Soon, however, he discovers that this is a trap set by a previously unknown nemesis named Syndrome, who, as an adolescent, aspired to be Mr. Incredible's sidekick until he was rebuffed and sent away.

While Mr. Incredible is endowed with "natural" super-powers, Syndrome acquired his powers through the use of technology, which he now harnesses to enrich himself, boost his ego, and obliterate as many former "supers" as he can find. Syndrome's objectives are partly self-serving and partly social engineering: His ultimate goal is to destroy social inequalities based on natural attributes, so as to level the playing field on which he unsuccessfully competed as an adolescent. "When everyone's super... no one will be," proclaims an indignant Syndrome, revealing a righteous sense of injustice underlying his evil ways.

But Syndrome is not the only one frustrated by the manner in which natural talents are allocated and utilized. Mr. Incredible's own son, Dash, endowed with super-speed, is forced to live his life in slow motion, just to fit in and "pass" as a normal kid. Dash hates it, and cannot understand why he is forbidden from using his special talents. His mother rationalizes that "everyone is special," but Dash will have none of this, pouting that this "is another way of saying no one is."

While not a central focus of the film, it is notable that in *The Incredibles*, the "good guys" are those whose powers are endowed naturally, while the "bad guy" (Syndrome) acquired his power through artificial technologic enhancement. This directorial choice of equating good with natural and evil with technological may be unintended, but it does reflect the long-held view in American society that people should succeed on their own merits. For instance, in his 1813 letter to John Adams,[1] Thomas Jefferson articulated such a belief in the context of who is best fit to lead, arguing, "there is a natural aristocracy among men. The grounds of this are virtue and talents." Jefferson then goes on to say that although "the invention of gunpowder has armed the weak as well as the strong," the natural aristocracy is most fit to govern.

Current thinkers who oppose enhancement technologies have a different reason for their unease; they fear that such technologies might be "dehumanizing" and that their use would undermine our human dignity: "To turn a man into a cockroach—as we don't need Kafka to show us—would be dehumanizing. To try to turn a man into more than a man might be so as well."[2] Of course, in a pluralistic society such as ours, such views about the inviolability of humanity's natural endowments are not universally held. Many see no problem with using technology for human advancement, and in fact embrace its use toward this end. The transhumanist movement, for example, holds that human nature can be improved through applied science, and that people should have broad discretion in determining how to use enhancement technologies for a wide range of health-related decisions that apply not only to themselves, but to their offspring as well.[3]

The Incredibles raises important questions about social equity and the role that medicine and technology should play in promoting a meritocratic society. Should individuals use technology to magnify their abilities, so that they can compete with those who naturally run faster, jump higher, or are endowed with greater strength? Or, is this somehow a form of "cheating," providing, as it were, some individuals with an unfair advantage that they do not deserve? Historically, medical professionals were hesitant to use their skills and resources to enhance healthy individuals, instead preferring to apply their expertise to the treatment of those with diseases. That is, when a "patient" had a problem that impaired so-called "normal" physiological functioning, then professionals willingly provided medications or surgical procedures in an attempt to restore his or her equilibrium. But, when a person who was *not* sick requested those same resources to enhance themselves, the profession balked, viewing such activities as outside the scope of legitimate professional activity and perhaps even an unjust use of resources. Of course, in these days of Viagra, cosmetic surgery, and steroid-enhancing drugs in sports, this pattern has changed. Now, advances that were originally aimed at the sick are quickly exported to the merely "needy," and soon after to anyone who is looking for an advantage.[4]

Such changes in medical practice reflect an underlying ambivalence about a number of concepts: (a) traditional notions of normalcy, (b) what it means to be authentic to oneself, and (c) how personal identity might be altered by technology. In actual practice, it is very difficult (and sometimes impossible) to distinguish normal from abnormal, or authentic from artificial, a problem that has implications for identifying who has a legitimate claim to medical treatment. Consider, for instance, an example provided by Allen and Fost in an article about whether growth hormone should be provided to nondiseased individuals.[5] Johnny and Billy are two hypothetical 11-year-old boys. Both are below the mean height for children their age, and both are predicted to reach a final adult height of 5 feet, 3 inches. While Johnny's short stature originates from a brain tumor that results in growth hormone deficiency, Billy secretes growth hormone normally. His only problem is that he has short parents. On what grounds can we justify providing growth hormone treatment to Johnny, but not to Billy? Neither bears personal responsibility for his small size, and both are at risk for encountering the same grade school taunting, economic disadvantages, and other drawbacks that can result from shortness.[5,6] In both cases, the desire for growth hormone treatment represents an equally reasonable response to a social world that often prefers tall people to short people. Is there any morally relevant reason why one should receive growth hormone while the other is denied it?

In part, this is a question about what it means to be authentic to oneself, and whether individuals remain authentic when they use medical technologies to alter and improve themselves. On the one hand, people have always aspired to improve themselves via external measures. People buy dietary supplements, choose the best schools, wear expensive clothes, put on makeup, and employ coaches. On the other hand, it would seem that at some point, externalities can so change a person that his or her identity is no longer the same. But establishing the precise point at which such interventions render one "untrue" to herself is not at all clear. Carl Elliott explores this theme in his provocative book *Better Than Well*,[7] using examples such as shyness, excessive blushing, and even unwanted regional dialects to illustrate the complexity of determining our authentic from inauthentic selves. Such conditions did not receive widespread medical attention nor warrant treatment until they were defined as clinical conditions (often by the pharmaceutical companies marketing drug therapies). But, after these conditions were articulated in clinical and/or pathological terms, then fixing them became a matter of restoring people to their authentic selves, and the profession embraced the task of treating these "maladies" without threats to their legitimacy.

While *The Incredibles* does not directly take on the culture war tensions of the enhancement/nonenhancement debate, it can be viewed as a modern-day morality play that reflects a particular perspective of good and evil. Ultimately, Syndrome is defeated, and along with him, his vision for a technologic-inspired egalitarian world. That viewers applaud this ending may reflect little more than a skillful portrayal of an unlikable villain who deserves to be defeated. Yet, this is not as simple as it seems. Despite the obvious wrongness of his methods, Syndrome's challenge to use one's intelligence and creativity to harness technology for improving upon native physical abilities is never seriously considered. This is a shame, because the issue deserves to be debated on its own merits without the connotations associated with a murderous, mad scientist cartoon character.

With this in mind, I have used *The Incredibles* for teaching fourth-year medical students during an Ethics and the Movies course. This film is an atypical offering for the class, as it is not overtly medical, it is youth-oriented, and is animated. Nonetheless, coupled with provocative readings about enhancement technologies, fairness, meritocracy, and justice, it has generated robust discussions about the appropriate role of the medical profession in mediating human enhancement, which segue into discussions about steroids in sports, and even into dialogues about the social construction of "normalcy" in our diverse society. For the ambitious, this film can be fruitfully paired with books such as Carl Elliott's *Better Than Well: American Medicine Meets the American Dream*,[7] or Leslie Fiedler's *Tyranny of the Normal: Essays on Bioethics, Theology & Myth*,[8] which both deal broadly (and differently) with the notion of normalcy. It can also be contrasted with other films, such as *Normal for Us: The Miller Twins*[9] a documentary about twin girls who, despite severe physical impairments, live fully functional lives as a result of architectural adaptations made to their family home by their ferociously dedicated parents. *The Incredibles* is a highly entertaining film, and with appropriate prodding, can challenge students and other viewers to examine their own views about human nature and to think more deeply about how we can (and should) harness technology in the service of humanity.

NOTES

    i. DVD Chapter 4 Scene 00:14:48 to 00:15:38
       You always say, "Do your best." But you don't really mean it. Why can't I do the best that I can do?"
       Right now, honey, the world just wants us to fit in, and to fit in, we just gotta be like everybody else.
       But dad always said our powers were nothing to be ashamed of. Our powers made us special.
       Everyone's special, Dash... .
       Which is another way of saying no one is.
    ii. Chapter 24: Scene 01:29:30 to 01:30:25
       Oh, I'm real. Real enough to defeat you! And I did it without your precious gifts, your oh-so-special powers... I'll give them the most spectacular heroics anyone's ever seen! And when I'm old and I've had my fun, I'll sell my inventions so that everyone can be superheroes. Everyone can be super! And when everyone's super...no one will be.

REFERENCES

1. Adams, J., Jefferson, T., Adams, A., and Cappon, L.J. 1988. Institute of Early American History and Culture (Williamsburg Va.). *The Adams-Jefferson letters: The*

complete correspondence between Thomas Jefferson and Abigail and John Adams. Published for the Institute of Early American History and Culture at Williamsburg, Virginia. Chapel Hill: University of North Carolina Press.

2. Kass, L.R. 2003. Ageless bodies, happy souls: Biotechnology and the pursuit of perfection. *New Atlantis* 1: 9–28.

3. Bostrom, N. 2005. In defense of posthuman dignity. *Bioethics* 19: 202–214.

4. Lawton, G. 2006. The new incredibles: Enhanced humans. *New Scientist Magazine* May 13, 2006.

5. Allen, D.B., and Fost, N.C. 1990. Growth hormone therapy for short stature: Panacea or Pandora's box? *Journal of Pediatrics* 17: 16–21.

6. Lee, J.M., Appugliese, D., Coleman, S.M., et al. Short stature in a population-based cohort: Social, emotional, and behavioral functioning. *Pediatrics* 124: 903–910.

7. Elliott, C. 2003. *Better than well: American medicine meets the American dream,* 1st ed. New York, NY: W.W. Norton.

8. Fiedler, L.A. 1996. *Tyranny of the normal: Essays on bioethics, theology & myth.* Boston, MA: D.R. Godine.

9. "Normal for us: The Miller twins." Cain, E. Oregon Public Broadcasting. Portland, OR: August, 2002. Retrieved from http://www.opb.org/programs/millertwins

emerging technologies: *artificial intelligence*

marcia santana fernandes

Artificial Intelligence (2002). William Hurt, Haley Joel Osment, Jude Law, Frances O'Connor. Directed by Steven Spielberg. Duration: 140 minutes.

Scene: DVD chapter 1 scene 00:03:06 to 00:04:40

ANY HEART IS CAPTURED BY the expression in the eyes of a child, especially because children remind us of our true soul. Thus, we cannot be indifferent to the look of Haley Joel Osment in the role of Meca-David in the film *Artificial Intelligence* (2002), directed by Steven Spielberg. The story of this 11-year-old artificial boy, David, reflects on our social existence. In a close look at the original scene, David's creator, Professor Hobby (William Hurt) tells his research team, the supernerds, that the invention was the realization of mankind's desire—a *Meca-child*, to give love without demands: he would need no food, no rest, no love in return. The Meca-child's feeling of love would be recorded in his subconscious, in his inner memory. When presented with David's qualities, a colleague asks Professor Hobby: What is the human responsibility for the Meca-child's feelings of love? This question can be paraphrased with an older question: What is our responsibility toward our own creations?

The illustrated scene from this film can be used as a starting point for a discussion of the slippery-slope principle.[1] We are responsible for our inventions and their corresponding consequences.[2] The blue fairies the Meca-David anxiously searches for in the film do not exist for mankind. There are no magic figures that can restore our lost sense of humanity and uniqueness.

A discussion of the ethics of emerging technologies can be extended to that of a foundation for human life and living—both natural and artificial. How can society deal with enhancement technologies applied to the human body? This discussion extends to areas including therapeutic limits in terminally ill patients; stem cell research and the use of human embryos; reproductive technology and the use of assisted reproduction, including methods to pseudo-design humans through the genetic alterations; and drugs to improve an individual's physical and mental capacity in sport and intellectual endeavors. These topics relate to health care as a social priority and are especially pertinent because emerging technologies are costly, individually invasive, and have a direct impact on social integration.[3]

To reflect upon these topics from a bioethical standpoint, we must keep an open mind and avoid preconceived ideas. Bioethics, here, is understood not as a discipline, but as a meeting ground for a number of disciplines, discourses, and organizations concerned with ethical, legal, and social questions raised by advances in medicine, science, law, and biotechnology.[4,2]

The complex bioethics model[2] provides an approach that situates ethics in reality. First, it is important to properly identify the problem being addressed, the facts and circumstances involved, the alternatives, and their consequences. Second, the ethical reflection should include a theoretical framework based on related cases. The theoretical framework could include different approaches from a virtue ethics, principles-based ethics, and human rights ethics. The related cases should introduce casuistry into the discussion. All these elements, from problem identification to prior knowledge and experiences, as well as analyses of possible benefits and risks, present opportunities for rational discussion. Finally, the complex bioethics model takes into consideration one's belief and values systems, and emotion, because these elements can interfere with rational decision-making. The limits to human actions cannot be listed linearly (with a beginning, middle, and end), but must instead be constantly adjusted to reflect changing social, cultural, and historical needs and desires. Because no mechanism can force us to reduce the risks of emerging technologies, careful reflections are key. For example, the indiscriminate use of human embryos in research is often based on the justification of scientific progress and on the assumption that such embryos are capable of neither reason nor love. This poses a pertinent question: Were we embryos? Certainly, the answer is "yes." However, we were not frozen embryos without a womb in which to develop. Does this fact somehow deny frozen embryos their humanity? In other words, are frozen embryos simply "pre-embryos" or "pure cells" or maybe "mecas"? Is that why they are disposable things, to be manipulated without questioning or control? In the same vein, emerging technologies have triggered the concerns of Hans Jonas[6] and Van Rensselaer Potter[7] about the limits of technology on human history. In all cases, the core issue is the principle of responsibility that lights the path to a balance between conservation, transformation, discovery, and (re)invention of (bio)technology. Hans Jonas[6] proposes this principle in order to block the tendency of humans to destroy what they dominate, because, as he believes, the actions in biological sciences "are irrevocable" and "what is done is done." Thus, certain actions must be a focus of ethical reflection: the tolerance for probable consequences, a retreat to a possible earlier state, changing direction, or maintaining the status quo. Similarly, Potter[7] associates a principle of responsibility with the feeling of humility—the recognition that, because all of us can make mistakes, we must exercise humility as scientists and professionals in our dealings with human life.

Responsibility and humility should guide medical activity, as illustrated in parts of the Hippocratic Oath.[8,9] Emerging technologies and their applications to health care, therefore, should not be subjected to wholesale legislative limitations, regardless of context or culture. Law-making must be interdisciplinary, intimately involved in the discussion of and reflection on bioethical issues, so that law makers and legislators can deal with their complexity as well as their social aspects and peculiarities in order to efficiently play their role—that is, to enforce and guarantee humans rights concerning our present and future generations.

In this film, humans come to terms with indifference and a tragic questioning of their own sense of humanity by transferring their frustrations to Mecas. Love is the sentiment chosen to define the difference between natural and artificial life; however, this love is unrecognizable, even in the eyes of an apparently human child, because even the look in the eye was artificially truthful. It is only through our appreciation of our humanity and uniqueness that we will find true, selfless love—what the Greeks called *agape*.[9]

REFERENCES

1. Schauer, F. 1985. Slippery slopes. *Harvard Law Review* 99: 361–383.
2. Goldim, J.R. 2006. Bioética: Origens e complexidade. *Revista HCPA, Porto Alegre* 26(2): 86–92. Retrieved from http://www.bioetica.ufrgs.br
3. Beck, U. 2009. *World at risk*. Cambridge, UK: Polity Press.
4. O'Neill, O. 2002. *Autonomy and trust in bioethics*, 1st ed. Cambridge, UK: Cambridge University Press.
5. Graves, R. 2000. *The Greek myths*, 1st ed., 8th edition, two volumes. London, UK: Folio Society.
6. Jonas, H. 1994. *Ética, medicina e ética*, 1st ed. Lisboa, PT: Vega–Passagens.
7. Potter, V.R. 1971. *Bioethics - Bridge to the future*, 1st ed. Hoboken, NJ: Prentice Hall.
8. Iserson, K.V., Sanders, A.B., and Mathieu, D. (Eds.). 1995. Hippocratic oath. In *Ethics in emergency medicine* (p. 493). Tucson AZ: Galen Press.
9. Aristotle. 1999. *The Nicomachean ethics*. Upper Saddle River, NJ: Prentice Hall.

5

human genetic engineering: *gattaca*

alexander m. capron

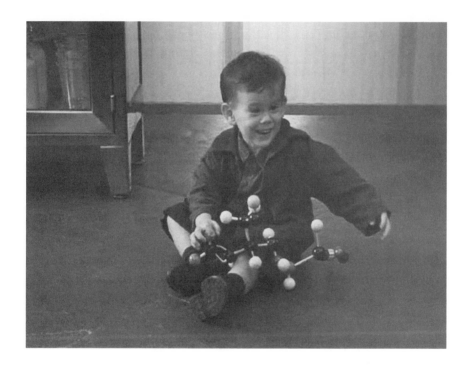

Gattaca (1997). Ethan Hawke, Uma Thurman, Alan Arkin, Jude Law, Gore Vidal, Blair Underwood, Tony Shalhoub, Xander Berkeley. Directed by Andrew Niccol. Duration: 107 minutes.

DVD chapter 4, scene 00:10:55 to scene 00:12:32

N THE SCIENCE FICTION GENRE, *Gattaca* is the quintessential bioethics film. (How many other films open with a quotation from Willard Gaylin, a founder of the field?) Unlike some science fiction, however, its science seems neither too fictional, nor is it the focus of the film, which might better be described as a police-procedural movie seen from the perpetrator's perspective. That said, it still raises significant issues far beyond asking what life would be like in a eugenic world. To mention but a few: genetic determinism versus free will, the proper limits of the artificial, human nature and worth, and the virtues of courage, honesty, and loyalty.

In the "not-too-distant future" (as a title card describes the time period), the Gattaca Aerospace Corp. launches numerous manned rocket ships every day, some aimed at interplanetary exploration. Yet, its employees wear smartly tailored business suits (even for space flights) rather than futuristic space outfits, drive cars that look like ours (although all electric), work on computers like ours in offices like ours, and otherwise go about a life very much like our own. With one exception: Some of them are *valids*, born from embryos that have been screened, selected, and genetically manipulated to be free of diseases and weaknesses, while others—those conceived the way babies have always been—are called *in-valids, faith births* or, more ominously, *de-gene-erates*.

While the film leaves the science of genetic manipulation vague, it repeatedly depicts the use of DNA for personal identification and prediction. The protagonist, Vincent Freeman (Hawke), is barely out of the womb before a delivery room nurse, having fed a drop of blood pricked from his heel into an analyzer, pronounces to his distressed father a long list of his firstborn's probable maladies, along with a predicted lifespan of 30.2 years. Vincent's mother, cradling him on the delivery bed, whispers a more hopeful view of his future ("I know he'll do something"), but her optimism is soon replaced by worry over his safety (every childish tumble is both a confirmation of his deficiencies and a cause for concern lest he further injure himself) and resignation over his marginalization by society (even the preschool won't accept him, for fear of liability).

So, in a scene near the beginning of the film, when Vincent's parents decide to have another child, they seek the help of a geneticist (Underwood) at the Eighth Day Center who meets their cosmetic wishes ("hazel eyes, dark hair,... and fair skin," the last pronounced with ironic amusement by the handsome Underwood, who has hazel eyes, dark hair but, of course, not fair skin). More to the point, he has also "taken the liberty of eliminating from the candidate embryos any potentially prejudicial conditions," from fatal diseases to milder burdens like myopia. To the parents' murmured suggestion that perhaps something should be left to chance, the doctor replies that "we want to give your child the best possible start," and then reassures them that "the child is still you, simply the best of you"—in contrast to the goofy-looking toddler Vincent, playing on the floor of the doctor's office, who serves as a reminder of all that is not the best of them.

Thus, the first of the eight significant relationships that frame *Gattaca* is the one Vincent has with the physician whose creation of Anton, Vincent's genetically perfected brother, symbolizes society's shunting aside of Vincent. Like all human relationships, each of the eight has its ambiguities and tensions, and hence opens up fascinating ethical dilemmas for discussion. For example, although the geneticist implicitly rejects Vincent, he does so with a benign smile; he means the child no harm, but he makes clear that Vincent's parents would be wrong to risk having another child like him. This introduces issues of prejudice and discrimination, as well as a utilitarian view of human worth.

The doctor appears to offer the parents choices (for example, letting them opt for a second son rather than a daughter), but it is clear that the contours of what counts as "the good" in human beings in this future world are not debatable. The message is clear: No responsible parent would fail to avoid any preventable burdens or even weaknesses; indeed, parents should provide their offspring with as many strengths and talents as possible. (In the original version of the scene, the doctor offers to insert genetic sequences "associated with enhanced musical or mathematical abilities," which the parents decline because the price is beyond their means.) This view is not new; it was eloquently expressed in 1974 by Joseph Fletcher:

> Should we leave the fruits of human reproduction to take shape at random, keeping our children dependent on the accidents of romance and genetic endowment, of sexual lottery or what one physician calls "the meiotic roulette of his parents' chromosomes"? Or should we be responsible about it, that is, exercise our rational and human choice, no longer submissively trusting to the blind worship of raw nature?[1]

Dual questions of virtue are thus raised. First, what constitutes being a good and loving parent? Fletcher asserts that such a parent will seek and use the means that science has created to perfect human beings. At the opposite extreme, Leon Kass argues that "making babies in laboratories—even 'perfect' babies—means a degradation of parenthood."[2] Kass denies that artificial techniques of the sort employed in *Gattaca* are even forms of *human* procreation. Daniel Callahan challenges this dichotomy between artificial and natural, since human beings naturally create culture, of which technology is a part.[3]

The second half of the virtue question is thus: What traits would a responsible parent select, or a good society encourage (or force) them to select for a child? Implicit in the manner in which people in the world of *Gattaca* answer that question is the understanding that virtues and capabilities reside in genetic endowment. The belief that DNA is destiny is clearly displayed in Vincent's second and third major relationships, namely with his parents and with Anton. The former take a fatalistic view of Vincent's limitations and try to quash his fascination with space travel, since his disabilities (discernible from the glasses he wears, as well as from a genetic test that any potential employer could easily, albeit surreptitiously and illegally, perform) means that the only time he's likely to see the inside of a space ship "is when you're cleaning one," as his father reminds him. Likewise, Anton—younger but soon stronger, taller, and braver—takes his superiority as a birthright. Finally, however, Vincent wins their long-running ocean-swimming competition, and indeed saves Anton from drowning: "It was the one moment in our lives when my brother was not as strong as he believed, and I was not as weak." Vincent takes that as his inspiration to leave home, with its constant reminders of his inherent shortcomings.

In all save one of Vincent's remaining five relationships, which occur after he first arrives at Gattaca as a maintenance worker, the DNA-as-destiny view is challenged to one degree or another. By dint of unending study and physical exercise, he begins a process of transformation that takes on a new dimension when he engages German, a shady character (Shalhoub) who specializes in helping people like Vincent take on the identity of valids, for when "a member of the elite falls on hard times" his or her genetic identity "becomes a valued commodity for the unscrupulous." The fallen in this case is Jerome Morrow (Law), a bitter young man in a wheel chair, paralyzed from the waist down by an attempted suicide, to which he was driven when, despite his peerless genetic endowment, he won only the silver medal, not the gold, in a major swim contest. In Vincent's relationship with his parents, we see what can happen when parents implicitly reject a child because of his perceived inborn weaknesses; in Jerome's life we see what can happen when a person dismisses his own accomplishments because of his failure to live up to his perceived inborn strengths.

The make-over Vincent receives at German's hands (the most radical aspect of which is his lower legs being cut and extended, to add two inches to his height) may be merely cosmetic but that is really all Vincent needs to get hired at Gattaca because it was not his own considerable abilities that the company's hiring standards measured but only Jerome's superior genes (delivered through blood samples under the fake fingertips on Vincent's hand and the urine in pouches strapped to his leg). As Jerome, by then known by his middle name, Eugene (one of the film's little jokes) explains to Vincent, by then called "Jerome," when the latter is panicking that a slip-up will cause them to be discovered, "When they look at you, they don't see you. They only see me."

This myopia is particularly prominent in Vincent's sixth relationship, with Josef, the director of Gattaca (Vidal), who regards him as the embodiment of eugenic perfection. Even when—during an investigation of the murder of another Gattaca official—it emerges that an unknown in-valid had infiltrated the space agency, Eugene is right that "They won't believe that one of their elite has suckered them all this time." Indeed, Josef is such a snob that he says sarcastically to Anton (who turns up as a police lieutenant to lead the murder investigation) that Gattaca has occasionally "had to accept candidates with minor shortcomings but nothing that would prohibit someone from working in a field such as law enforcement."

Besides his relationship with Eugene, Vincent's most complex relationship is with a co-worker, Irene Cassini (Thurman), who shares his ambitions but whose genome is not quite as perfect as Jerome's, for her heart is too weak to allow her to travel to Titan (a moon of Saturn) as "Jerome" is scheduled to. Early in their relationship, she finds a hair of Jerome's on a comb (actually planted by Vincent for this purpose), which she takes to a facility where people can have genetic profiles run anonymously—a quick way of finding out whether one's date possesses impressive potential as a mate. At this point, she seems as committed to the genes-as-destiny view as Josef, yet by the end of the film, as she becomes aware of Vincent's deception, her admiration for his accomplishments and aspirations leads her not to turn him in to Anton and his assistant, Detective Hugo (Arkin) who believes that the murder was committed by an in-valid. This willingness to look beyond genes in judging ability is also seen in the eighth relationship, that with Gattaca's medical officer, Dr. Lamar (Berkeley). Just before Vincent's rocket is ready to launch, an unexpected urine test produces an "in-valid" result, but Dr. Lamar covers it up; it turns out that he has known all along that "Jerome" was what is called a "borrowed ladder," but kept quiet because his son, who also wants to be an astronaut despite having a disqualifying defect, admires Vincent.

Students are thus left with the ambiguity in Gaylin's epigram[i]: "I not only think that we will tamper with Mother Nature. I think Mother wants us to." Who is tampering? Only the geneticists, or Vincent as well? Can a man refuse to play the hand he was dealt? Is Josef wrong when he says, "No one exceeds his potential"? Even Jerome grows spiritually. When Vincent thanks him, he replies, "I only lent you my body. You lent me your dream." Does this mean that free will triumphs in the end over the genetic determinism that held Vincent's parents in its grasp, back in the doctor's office, when they ordered up Anton? Is being "natural" a virtue in itself, or is nature itself too malleable to provide a moral grounding for action? Rather than a simple story of right and wrong, Gattaca provides a means of addressing a virtually endless range of issues in bioethics.

NOTE

i. Dr. Willard Gaylin, along with William Callahan, founded the Hastings Center in 1969. This epigram is found in the opening credits of the movie *Gattaca*.

REFERENCES

1. Fletcher, J. 1974. *The ethics of genetic control: Ending re- productive roulette*, p. 36. Garden City, NY: Anchor Press/Doubleday.
2. Kass, L.R. Winter, 1972. Making babies: The new biology and the "old" morality. *Public Interest* 32: 49.
3. Callahan, D. 1972. New beginning in life: A philosopher's response. In M.P. Hamilton (Ed.), *The new genetics and the future of man*, pp. 100–101. Grand Rapids, MI: Eerdmans.

reproductive cloning: *multiplicity*

stephen r. latham

Multiplicity (US, 1996). Michael Keaton, Andie MacDowell.
Directed by Harold Ramis. Duration: 117 minutes.

DVD Chapter 1 Scene 00:19.45 to 00:22:37

DOUG KINNEY (MICHAEL KEATON), A busy building contractor, has no time for his wife (Andie MacDowell) and children. While working construction at a mysterious scientific research facility, Doug meets Dr. Leeds, who offers Doug a most unusual method of finding more time: He will create a clone of Doug who can do his work, leaving Doug to spend more time with his family. The clone is created—and later, another, and still more—but things don't work out as planned. By the film's climax, Doug appears to have lost both his job and his family to the confusion caused by mix-ups among the clones. Finally, though, with help from the clones, Doug turns the situation around in time for a happy ending. The clones ride off into the sunset, leaving a chastened but happy Doug to contemplate the lessons he's learned about priority-setting, work–family balance, and unity of character.

The scene in which Doug meets his clone for the first time is probably just what the term "cloning" brings to mind in pop culture: twin adults, face to face with one another, so identical as to be confused even about who is the copy and who the original. But this fantasy has little to do with what real reproductive cloning would actually entail.[1] Cloning—the real kind, of the sort that gave us Scotland's famous Dolly the Sheep—begins with a donated egg. The nucleus of that egg, containing the entire nuclear DNA, is removed and replaced with the nuclear material from a donor's adult cell—the donor being the person to be cloned. (In the case of Dolly, nuclear material was taken from one of her mother's mammary cells.) The egg, with its newly acquired nucleus, is stimulated chemically or electronically to begin cellular division; if that process begins, the egg starts becoming a blastocyst.

In *therapeutic cloning*, the blastocyst is dismantled in order to propagate stem cell lines, from which tissue for therapies may be derived. But in *reproductive cloning*, the blastocyst is transferred into the uterus of a potential mother, there to implant and be carried until birth. The cloned baby will be born with nuclear DNA identical to that of the adult cell donor, although with mitochondrial DNA from the egg donor, since mitochondrial DNA is carried in the cytoplasm around the nucleus (the "white") and not in the nucleus itself (the "yolk"). The child

will be genetically identical to its donor-parent, except to the extent that mater-
nally inherited mitochondrial DNA may affect its metabolism or carry risk of
certain genetic diseases. Of course, the child will be different from the donor-
parent in other quite fundamental senses: From its earliest development in the
womb, it will have been exposed to a different biochemical and social environment. Its mother will have had a different diet from that of the adult-cell nucleus
donor; it will be exposed in utero to different levels and types of stress, nutrients,
hormones, and stimuli. These factors alone will cause its genes to express differently than those of the adult donor. Of course, from the moment of its birth, the
newborn clone will be exposed to a radically different environment from that in
which its donor-parent was raised. Not least of these differences will be the fact
that the cloned donor-parent will be a live, middle-aged adult. In short, the clone
will not be identical to its clone-parent because it will have different mitochondrial DNA, different environmental exposures during its prenatal development,
and vastly different experiences throughout its life. It won't even look identical to
its clone-parent, except in the sense that it will look rather like the clone-parent
looked back when the clone-parent was the clone's age.

Dolly and a number of other mammals have been cloned in this manner, but
no human being ever has. Many people believe that it would be immoral to
engage in human reproductive cloning; even those who approve of creating
cloned human embryos for stem cell research and other therapeutic purposes
draw the line at cloning to produce a live, human baby. In fact, human reproductive cloning is outlawed in much of the world. Given that we regularly create
babies via in vitro fertilization, what makes cloning a new baby different enough
to be morally wrong?

The first and simplest answer is that it would be wrong to conduct the
experiments necessary to perfect the process of human reproductive cloning.
Dolly the Sheep was only born after 277 earlier failures, including numerous
miscarriages and sheep born with birth defects, many of whom led short,
miserable lives. Surely it would be immoral and cruel to go through a comparable
experimental phase with human mothers, fetuses, and babies. But some bioethicists have gone further, claiming that human reproductive cloning would be
wrong even if it could be conducted safely and effectively, producing only healthy
babies. One set of arguments against human reproductive cloning concentrates
on the clones themselves.

Leon Kass, for example, has argued that a clone—since it will be born with a set
of genes that has already lived—might have so much of its independence subverted
by its method of manufacture that it may even lack the basic human capacity for
moral agency.[i]

Others have argued, in a similar vein, that cloning would deprive the clone of
an "open future."[2] But these arguments, like the pop culture argument that clones
would somehow lack "souls" of their own,[3] seem to depend on an elementary and
incorrect genetic determinism. We are not our genes; neither our moral agency

nor our personal future consists in the mechanical unfolding of a genetically predetermined character. Only a thoroughgoing genetic determinist would think that a cloned baby is doomed to be a rerun of its donor-parent.

A second, and considerably more fruitful, line of moral objection to human cloning focuses not on the capacities of the clone, but on the model of parenting that cloning seems to imply—and on some of the psychological consequences of adopting that model. Michael Sandel, for example, has argued that genetic engineering—of which cloning is one form—would fundamentally transform the process of having children,[4] elevating "dominion over reverence." The parent who clones a child seems to regard that child as an object to be mastered technologically. Parents of cloned children will fail to develop the kind of humility that comes from the realization, common enough in ordinary parenting, that one can't have just the children one wants. Ordinary parenting requires one to accept the unknown and the unbidden, and to love it unconditionally. Will parents of made-to-order children experience that same love? Additionally, Sandel argues, such parents may be burdened with an unprecedented sense of responsibility for the fates of the children they've engineered. Finally, the engineering of children may diminish our sense of social solidarity, by undermining our conviction that misfortunes are undeserved. If others' misfortunes are the result not of some random genetic lottery, but of their own poor genetic planning, why come to their aid?

Like the earlier arguments, however, these psychological objections to cloning seem predicated upon an unrealistic genetic determinism. Surely, the fact that a cloned child shares one of its parents' genes does not make it impossible for that child to surprise its parents, or to emerge as something new and unexpected! After all, even identical twins, who share not only the same genes but also the same age and very nearly the same environment, become distinct individuals, often in surprising ways. Why wouldn't a cloned child be just as "new" to its parents as any other? Would a clone's parents really be hobbled by an unprecedented sense of responsibility for their children's failures? Only if those failures had been written into their children's genes. In a world where reproductive cloning was common, would the idea of undeserved misfortune really disappear? Only if all misfortune were genetic.

But our fates are not in our genes. We live and grow and change, each of us, in a world; and then we leave it. A human clone, if we were ever to make one, would not be a do-over, or a chance at immortality, or a cheap reproduction, or a precious duplicate. It would be a baby.

NOTE

i. Leon R. Kass MD, a known opponent of cloning, is a former chairman of the President's Council on Bioethics (2001-2005). He discusses this and many other issues in his book Life, Liberty and the Defense of Dignity: The Challenge of Bioethics, Encounter Books, San Francisco, 2002.

REFERENCES

1. US Department of Energy. *Human genome project information: Cloning fact sheet.* Retrieved from http://www.ornl.gov/sci/techresources/Human_Genome/elsi/cloning.shtml
2. Brock, D.W. 2002. Human cloning and our sense of self. *Science* 5566: 314–316.
3. Ishiguro, K. 2006. *Never let me go.* New York: Random House Vintage International.
4. Sandel, M.J. 2007. *The case against perfection.* Cambridge, MA: Harvard University Press.

7

therapeutic cloning: *the 6th day*

cristiane avancini alves

The 6th Day (2000). Arnold Schwarzenegger, Robert Duvall, Tony Goldwyn.
Directed by Roger Spottiswoode. Duration: 124 minutes.

DVD Chapter 10 Scene 00:31:31 to 00:33:40

"GOD CREATED MAN IN HIS own image, and behold, it was very good.
And the evening and the morning were the sixth day." This passage of
Genesis 1:27,31 is the opening of the movie starring Arnold
Schwarzenegger, who is cloned by mistake. This "error" left two identical persons
(at least, physically equal) alive. "There's been a Sixth Day violation. A human was
cloned," explains one of the characters. According to the film, ten years before its
context and time (the initial scenes refer to a "near future") a human was cloned.
The Supreme Court imposed the "destruction" of that clone, and the Sixth Day
Law banning human cloning was established.

In the analyzed scene, this decision is discussed during the inauguration of a
modern reproductive center, where groups protesting against cloning were also
present. The speech of Dr. Wier (Robert Duvall), the director of the institution,
explains that human cloning is not only illegal (referring to the Sixth Day Law) but
also that scientists remain years away from possessing the technology to do it.
When asked by a journalist if he wanted this law repealed, the mentor of the
project, Michael Drucker (Tony Goldwyn), answers in his place: "Dr. Weir is interested in medicine, not in politics." The movie context reveals the existence of
many "RePet" stores, since animal cloning is allowed. Publicity and marketing
instruments give the public the idea that cloning their pet is a sweet and lovable
alternative, especially for their children's emotional happiness. Another journalist,
during the interview, says provocatively to Drucker that protesters claim that he
uses "RePet" shops to soften people up to the idea of human cloning.

Even if the movie context is surrounded by a technologic and futuristic world,
and even if cloning is considered as a recent laboratory phenomenon, the word
itself derives from antiquity: from the Greek word for "twig." Initial use of the
term applied to early 20th-century botany, designating plant grafts. "Clone" eventually came to be used for microorganisms as well. By the 1970s, the word came to
designate a viable human or animal generated from a single parent. Over the last
few years, cloning has come to mean any artificial, identical genetic copy of an
existing life form. In the natural course of reproduction, the male sperm fertilizes

a female egg, forming an embryo. The embryo's genetic structure is located in the chromosomes found in the nucleus of every embryonic cell. The new organism obtains one half of its genes from the mother's egg and the other half from the father's sperm. In cloning by nuclear transfer, the egg nucleus is removed through a microscopic laboratory procedure and replaced with a donor's nucleus, containing the unique genes of that individual. The egg, which grows into an embryo, therefore contains only the donor's genes. The cloned organism emerges as a near genetic copy of its sole "parent" rather than a random genetic combination of two parents.

The pioneer era of cloning dates to 1952, with the work of biologists Robert Briggs and Thomas King in Philadelphia. They tried to clone vertebrates. Around the 1970s, the British biologist John Gurdon successfully cloned a tadpole from a somatic cell, proving that a developed embryo or differentiated cells can be reactivated and produce a new life. However, to accomplish the same feat on mammals appeared difficult, especially the transfer of embryos that must be transplanted into a womb and result in pregnancy. This situation changed in early 1997, when a Scottish team announced the birth of Dolly, a lamb cloned from an adult sheep. After many failed attempts, the veterinary researcher Ian Wilmut and his colleagues managed to obtain an egg cell that began dividing normally, and this was implanted into a surrogate Scottish Blackface ewe. After a normal gestation period of about five months, Dolly was born.

Since Dolly, the cloning of several mammal species has resulted in many live births, but scientists are far from perfectly controlling the results, and they observe a wide range of abnormalities and defects in cloned animals. As might be expected, the possibility of cloning animals opened the debate regarding human cloning; here, it is important to understand the differentiation between *reproductive cloning* and *therapeutic cloning*. First of all, "therapeutic cloning" is not an appropriate term because it suggests possible beneficial applications of cloning, which presently seem completely unjustified. Instead of "therapeutic," scientists internationally recommend the use of the term *research cloning*.[1] In "reproductive cloning," the aim of somatic cell nuclear transfer is to create an embryo carrying the same genetic information as the progenitor and to implant this embryo into a womb to generate a pregnancy, and then a baby. The aim of research cloning, however, is not to produce a child but to derive embryonic stem cells that contain genetic characteristics identical to the progenitor. It can be done by cell nuclear replacement (CNR), or by the use of surplus embryos originated from in vitro fertilization (IVF).

Unavoidably, this process destroys the embryo. Because of that, ethical and legal dilemmas arise concerning the status of the embryo and its use for research. Ethically, for those who consider that an embryo should be protected from the instant of conception, its destruction for research cannot be justified. Legally, then, scientists face conflict in conferring the status of person upon a human embryo because it carries rights and duties defined normatively. For others, however, the embryo does deserve protection and a certain respect, but not to the same extent as fully developed babies, so its destruction can be justified to provide treatment for patients.

At the international level, two declarations from the United Nations and a resolution from the World Health Organization presently govern human cloning.[2] Reproductive cloning is considered ethically unacceptable and against human dignity and integrity. Ian Wilmut himself affirmed that cloning a mammal resulted in a high failure rate: from 277 of his "reconstructed" embryos only 29 were implanted in ewes and only one developed successfully; he concluded that similar experiments with humans would be totally disapproved. Nevertheless, research cloning remains a controversial field. On one hand, it holds the possibility of new therapeutic alternatives in biomedical assistance and research, while on the other hand, risks clearly exist in using research cloning because of the unknown harms that this technique could bring into the world.

The 6th Day mixes these elements and presents an interposition among reproductive cloning and research cloning. It is important to clarify the difference between these two concepts. An article indicates that, after Dolly's birth, the ingredients for a "media and consumerist spectacle" were served: sons à la carte and the old dream—or nightmare—of perpetuation and reproduction as self-repetition.[3] The author explains that media influence can give, for instance, an unfavorable emotional weight to the term "cloning" due to the ban on reproductive cloning by the international community, whereas research cloning can be an alternative source of biomedical development. A prime example of this media influence and its impact on political issues was the announcement of a cloned human blastocyst. Ultimately known as the "Korean cloning fraud," this event occurred when a South Korean researcher, Hwang Woo-suk, claimed to have created human embryonic stem cells by cloning. Woo-suk later admitted fabricating data, but irresponsible reporting and unfounded speculation by scientists created misconceptions and false hopes within the general public.[4] The researcher had his picture plastered on public transport, and posters were released proclaiming that he would change the world. He faced further pressure to succeed because the nationalistic ethos of South Korea meant that his fame reflected well on the government.

This scenario is part of the international discussion concerning human cloning, since many countries, in particular developing ones, still lack specific regulations on human cloning, a context that makes people vulnerable to external and profit-driven scientific and technologic research. The example of Hwang Woo-suk suggests that nothing is truly forbidden, and everything remains in the realm of possibilities. This could be a favorable situation for some researchers, since it means that stem cell research is better funded and thus remains transparent, rather than being carried out in countries with few or no controls.[5] The human cloning debate "makes us aware of the need to foster a genuine and world-wide discussion on bioethical issues (rather than leaving the field to political power games), which may be even more important than reaching immediate substantive conclusions."[6]

On the seventh day, Genesis states that God rested after contemplating His creation. A movie is a particular and special form of human creation that challenges our imagination and thoughts. The hopes raised by the bioethical analysis of a work of fiction recognizes our humanity and expands our knowledge, because only a well-educated and informed society can freely decide its destiny and contribute to a deep and sensible debate concerning life issues.

REFERENCES

1. UNESCO. 2005. *Human cloning–ethical issues*. Retrieved June 6, 2009 from http://www.unesco.org
2. UNESCO. June 9, 2009. *Report of IBC (International Bioethics Committee) on Human Cloning and International Governance*. Retrieved August 29, 2009 from http://www.unesco.org
3. Casado, M. 2009. Clonagem: uma questão de responsabilidade. In J. Martins-Costa, L. Ludwig Möller (Eds.), *Bioética e Responsabilidade*. Rio de Janeiro: Editora Forense.
4. Saunders, R., and Savulescu, J. 2008. Research ethics and lessons from Hwanggate: What can we learn from the Korean cloning fraud? *Journal of Medical Ethics* 34: 214–221.
5. Lenoir, N. 2006. Biotechnology, bioethics and law: Europe's 21st century challenge. *The Modern Law Review* 69: 1–6.
6. Biller-Andorno, N. 2005. It's cloning again! *Journal of Medical Ethics* 31: 63.

8

transgender/transsexual health care: *southern comfort*

april m. herndon

Southern Comfort (2001). Robert Eads, Lola Cola, Maxwell Scott Anderson, Cas Piotrowski. Directed by Kate Davis. Duration: 90 minutes.

DVD Chapter 4: Time Is Running Out, Scene 13:15–15:31

THE DOCUMENTARY *SOUTHERN COMFORT* TELLS the story of Robert Eads, a female-to-male (FtM) transsexual man living in rural Georgia, surrounded by a community of transsexual friends, his male-to-female (MtF) partner Lola Cola, and cisgendered[i] allies. Tragically, Robert is living his last days with friends and family as terminal cancer of the cervix, ovaries, and uterus—the last remaining parts of his female body—claims his life. He hopes to live long enough to walk Lola Cola down the aisle and to attend one last Southern Comfort Conference, an annual trans-based conference held in Georgia. Robert makes it to one last Southern Comfort conference, but the cancer claims his life shortly after.

In this particular scene, Robert talks about waking up feeling ill the previous January and tells the audience that it took three weeks for him to find a doctor who would treat him. After finally seeing a doctor, Robert was told he had terminal cancer of the cervix, ovaries, and uterus, which he finds particularly ironic since he asked for a hysterectomy when he began transitioning and was told not to worry about it because of his age.

Robert's friends Tom and Debbie speak candidly about their experiences while trying to obtain medical care for Robert when he fell ill while staying in their home. Tom and Debbie explain that Robert woke up very ill and in a "pool of blood" one morning; yet they struggled to find medical care. When they began calling doctors, they were asked if Robert had insurance, and they replied that Robert was uninsured but they would pay the bill. Debbie says the bigger issue was Robert's gender identity. She said to one hospital: "Well, here's another thing. He's trans." The hospital representative replied, "Well, maybe you'd better go [elsewhere]." In the end, Tom and Debbie claim they called over 20 doctors and "don't know how many hospitals." All refused to treat Robert, with two or three doctors admitting they couldn't treat him because it would be embarrassing to their other (read: female) patients.

In teaching Women's and Gender Studies and Bioethics classes, I use *Southern Comfort* to educate students about the humanity of transgender and transsexual people and to prompt discussions about the challenges transgender and transsexual people encounter when trying to access healthcare. Like many marginalized groups, trans people are often underinsured; yet, Robert's story primarily enables discussions of the bias and fear that sometimes prohibit trans-identified patients from accessing even urgently needed care. His story offers powerful lessons about the need for sensitivity to and consideration of birth sex in providing trans-identified patients with appropriate care, the importance of patient autonomy where gender identity is concerned, and the beneficence required to act in an ethically responsible manner.

Discrimination of trans-identified people in a variety of social settings is well documented. Although statistics can be challenging to gather and assess because individuals who transition sometimes fully assimilate and no longer identify as trans, available statistics suggest that significant numbers of trans people live in poverty, suffer employment discrimination, and are the victims of hate crimes.[1] Several state, city, and county jurisdictions recently passed legislation and initiatives to protect trans-identified people from discrimination, but gender identity is still not recognized as a protected category in the same way that race has been recognized.[2]

Like all people, trans-identified people sometimes require medical care for general problems (such as broken bones) and sometimes require medical care more focused on their individual needs (such as Pap smears for those who still have female reproductive organs in spite of a male gender expression or identity). In both cases, trans people may encounter difficulties in accessing necessary care. In Robert's case, he was refused care specifically because of his identity as a trans man and a lack of sensitivity to him as a person and his needs.

Robert has a set of health needs not unlike many people in the process of transitioning or who have already transitioned. At the time of filming, Robert has been living as a man for some time. Although his outward and social transition from female to male is complete, Robert did not undergo what many trans people call "bottom surgery" (the reconstruction of the sex organs to match one's chosen gender identity) or have a hysterectomy. Robert's reproductive and sex organs being at odds with his chosen gender identity is not, however, unusual among the trans community. The cost of undergoing full sex reassignment surgery is profound, especially given that many insurance companies will not pay for these procedures. With a price tag of upwards of $50,000 for FtM surgeries and from $7,000 to $14,000 for male-to-female (MtF) surgeries, many trans people simply cannot afford to undergo full sex reassignment.[3] The results of the surgeries, especially phalloplasty techniques, may also be a factor; as Max notes earlier in the film, "any phalloplasty" today will be recognized by people as "not God made but man made."

Also, many in the trans community believe that expressing one's true gender identity doesn't always necessitate "bottom surgery," a sentiment echoed by several trans people in the film who have not undergone full sex reassignment surgeries. For example, Robert had his breasts removed and has undergone testosterone therapy, so that observers read him as male, but insists that he doesn't need something "swinging between his legs" to make him a man.

Given the prohibitive costs and some people's belief that full sex reassignment surgery is unnecessary or has less than desirable results, many trans-identified people may still have sexual and/or reproductive anatomy at odds with their gender expression, which seems to be part of the reason Robert is denied care. Robert notes that two or three doctors (presumably Ob/Gyns) said that it would be "too embarrassing" to have Robert in their offices. Of course, one does usually see women rather than men in Ob/Gyn offices, but it's not totally unheard of to see men in Ob/Gyn offices, as many often accompany their wives. This embarrassment should not, of course, prohibit treatment.

Even within the cisgendered population, people sometimes develop conditions that seem to be at odds with their gender identity. Take, for example, the case of men with breast cancer. While oncologist's offices may not necessarily be gender specific, one can certainly imagine a situation in which the best oncologist in the area only treated breast cancer, and a male might need to enter a waiting room and an examination office where only women have been previously seen. The ethical course of action is, of course, to see a patient in need, regardless of his or her gender identity.

Robert's situation highlights another health concern for people who are transitioning or have already transitioned, especially those who might still have reproductive and/or sexual anatomy at odds with their gender identity. For Robert in particular, it's possible that his testosterone therapy contributed to his cancer of the cervix, ovaries, and uterus, and physicians need to be aware of this risk, even though the trans population is poorly studied.[4]

There are also health risks from lack of preventative care. Trans-identified people sometimes avoid medical care due to stigma or have difficulty finding a doctor who will treat them for concerns related to a birth sex that may be at odds with their gender expression. For example, in *Principles of Transgender Medicine and Surgery*, Ettner, Monstrey, and Eyler suggest that transsexual women who still have prostates and no history of estrogen use should still get PSA screenings and digital rectal exams. Transsexual women with a history of estrogen use need not be given PSA screenings because estrogen use can skew the results but should still receive digital exams.[5] The American Cancer Society also notes that FtM individuals, even those who have had their breasts removed, are still at risk for breast cancer because not all of the tissue has been removed.[6] All of these situations necessitate health care providers sensitive to the needs of patients who have transitioned—or even those who haven't transitioned but have an outward gender expression different from their birth sex and/or sexual or reproductive anatomy.

Most poignantly, Robert's story underscores the prejudice that may prohibit trans people from receiving any care, much less care sensitive to the needs of their birth sex. A touchstone case exhibiting the prejudice that trans people often face is that of Tyra Hunter, a trans woman severely hurt in a car accident in Washington,

D.C. and who eventually died from her injuries. According to witnesses, who later testified in a wrongful death suit filed by Hunter's mother, the emergency medical technicians stopped working on Tyra at the roadside once they had to remove her pants and discovered that she still had male sexual anatomy.[7]

In "A Bill of Transsexual Rights," Dr. James Cantor outlines the basic issues of respect and sensitivity necessary for the just and ethical treatment of trans-identified people, such as the right to be recognized as one's chosen gender, including in health care settings, and a basic right to respect.[8] Without this basic respect, autonomy and beneficence, two cornerstones of ethical health care practices,[9] are strained. Ultimately, trans-identified patients like Robert have the right to health care that is timely and respectfully provided, just as one would expect it be for cisgendered patients.

NOTE

i. *Cisgender* is a term used to refer to people for whom there seems to be a match between their birth sex and their gender identity, and who are comfortable with the gender assigned them at birth.

REFERENCES

1. Human Rights Campaign. How do transgender people suffer from discrimination? Retrieved July 17, 2009 from http://www.hrc.org/issues/1508.htm
2. Transgender Law and Policy Institute. Non-discrimination laws that include gender identity and expression. Retrieved July 17, 2009 from http://www.transgenderlaw.org/ndlaws/index.htm
3. Sex Reassignment Surgery. *Encyclopedia of surgery: A guide for patients and caregivers.* Retrieved July 17, 2009 from http://www.surgeryencyclopedia.com/Pa-St/Sex-Reassignment-Surgery.htmls
4. Dizon, D.S., Tejada-Burges, T., Koelliker, S., Steinhoff, M., and Grainai, C.O. 2006. Ovarian cancer associated with testosterone supplementation in a female-to-male transsexual patient. *Gynecologic and Obstetric Investigation* 62: 226–228.
5. Ettner, R., Monstrey, S., and Evan Eyler, A. 2007. *Principles of transgender medicine and surgery.* Philadelphia, PA: Hayworth Press.
6. American Cancer Society. Transgender and transsexual individuals fact sheet: Access to care and cancer disparity fact sheet. Retrieved July 17, 2009 from http://www.glbthealth.org/documents/FactSheetRevised-TransgenderedIndividuals.pdf
7. Feinberg, L. Trans health crisis: For us it's life and death. *American Journal of Public Health* 91: 897–900.
8. Cantor, J. A bill of transsexual rights. Retrieved July 22, 2009 from http://individual.utoronto.ca/james_cantor/blog9.html
9. Beauchamp, T., and Childress, J. 2008. *Principles of biomedical ethics.* New York: Oxford University Press.

coming of age with intersex: *xxy*

elizabeth reis

XXY (2007). Inés Efron, Martín Piroyansky, Ricardo Darin, Valeria Bertuccelli. Directed by Lucia Puenzo. Duration: 91 minutes.

DVD Chapter 7 Scene 47:24 to 50:44

XXY IS SET IN URUGUAY AND tells the story of 15-year-old Alex and her parents as they confront Alex's intersex condition. Intersex used to be called hermaphroditism and lately has been renamed disorders of sex development (DSD) in medical circles; it is an umbrella term that describes incongruity between external genitalia, internal reproductive anatomy, hormonal levels, and chromosomes. Typically, such conditions have been medically treated (but not eliminated) with a combination of hormones and surgery; such controversial management raises ethical questions about autonomy and consent, issues highlighted in this film. Alex's body is not typically female, and she has been taking hormones to curtail masculinization and to foster female secondary sex characteristics. Her parents avoided so-called normalizing surgery for her as an infant and small child, ultimately moving to a coastal village to escape the prying eyes and opinions of busy-bodies. When Alex is 15, her mother invites a family friend—a surgeon, who brings his wife, and teenage son—to evaluate Alex and discuss the possibility of surgery, feminizing what seems to be a phallus-like enlarged clitoris. This encounter makes the family face questions about Alex's identity: Is Alex a girl or a boy? Is she sexually attracted to girls or boys? Throughout *XXY*, Alex takes steps to evade further medicalization of any sort and begins to decide for herself not only her sexual identity but her gender identity as well.

In this scene, Alex's father visits someone (*una hermafrodita*) he has read about in the local newspaper who was born with ambiguous genitalia, raised as a girl, and who decided as a teenager to become a man. We are led to suppose that Alex's father is considering the possibility that Alex may also choose such a transition to manhood. The man he meets is quite content with his new life and gender. He warmly explains to Alex's father that he endured a childhood of invasive medical observation and intervention. Finally, at 16, he could no longer tolerate efforts to keep him female; he began taking testosterone, had another surgery (presumably a mastectomy, although the viewer is not given specifics), and started living as a man. Six months later, he met a woman whom he ultimately married, and they adopted a child. The story he conveys is that his life is "normal," not freakish, and he seems happy. Alex's father wonders aloud if he and his wife made the right decision to avoid surgery when Alex was an infant. Recalling infant surgeries, hospital visits, and feelings of shame, the man offers comforting words: "Making her afraid of her own body is the worst thing you can do to a child." The father leaves reassured in the decision to let Alex be, allowing her to decide for herself what she wants to do with her body and her life.

When I show *XXY* in class, I point out that most children born with ambiguous genitalia in the United States do not escape medical intervention. Most endure "normalizing" surgery to reshape their genitals to more closely match their intended gender of rearing, which doctors determine after assessing the gonads, hormone levels, chromosomes, and the look of the ambiguous external organs. A baby girl born, like Alex, with an enlarged clitoris, would typically have surgery to reduce the clitoris in size so that it looked less phallic; a baby boy with a penis considered too small (judged to be inadequate to allow, ultimately, sexual penetration) might be reshaped to resemble a baby girl, with his testes removed. An infant assigned to be female might have surgery to create, enlarge, or elongate her vagina so that, when she was older, it could accommodate heterosexual intercourse.[1] Johns Hopkins psychologist John Money, who was a leading expert in the field beginning in the 1950s, advised "that sex be assigned primarily on the basis of the external genitals and how well they lend themselves to surgical reconstruction in conformity with assigned sex, due allowance being made for a program of hormonal intervention."[2]

John Money's rationale for choosing a child's gender defined intersex management for the next 50 years. Although physicians understood the importance of chromosomes and hormones, most followed Money's advice, elevating external genital morphology as the single most important criterion in deciding how to treat intersex people. Money firmly believed that, in spite of confounding indicators, social gender could be created to match genital shape. At first glance, this protocol might seem like a good idea. It was conceived as a way to provide children with a stable gender identity and to ease their parents' distress. Parents could not raise a child unequivocally as male or female, Money and his colleagues believed, if the genitals did not match the baby's gender. Doctors in the 1920s and 1930s had worried that patients were living their lives as the wrong sex, and so Money's efforts were meant to guarantee that the correct gender was chosen during infancy. But, as countless cases suggested, no sure way exists to choose the gender of an infant born with ambiguous genitalia, particularly one with mixed gonadal status, chromosomes, and hormone levels.[3]

Before John Money's protocols took hold, doctors debated the deciding factors that should determine a person's sex, but neither the gonads nor the chromosomes proved to be reliable indicators. A woman with androgen insensitivity syndrome (AIS), for example, has an XY karyotype, which typically would indicate maleness; however, her body, unable to process the androgens she makes, develops physically as a girl. Women with AIS look completely female, although they have internal testes.[1] In the past, doctors wondered: Should such patients be told they were "really men" despite the way they looked and felt about themselves? By the mid-20th century, when John Money and his colleagues wrote a series of influential articles on the intersex management of infants, doctors were doubtless relieved to have a set of guidelines to follow. Money's work made it seem easier to surgically reshape bodies and influence the gender of babies, particularly because his protocols assured parents that gender could be successfully manipulated before 18 months of age.[3]

Since the mid-1990s, however, intersex activists have pointed out serious problems with Money's approach of surgically shaping children, including scarring, fistulas necessitating further surgeries, incontinence, lack of sexual sensation, and, perhaps most important, the sense of shame and the consequences of secrecy that often attends genital medical intervention. Intersex activists have made serious headway in convincing doctors (and parents) that children should not have to undergo painful surgeries that are often cosmetic rather than medically necessary.[4] Intersex protocols are, in fact, changing. In 2005, a group of doctors, therapists, and intersex adults issued a consensus statement that cautioned against early surgery and advised waiting, as Alex's parents did in the film, until the child is old enough to decide for his- or herself.[5] Choose a gender, everyone advises, but do not do anything irreparable to the genitals.[6] Some surgeries, like constructing a vagina deep enough to accommodate penile penetration, for example, require months of painful postsurgical dilation to prevent collapse. Why put a small child through such an ordeal if, when she is old enough for sexual relations, she might choose other means to sexual satisfaction? Why reduce an enlarged clitoris if the surgery will cause scarring and reduce or eliminate sexual sensation forever? As Suzanne Kessler, Lessons from the Intersexed, points out, "Gender ambiguity is 'corrected,' not because it is threatening to the infant's life, but because it is threatening to the infant's culture."[7]

Perhaps, in the future, we will see genetic testing playing a bigger role in intersex management. For now, testing is limited because prenatal sex development involves many genes, not just those on the X and Y chromosomes, and companies that develop genetic tests focus on anomalies that occur more frequently. Prenatal treatments for some conditions, such as congenital adrenal hyperplasia, which affects the adrenal glands and can cause masculinization in girls, raise ethical concerns. The insistence on normative bodies perpetuates the longstanding negative ways that intersex bodies have been scrutinized and pathologized, based on social anxieties about marriage and heterosexuality, rather than on medical necessity. The prevention of homosexuality has long motivated surgical and nonsurgical sex assignment, for example, and even today the use of the prenatal drug dexamethasone as a treatment for congenital adrenal hyperplasia may be linked to its deterrence.[8]

XXY is a rich and complicated plot that explores the difficulties of coming of age with intersex, with or without medical intervention. The film is elliptical in terms of Alex's precise condition. This is useful, as there are several that raise similar issues of autonomy and consent. Whatever the condition, the broader message is to let the patient decide for her- or himself what (if anything) should be done. In the film, Alex's father explains to the visiting surgeon that although he knew of Alex's intersex condition two months before her birth, when he laid eyes on her, he saw only perfection. Why not just let Alex, and all such affected children, be? Why not encourage them to love their bodies the way they are, and, if they do not, let them opt for surgery when they are older and can decide for themselves?[i]

NOTE

i. For further information on intersex, the reader is directed to the following books:

Dreger, A.D. 1999. *Intersex in the age of ethics*. Hagerstown, MD: University Group.

Holmes, M. 2008. *Intersex: A perilous difference*. Selinsgrove, PA: Susquehanna University Press.

Hughes, I.A., Houk, C., Ahmed, S.F., and Lee, P.A. 2005. Consensus statement on management of intersex disorders. *Archives of Disease in Childhood* 91: 554–563.

Preves, S.E. 2003. *Intersex and identity: The contested self*. New Brunswick, NJ: Rutgers University Press.

REFERENCES

1. Karkazis, K.A. 2008. *Fixing sex: Intersex, medical authority, and lived experience*. Durham, NC: Duke University Press.
2. Money, J., Hampson, J.G., and Hampson, J.L. 1957. Imprinting and the establishment of gender role. *AMA Archives of Neurology and Psychology* 77: 333–336.
3. Reis, E. 2009. *Bodies in doubt: An American history of intersex* pp. 55-81. Baltimore, MD: Johns Hopkins University Press.
4. Chase, C. Hermaphrodites with attitude: Mapping the emergence of intersex political activism. *GLQ: A Journal of Lesbian and Gay Studies* 4: 189–211.
5. Hughes, I.A., Houk, C., Ahmed, S.F., and Lee, P.A. 2005. Consensus statement on management of intersex disorders. *Archives of Disease in Childhood* 91: 554–556.
6. Consortium on the Management of Disorders of Sex Development. 2006. *Clinical guidelines for the management of disorders of sex development in childhood*. Rohnert Park, CA: Intersex Society of North America. Retrieved from www.dsdguidelines.org
7. Kessler, S. 1998. *Lessons from the intersexed*, p. 32. New Brunswick, NJ: Rutgers University Press.
8. Meyer-Bahlburg, H.F.L. 1999. What causes low rates of child-bearing in congenital adrenal hyperplasia? *Journal of Clinical and Endocrinological Metabolism* 84: 1844–1847.

women's rights: *a private matter*

toby l. schonfeld

A Private Matter (1992). Sissy Spacek, Aidan Quinn, Estelle Parsons.
Directed by Joan Micklin Silver. Duration: 92 minutes.

DVD Chapter 2 Scene 00.13:45 to 00.16:58

A PRIVATE MATTER RECOUNTS THE TRUE story of Sherri Finkbine (Sissy Spacek), host of Romper Room and happily married mother of four, who is in the first trimester of her fifth pregnancy in 1962. Finkbine confronts issues of reproductive choice as she learns that the tranquilizers she took as sleep aids have been shown to cause birth defects when taken during pregnancy. While she does not waiver on the decision to have an abortion, she struggles against the need for secrecy throughout the process. As she waits for the day of the termination to draw near, the media learn of Finkbine's decision to terminate the pregnancy and become a malingering, pervasive presence throughout the film. The Finkbines must eventually travel overseas to have the pregnancy terminated.

This scene introduces the malignancy of silence that permeates the film. Dr. Werner (Richard Venture) tells Sherri and her husband Bob (Aidan Quinn) about the likelihood of significant malformations in the fetus and takes Bob out of the room as Sherri is processing the information. Once in the anteroom, Dr. Werner assures Bob that the right decision is to terminate the pregnancy and informs him that while he won't "break the law," he will arrange a termination but keep it quiet. They return to the office and inform Sherri that the pregnancy must be terminated, and Bob schedules the operation with Dr. Werner for the following week. Dr. Werner reassures Sherri that she lacks culpability in this decision, saying: "You've done nothing wrong, Sherri; it's the drug. You've done nothing wrong."

While ostensibly about abortion, the legitimacy of the woman as a moral agent[i] and the harms caused by silence and selective disclosure dominate the moral considerations of the film. Depriving the woman of the choice about what will happen to her own body and to a wanted pregnancy demonstrates the harms that can be inflicted even when malicious intent is absent. Women have been particularly singled out as patients who are less likely to be able to handle difficult decisions,[1] when often acting in the patient's "best interests" simply served to continue the cycle of oppression that characterized the practice of health care. Gender disparities remain a problem in clinical medicine, in part because women were excluded from most clinical research until quite recently. This is not just a U.S. phenomenon; attempts to address gender disparity in medical research have been introduced in several countries.[2] Yet, the notion that a woman's body is both sufficiently like a man's body to justify similar treatment regimens, and yet different enough to discourage its inclusion in clinical trials, demonstrates how biological mechanisms may confound clinical care.

It is not just in physical medicine where gender disparities are apparent. The filmmakers imply that Sherri's continuing emotional distress over the decision to terminate the pregnancy reinforces her lack of fitness as a moral agent, a common way of disempowering women: By viewing women as "overly emotional," their concerns are easier to relegate as nonessential. However, it is fallacious to think that moral choice is necessarily free of remainders. Moral distress generally occurs when an agent knows the right choice but is unable to act on it,[3] yet some decisions leave moral remainders even when the right action has been performed.[4] Consider the proverbial *Sophie's Choice*, in which there is no good option. Women in situations similar to Sherri's may have just such an experience, one in which any choice leaves feelings of anguish. Providers must attend to the fact that different individuals may process information differently, and they must exercise respect for patient autonomy. This kind of sensitivity, central in discussions of cultural diversity, applies not just to women as a group, but in fact to particular individuals who may have idiosyncratic ways of approaching moral choices.

The way that Dr. Werner and Bob manage the situation during the consultation makes clear their judgment about how Sherri should act. This paternalistic—and unethical—imposition of others' values and priorities on the moral agent is not limited to decisions about abortion. Rather, examples of such value judgments can be seen in family planning more generally. Consider the refusal of pharmacists to provide emergency contraception (Plan B) to patients who request it, or physicians who fail to inform concerned women that this is a legitimate health care option. Respect for patient autonomy requires that health care providers ascertain the values, goals, and priorities of their patients and make recommendations according to those values, rather than according to their own.

In *A Private Matter*, it is the need to keep the decision secret that weighs most heavily on the protagonist—in a sense, the required secrecy serves as the antagonist in this drama. The hospital in the film routinely performed 300–400 pregnancy terminations per year, unbeknownst to the public and much of the staff, because of the required silence. Sherri commented that one never knows if these situations happen to other people, "…because everyone keeps it a secret." The most troubling aspect of this process for Sherri was the silence: "What I hate most about it is that it has to be a secret. It's like I'm doing something dirty." Kumar, et al.[5] note that "Stigmatised behaviours need not be visible to be stigmatized." One might think that making abortion legal in the United States would remove the stigma, yet this has not proven to be the case. The social stigma against women who undergo abortions persists. When she was leaving the hospital after being told the abortion could not proceed, Sherri displays her frustration with the required silence by saying, "I can do it if I think I'm wrong, but if I think I'm right, I have to be stopped… It's like I'm contagious." This view conforms to the notion by Das that "stigma is seen as contagious."[6] In the case of abortion, highly contextualized decisions are oversimplified, and the prevalence of abortion is misrepresented, so that the practice itself becomes "exceptional."[4] Once this has occurred, it becomes relatively easy to stereotype the woman who has selected pregnancy termination.

Kumar et al. theorize that the normalization of the abortion stigma is due to the fact that the practice flouts three cultural expectations for women: "perpetual fecundity; the inevitability of motherhood; and instinctive nurturing"[5]—all of which are also confounded by contraception and other forms of family planning. Yet, A Private Matter succeeds in demonstrating challenges to each one of these ideals: Sherri has four children and goes on to have two more in the years following the abortion. She is an exemplary mother who loves children in general (e.g., her job as host of a children's television program), and her struggle about the abortion is precisely because of her nurturing instinct: She simply extends that instinct toward all of her children, rather than merely toward the fetus she is carrying. In this way, the film challenges viewers to analyze critically the social expectations for women in society.

Secrecy and silence are not only issues relevant to pregnancy choices. Failure to discuss topics considered sensitive by the public can have negative personal and public health consequences. Consider the situation of abstinence-only education in the public schools that, until recently, was the government's requirement in the United States. Former U.S. Surgeon General M. Jocelyn Elders describes the results of this system of values: "On an individual level, preventable health-risk behaviors among sexually active adolescents can expose them to lifelong consequences about which they are ill informed. On a national level, the result of withheld information and distribution of misinformation is America's sexual dysfunction, which can be measured by rates of unintended pregnancy and sexually transmitted infections (STIs) that are higher than those of virtually every other Western country. This dysfunction threatens public health, disrupts family life, and generally imposes a high societal cost through poverty—and the misery that poverty invariably brings."[7]

Negative personal and public health consequences have also been reported for those with HIV and AIDS, and for those women who are victims of domestic violence. Studies have shown that members of these groups in particular do not trust the confidentiality protections in place and therefore independently withhold information from their care providers for fear of disclosure.[8] This is, in some ways, the paradox of medical confidentiality: We must respect a patient's right to decide who has access to her personal health information, and yet we have created health care systems that make it difficult for that information to remain private in a fundamental way.[9]

Interestingly, the silence demonstrated in this film goes beyond the traditional physician–patient relationship. By having to practice medicine "on the sly," Dr. Werner's professional integrity is challenged by the requirement that no one "extraneous" find out about the abortion. Members of the Ethics Committee assembled at the hospital to discuss Sherri's case are astounded to learn of the number of abortions performed routinely at the hospital, and the committee ultimately decides against the provision of the abortion, not on medical grounds, but on the fear of liability against each of them individually.

Finally, the silence of women as a group is exemplified by the portrayal of the issues in this film. The Ethics Committee of the hospital is composed entirely of men. Bob and Dr. Warner continue to discuss the options independently of Sherri, even after the hospital refuses permission for the termination. The executives at the television station who make decisions about Sherri's job are men. All of the reporters are men. The one other significant female character in the film, Sherri's mother (Estelle Parsons), is portrayed as a person who can't understand this decision, and whose approach is to deny the current crisis and focus on her characterization of her daughter as a "good person" about whom she has always been proud.

A partial explanation for this male exclusivity is the era portrayed in the movie (the 1960s). Yet, it is not clear that the current decade, with its increase of female physicians, will reflect a change in the way that providers, patients, and families interrelate. To the extent that the social expectations of women continue largely unchanged,[10] women as a group are likely to continue to struggle in health care settings. Consider further the way women in the media are portrayed today: Even those dramas that feature women in health care usually show the woman providers as subservient to men in the health care hierarchy. This accurate reflection of the current power structure in academic medical centers and health care facilities demonstrates the challenges to women's rights in health care. In its own way, *A Private Matter* demonstrates the disempowerment of women in all areas of the moral life, and displays the harms that can ensue both to the woman herself and to society at large.

NOTE

i. A "moral agent" is an individual who has the capacity to make a choice or take an action, and by virtue of this capacity is responsible for the rightness or wrongness of the action taken or decision made.

REFERENCES

1. Sherwin, S. 1991. *No longer patient*. Philadelphia, PA: Temple University Press.
2. Bennett, B., and Karpin, I. 2008. Regulatory options for gender equity in health research. *International Journal of Feminist Approaches to Bioethics* 1(2): 80–99.

3. McCarthy, J., and Deady, R. 2008. Moral distress reconsidered. *Nursing Ethics* 15: 254–262.

4. Gowans, C. 1994. *Innocence lost: An examination of inescapable moral wrongdoing.* New York: Oxford University Press.

5. Kumar, A., Hessini, L., and Mitchell, E.M.H. 2009. Conceptualising abortion stigma. *Culture, Health and Sexuality* 11(6): 625–639.

6. Das, V. *Stigma, contagion, defect: Issues in anthropology of public health* (paper presented at US National Institutes of Health conference on Stigma and Global Health: Developing a Research Agenda. Bethesda, MD, 2001). Retrieved July 31, 2009 from http://www.stigmaconference.nih.gov/FinalDasPaper.htm

7. Elders, M.J. 2008. Contraceptive availability to adolescents: Do American values violate our most vulnerable? *Clinical Pharmacology and Therapeutics* 84(6): 741–745.

8. Sankar, P., Moran, S., Merz, J.F., and Jones, N.L. 2003. Patient perspectives on medical confidentiality. *Journal of General Internal Medicine* 18: 659–669.

9. Siegler, M. 1982. Confidentiality in medicine: A decrepit concept. *New England Journal of Medicine* 307: 1518–1521.

10. Schmid Mast, M., Hall, J.A., Klöckner, C., and Choi, E. 2008. Physician gender affects how physician nonverbal behavior is related to patient satisfaction. *Medical Care* 46(12): 1212–1218.

part eight

end of life and right to die

advance directives and living wills: *autumn in new york*

alister browne

Autumn in New York (2000). Richard Gere, Winona Ryder, Anthony LaPaglia,
Elaine Stritch. Directed by Joan Chen. Duration: 103 minutes.

DVD Chapter 13 Scene 01.24.47 to 01.27.27

I N *AUTUMN IN NEW YORK*, Charlotte Fielding (Winona Ryder) is dying. She has
a tumour causing cardiac problems, and her all-business physician bluntly
tells her that she will get progressively weaker and suffer collapses of increasing
severity. High-risk surgery could perhaps be tried as a final effort, but she does not
recommend that. In light of this, Charlotte writes an advance directive (AD)
refusing the surgery. Then she meets Will Keane (Richard Gere), a rich, sophisticated chef and playboy, twice her 22 years; She falls in love and changes her mind
about her AD. She decides she wants to try everything that could extend her life
and requests the surgery. The surgery is done but, alas, to no avail. Her relationship with Will begins when leaves are falling and ends with snow on the ground.

This scene depicts Charlotte's change of heart. Will has just returned from
Ohio, where (unbeknownst to Charlotte) he has found a surgeon who will
operate. Charlotte finds this out from a chance remark and is furious. What Will
arranged, she tells him, is exactly what she did not want and made her AD to
prevent. But Will's despair at the thought of losing her without trying everything
wins her over, and she comes to realize that she does not want to leave him either.
Charlotte tears up her AD and tells Will that she will instruct her doctors to do
what he says.

I use this plot line as a launching pad for a discussion of ADs. The basic idea of
ADs is to allow individuals to project their health care preferences into a time
when they can no longer make decisions for themselves. As such, these directives
promise to make clear the wishes of incapable patients and take a lot of pressure
off physicians. Sometimes ADs fulfill this promise, but sometimes they do exactly
the opposite.

Advance directives came into being the in late 1960s, with the shift from a
Hippocratic model of health care, in which physicians made decisions, to an
autonomy model, in which decisions are left as much as possible to patients. Their
rise to popularity stems partly from respect for autonomy and, since they primarily
refuse health care, partly from the hope that they will conserve money and health
care resources.

The hoped-for cost saving has not materialized. Few people have ADs (10% Canadians, 20% Americans), they are frequently not followed, and the start up and administrative costs of programs such as the U.S. Patient Self-Determination Act are enormous.[1] This may change, but for the present, the value of ADs must reside in the promotion of patient autonomy. It will be best, however, to begin with some distinctions. Advance directives come in two kinds. The first are *proxy directives* (also called *durable powers of attorney*). The second are *instructional directives* (also called *living wills*). Most jurisdictions in the Western world allow for both forms of ADs, but they vary on what is needed to give them legal force. In some, an unwitnessed note written in private is binding; in others, a specific form filled out by a lawyer and signed in the presence of witnesses is necessary—and everything in between may be required by other jurisdictions.

Proxy directives allow individuals to designate who they would like to make end-of-life decisions for them, and (in some jurisdictions) specify the extent of that person's authority. Absent a proxy directive, the decision maker will be drawn from a legal line that traditionally begins with "spouse, adult child, parents," and continues on. If this line does not uniquely identify an individual, or if the identi-fied person is not available or willing to act as the decision maker, some public official becomes the person to make the decisions. Sometimes proxies have the same authority that the persons themselves have, namely the ability to refuse any treatment whatsoever. But sometimes this is limited. Thus, if individuals want someone not on the legal line to make the decisions, or want to give the decision-maker unbridled authority, they can bring this about by a proxy directive.

So, if Charlotte wants to be sure that Will is her decision maker, she had better marry him or make a proxy directive. Charlotte does not make Will her proxy. But if she wants her physicians to follow Will's instructions, she would be well-advised to do so. For, as long as he does not marry her, and without such a directive, he has no legal standing. Her physicians may follow his instructions, but they are under no obligation to, and may well not if someone else requests something different. Charlotte, for instance, may be well-advised not to give Will unrestricted authority, given that he has revealed himself to be a womanizer with a short attention span for his current loves. But when one is luckier with partners, one may want them rather than physicians to have the final say. Proxy directives require careful thought, but instructional directives cause the most controversy.

There are two species of instructional directives. The most common one is what we might call "means-directed." These give individuals an opportunity to say what treatment they want or do not want under what health conditions. They can be simple, like the "Levels of Intervention" directives common in long-term care, which invite individuals to choose whether, in the event of a life-threatening crisis, they would like comfort care only, maximum care within the confines of the facility, transfer to acute care but no attempt at cardiopulmonary resuscitation (CPR) or admission to the intensive care unit, or maximum care. There are also more complex varieties that enable one to make finer-grained choices. These give individuals the opportunity to say, for example, whether they want CPR, ventilation, dialysis, life-saving surgery, blood transfusion, life-saving antibiotics, and tube-feeding, if they are in their current health, have a mild stroke, moderate stroke, severe stroke, have mild dementia, moderate dementia, severe dementia, are in a permanent coma, or have a terminal illness.[2] Some instructional directives, in addition, invite individuals to say what they would want if their conditions are reversible or irreversible.[3]

The other species of instructional directives is "end-directed." These are made for individuals who do not particularly care about specific treatments, but do worry about outcomes. By means of these directives, individuals can direct physicians to do everything they can as long as there is a reasonable chance of achieving an acceptable outcome, and say what outcomes they consider acceptable and unacceptable. A common one simply directs physicians to forgo treatment if "there is no longer any possibility of a rational existence." Others allow individuals to be more discriminating, and to decline treatment when they are in a permanently unconscious state, or can no longer communicate, or can no longer take care of themselves, and so on.[4] These two species are not mutually exclusive, and some AD forms combine them. Individuals also do not have to make instructional directives by filling out any premade form. They can simply write out what they want, or use a form and modify it in any way they please.

There is reason to be skeptical about whether instructional directives succeed in getting patients the care they want. Studies show that the preferences of patients do not tend to be stable over time, and hence that their predictions about what they would want in the future are far from certain. They also show that it is difficult for patients to articulate those preferences in a way that cannot be misunderstood.[5] Some have concluded from this that instructional ADs are not a good idea; a more nuanced position, however, is to distinguish between circumstances in which they are and are not likely to be helpful.

Instructional directives are substitutes for patients making decisions in real time and in consultation with their physicians. They work best when they most closely approximate these circumstances, and they do this when patients unambiguously identify what care they want when, and are unlikely to change their minds about that. Thus, patients can be advised to make means-directed instructional directives if they have firm views about certain procedures for ideological reasons (e.g., no blood because they are Jehovah's Witnesses), or have had experiences with specific health care (e.g., ventilation) they would not like to repeat. Similarly, these directives are helpful if patients are visibly disabled and want the care that anyone without that condition would receive, but fear that physicians may not provide it, or if they have health conditions that enable them to predict with some accuracy what the future holds, as in Charlotte's case. Charlotte has to make up her mind whether she wants aggressive treatment when the time comes. This may not be easy to do, but once she decides what she wants, instructional directives are tailor-made to communicate that information.

But, as individuals deviate from those conditions, it becomes increasingly difficult to be confident that they will be well-served by such a directive. Suppose, for example, that after Charlotte made her AD she turned to Will and suggested that he make one too. He seems healthy enough, but is middle-aged, regularly dines on French cuisine, has a type-A personality, and makes love a lot. Maybe, Charlotte would suggest he should have an instructional directive in his life-planning documents. Would Will be well-advised to take up the suggestion?

We can begin to see the difficulties Will would encounter by considering the situation of essentially healthy patients asked to designate a Level of Intervention upon entering a hospital. Anything they say puts them in potential jeopardy. They will not want comfort care only if a life-threatening crisis is fully reversible by maximum care, or maximum care if they have a devastating stroke, and the in-between levels may likewise be not enough or too much. The finer-grained versions do better, but there is still risk. For example, how confidently can healthy individuals say that they would (or would not) want dialysis if they had a moderate stroke? Wouldn't that depend on how the stroke had affected them (e.g., whether they could think, speak, walk, swallow, etc.), whether the condition is reversible, and if so, how sure, quick, and full the recovery would be? Nor would it be easy to add the qualifications necessary to ensure that they get exactly what they want. End-directed instructional directives are better suited to the healthy, for judgments about ends tend to be firmer than those about means. But, even here, it is difficult to make accurate estimates of acceptable conditions one has never experienced. *Now* one may not want this or that; *then*, when the alternative of death is near, one may change his or her mind.

Instructional directives thus carry some risk for the healthy, and Will may rather take his chances with decisions made by others at the time of need. But let us suppose that he is willing to brave the risk. How would he, as a reasonable and prudent person, want physicians to treat his directive? Would he want them to stick to the letter of what he says and do exactly that? Or, would he prefer them to exercise discretion, ask whether that is what he would really want in these circumstances, and set the instructions aside if they think it is not?

The interventions one would want in a medical crisis depend on the effects one has suffered, the extent, probability, and speed of their reversibility, and the burdensomeness of care. Means-directed instructional directives cannot be sufficiently sensitive to these factors to ensure that they will help patients get the care they want. End-directed instructional directives may be better suited to this population, for judgments about ends tend to be firmer than those about means. But they share with means-directed directives the problem of making accurate estimates of what conditions are acceptable when one has never experienced them. Now, one may not want this or that; then, one may have a different opinion. It is notorious that quadriplegics often (to their great surprise) satisfactorily adjust to their condition, and individuals who suffer dementia sometimes seem quite happy. Given all this, healthy individuals with no ideological commitments or history of health problems may reject instructional directives in favor of decisions made by their loved ones in consultation with physicians at the time of need.[6]

The danger of a mismatch between what instructional directives literally say and what their authors would have chosen raises the question of whether physicians should always follow them. For example, does "no surgery" mean that patients do not want a hip pinned or a pacemaker implanted if those things would be comfort measures? Does "no life-preserving treatment if demented" mean that patients do not want to be kept alive when they are only pleasantly confused? Does a patient who stipulates "no electroconvulsive therapy" (because he believes ECT usually turns people into vegetables) mean that the patient does not want ECT when it is a safe and effective life-saving treatment? Such doubts must make us hesitate to say that physicians should always do what instructional directives literally say. "No" means no, but what "No" refers to may not be clear.

Given this, how should AD legislation be written? If it stipulates penalties for noncompliance, physicians will be encouraged to practice defensive medicine and do what instructional directives literally say, with the consequence that patients will sometimes not get the health care they want. On the other hand, if no such penalties exist, that will encourage physicians to exercise discretion, and that will again mean that patients will sometimes not get the health care they want. Some jurisdictions have penalties (fines, suspensions, or revocations of licenses) for non-compliance. Others allow physicians to exercise discretion, permitting them to disregard ADs refusing the provision of life support when there is a good faith belief that continuing life support serves the patient's interests.[7] Whichever policy is adopted, patients will sometimes certainly not get the health care they would have chosen, and there is no evidence that one alternative will promote patient autonomy better than the other. It thus remains an open question as to how the legislation should be written, and however it is, what the moral obligation of a physician is when faced with an instructional directive that the physician has reason to think the patient would not want followed.

Contemporary Western health care differs from Hippocratic in that the goal is not to provide patients with the best care, but with the care they want. Thus, the idea of ADs must be attractive to all those who line up with this philosophy. But if the above arguments are right, ADs cannot be recommended for everyone. Proxy directives are a good idea when people have special views about who should make their decisions or the authority they want their decision makers to have. So are instructional directives, in which patients have fixed views or a foreseeable future. But when neither of the former is so, proxy directives are pointless; and when neither of the latter is, one has to be feeling lucky to make an instructional directive.

REFERENCES

1. Singer, P.A., Robertson, G., and Roy, D.J. Advance care planning. 1998. In P.A. Singer (Ed.) *Bioethics at the Bedside* p. 41. Ottawa: Canadian Medical Association. Also,

Fagerlin, A., and Schneider, C.E. Enough: The failure of the living will. *Hastings Center Report* 34(2): 30–42.

2. University of Toronto Joint Centre for Bioethics. "Living Will." Retrieved from www.utoronto.ca/jcb

3. Molloy, W. *Let me decide: The health-care directive that speaks for you when you can't.* Toronto: Penguin Canada.

4. Browne, A., and Sullivan, W.J. 1999. Advance directives: A third option. *Annals of the Royal College of the Physicians and Surgeons of Canada (RCPSC)* 32(6): 352–354.

5. Fagerlin, A., and Schneider, C.E. 2004. *Hastings Center Report* 34 (2) 30–42.

6. Lynn, J. 1991. Why I don't have a living will. *Law, Medicine & Health Care* 19(1–2): 101–104.

7. Olick, R.S. 2001. *Taking advance directives seriously: Prospective autonomy and decisions near the end of life* p. 28. Washington, DC: Georgetown University Press.

2

brain death: *steel magnolias*

andrew fenton

Steel Magnolias (1989). Sally Field, Dolly Parton, Shirley MacLaine, Daryl Hannah, Olympia Dukakis, Julia Roberts. Directed by Herbert Ross. Duration: 117 minutes.

DVD chapter 24 scene 01.28:28 to 01.33.48

REVOLVING AROUND THE ORDINARY LIVES of several women in small-town Louisiana, *Steel Magnolias* contains a number of themes notewor-thy for their political and ethical significance (e.g., communal parenting, gender essentialism, organ transplantation, parents outliving their children, pro-natalism, pronutpialism). It also spotlights the brain death of one key character.

Shelby Eatenton's (Julia Roberts) marriage sets the context for the beginning scenes of the movie. Because she is diabetic, Shelby's choice to have a child is implicated, albeit vaguely, in her subsequent ill health (i.e., renal failure). Although she receives a kidney transplant, donated by her mother M'Lynn Eatenton (Sally Fields), and, for a time, seems healthy, Shelby suddenly deteriorates. While at home caring for her son, Shelby collapses and never recovers consciousness. Several scenes set in the hospital follow the family in crisis, particularly M'Lynn. However, curiously few—either leading up to Shelby's hospitalization or up to her husband Jackson Latcherie (Dylan McDermott) consenting to the removal of life support—detail her changing medical condition or the decision process to have the life support removed. The relative invisibility of these medical details probably reflects an unwillingness to introduce material that would change the overall "feel" of the movie. It may also reflect the difficulty of taking on such topics as brain death in film.

Brain death—a condition that is not to be confused with either vegetative or minimally conscious state—has been defined as the irreversible "loss of all clinical brain function,"[1] including the capacities for phenomenal consciousness and to breathe on one's own.[2] This reflects a longstanding view of brain death as the irreversible cessation of those brain functions that integrate the functioning of the organism as a whole.[3,4] This can occur without the complete absence of what qual-ifies as organic life within the body of an organism, including some of the brain.

Historically speaking, the clinical importance of brain death is tied to two events in the 2oth century: (a) the ability to artificially maintain cardiopulmonary function; (b) the development of efficient organ transplantation.[1,5] In contemporary medicine, death occurs with the irreversible cessation of all biological functions critical for the continued functioning of the individual, although this can be variously understood. Traditionally, the irreversible cessation of cardiopulmonary function[3] determined this. However, in an age of artificial ventilation, the patient can outlive his capacity to breathe unassisted. The inadequacy of the traditional criterion for death in the wake of this medical advance motivated responses from such diverse groups as the Harvard Ad Hoc Committee[6] (in 1968), the National Conference of Commissioners on Uniform State Laws[3] (in 1980), and the President's Commission for the Study of Ethical Problems in Medicine and Biomedical and Behavioral Research[4] (in 1981). Around the world, brain death is commonly regarded as the criterion of death in those minority of cases in which a patient is artificially ventilated and yet lacks brainstem reflexes.[5] Although it remains controversial to highlight the importance of organ transplantation in the rise to prominence of brain death as a clinical indicator of death,[i] clearly, in a context in which a patient's cardiopulmonary functions can be artificially maintained but his or her critical brain functions have ceased, the traditional cardiopulmonary criterion for the death of that patient is no longer relevant.[2]

When discussing brain death in the context of medical ethics, several things are noteworthy from the outset. First, the nature, moment, and significance of death, as discussed in this context, are neither straightforward nor decided by the relevant biological sciences. As noted by Barbara Koenig and Patricia Marshall,[7] "[d]eath is a fact of life, but awareness of mortality is a social, not a biological reality. Knowledge about death and its meaning and value is socially constructed."[ii] Second, as noted by Sam Shemie et al.,[1] brain death "implies a notion of irreversible loss of personhood and integrative functions of the brain." The first conjunct, the irreversible loss of personhood, probably implicates metaphysics, such as philosophical reflections on the nature of observer-independent reality. Although there are moral and legal senses of "person" or "personhood" that are important here, particularly for health practitioners, it is primarily the metaphysical sense of these terms—what it really means to be a person, independent of how we tend to understand personhood—that will track those concerns informing how patients, their loved ones, and caregivers make decisions about, or understand, death.[iii] Knowledge contained in the relevant biological sciences about human anatomy, physiology, and neurology will be of limited use when tackling many metaphysical views of the human person, including his or her death. Third, and in consequence of the preceding, brain death will enjoy varying significance or weight in judgments about the final death of a person.[iv] Fourth, as disagreements in metaphysics are notoriously difficult to rationally resolve, health practitioners and bioethicists should be wary, when engaged in the pursuit of medical care, of making blanket declarations about when an individual has truly, or really, died. Although it may befall a health care practitioner to make a final decision as to the moment of a patient's death, he or she should be mindful that such a judgment is neither straightforwardly verifiable nor incontestable.

A patient's death can be understood in at least one of three ways: (a) animal or organismic death; (b) the death of a human being; (c) the death of a person.[v] Each of these ways of understanding a patient's death has different ontological, ethical, and social significance.

Animal death falls squarely under the domain of the biological sciences and contrasts with what we might call animal life—consisting in such characteristics as cell reproduction, homeostasis, metabolism, and growth. We should take care to distinguish between animal death understood as the death of the whole animal (or organic death) and the death of the animal as a whole (or organismic death). Organic death implicates the cessation of all of those characteristics constituting life (e.g., cell reproduction, homeostasis, metabolism, growth). However, organismic death implicates the cessation of somatically integrative functions broadly construed.[2,8] If we understand a patient's death as animal death, and animal death as organic death, then brain death does not mark an individual's final, or absolute, death as a biological entity. Subsequent to brain death, certain organic functions remain.[9] Interestingly, the body is still capable of behavior even subsequent to the respiratory failure of a brain dead patient after ventilation is removed. The *Lazarus sign* is a dramatic example here, in which the arms can spontaneously cross over the chest or move in response to noxious stimuli, such as painful stimulus to an upper arm.[10] Life, in some broad sense of continued electrical activity, is not totally absent subsequent to brain death. Alternatively, if we understand a patient's death as animal death, and animal death as organismic death, brain death *may not* mark an individual's final, or absolute, death as an organism (or biological entity). The functions that remain after brain death may still be properly regarded as integrative in nature and critical to organismic life (e.g., hemodynamic stability). Brain death is only relevant under this understanding of animal death if brain death implicates the cessation of somatically integrative functions.[6]

The death of a human being and death of a person are the possible types of patient death that bring more philosophical discussions of brain death to the foreground.[11] For an individual to enjoy beinghood, they must have the capacity for subjective experiences (e.g., pleasure and pain), and it must be possible for them to fare well or badly from their perspective.[12,vi] To distinguish beinghood from personhood, note that we are not the only animals to enjoy beinghood, even if such animals are not persons. Many domestic pets, like cats and dogs, are good examples of beings—although *perhaps* not metaphysical persons—whose lives can fare well or badly depending on what happens to them. Traditionally, for an individual to enjoy autonomous personhood, he must have the ability to choose what is best for himself and have the capacity for complex thought and self-awareness, and these capacities must be implicated in what it is for them to fare well or badly from their perspective.[12] That, from her perspective, an individual's life can fare well or badly underlies the ascription of interests to that individual and the attendant capacity to be harmed.[13] "Doing no harm" is one of the paramount moral commitments of medical practice. As a functioning, reasonably developed, central nervous system is a necessary condition for either beinghood or personhood in mammals such as humans, the death of the brain marks the death of the being or person.[vii] The death of a being or person marks the boundary of possibly doing harm to the relevant individual. Thus, the death of a being or person is critical in many discussions in bioethics (e.g., abortion, euthanasia).

Brain death can be understood in at least three ways: (a) cessation of activity in those cortical or subcortical regions implicated in so-called higher cognitive functions[5]; (b) cessation of general, somatically integrative brain functions[5]; and (c) cessation of activity in the brainstem.[2] Each of these ways of understanding brain death requires different criteria for its determination.[viii] Also, each understanding of brain death has attendant problems. Even for those inclined toward understanding patient death as death of the human being or person, the first criterion (a) may not track what is of ethical importance. That is to say, a possible criticism of the first criterion is that a cessation of so-called higher cognitive functions may still leave a patient with his beinghood intact, depending on what qualifies as higher cognitive functions. Consequently, his medical treatment may still require equal consideration of his right to continue to live, to bodily integrity, and to a life free of unnecessary pain or discomfort. The second criterion (b) has been criticized because not all brain functions must cease for a patient to be judged brain dead. Such an understanding of brain death does not track the practice of determining brain death, and not all somatically integrated functions are brain mediated.[8,14] The third criterion (c) has been criticized because certain brain functions, and perhaps phenomenal consciousness, can survive the cessation of brainstem function.[5]

Many defenders and critics of brain death continue to contend that organismic death (i.e., death of the organism as a whole) is the ethically relevant understanding of death for dealing with end-of-life medical care.[5,8] This perspective is problematic. For example, there is a danger of confusing the different senses of patient death outlined above, senses that, contra bioethicists like Bernat, are socially significant to those involved. It is difficult to shake the impression that the emphasis on organismic death as that which is of final clinical importance forgets the foundations for the claim to medical care that each community member can make on his or her greater society. An equal respect and regard for persons who enjoy a high moral status and whose life can fare well or badly is surely one important way to understand this foundation. Arguably, we risk losing the focus on this foundation and of patients as persons if we focus on patients as organisms.

Unfortunately, many health care workers will, at some point in their career, face the death of a patient. Ascertaining when a patient has died, particularly when he or she is concurrently receiving basic medical care and are ventilated, can be difficult for the relevant families and health care practitioners alike. In *Steel Magnolias*, the obvious physical and psychological toll of M'Lynn Eatenton's hospital-bed vigil is but one way in which the circumstances surrounding a patient's brain death can be difficult. M'lynn's expressed grief in the cemetery following Shelby's funeral implies that M'lynn regarded her vigil with Shelby—until there were no "life signs"—as completing a circle that began with Shelby's birth. As she says, "I was there when that wonderful creature drifted into my life, and I was there when she drifted out." This, perhaps, reflects the difficulty of coming to terms with when a family member has died. Alternatively, this reflects the difficulty of deciding when a family member has died. Difficulties for health care practitioners can parallel M'lynn's difficulty with what medicine commonly regards as the "real" moment of death.

There is a literature which, in discussing the spinal reflexes and automatisms that can remain for hours after a patient's brain death, is clearly directed toward better preparing health care practitioners for the expression of behavior (e.g., Lazarus sign) that is not "life indicative."[15] In the context of discussing organ donation, brain dead patients are commonly described as cadavers (e.g., heart-beating cadaver donors), perhaps as a way to disambiguate these "signs of life" from the genuine articles.[16] That there is organic life still present (think here of spinal reflexes) troubles this suggested locution. Arguably, the three senses of patient death mentioned above can help heath care practitioners and family members navigate this complex terrain. Understanding that a patient has irreversibly lost his or her capacity for phenomenal consciousness and very simple mental states correlated to neural responses to visual or tactile stimuli can hasten the grieving process. Understanding the distinction between organic and organismic life may also aid families in recognizing that what remains after brain death is no longer their mother or sister, qua the person they have known and loved. Families may find it reassuring to think that their difficulties in recognizing the death of a loved one may be tracking the different senses in which their loved can be understood to be dead (or living). This, in turn, may help families to see the significance of what heath care practitioners are communicating about their loved one and deepen the trust that is so crucial to a decision to discontinue life support that is free of coercion, or even the appearance of coercion. Remembering, however, that how we understand patient death is neither always straightforward nor incontestable can underwrite a deep understanding of the struggles of the relevant family members or caregivers and a sense of humility in the face of such a profound event.

ACKNOWLEDGMENTS

The writing of this chapter was funded by a grant from the Canadian Institutes of Health Research.

NOTES

i. Although, see a recent *Nature* editorial which does just that.[9]

ii. This is, of course, no less true at the beginning of life. Interminable debates over the moral status of abortion evidence this.

iii. Under legal conceptions of personhood, which extend over those ordinarily understood to be persons (i.e., this author and the readers), corporations can also qualify as persons. That is, corporations can enjoy a certain standing within society—they can possess certain rights, as well as responsibilities and obligations. Similarly, although moral conceptions of personhood extend over this author and the readers, it is primarily concerned with a certain moral standing within the relevant moral community (i.e., that the relevant individuals enjoy a right to life or existence, bodily or physical integrity, autonomy, and the like). Such extensions of the notion of personhood do not require that the recipients possess certain features ordinarily associated with being a person (e.g., self-consciousness). Consequently, neither of these conceptions of personhood entirely captures what is at stake when talking of patient death. For a useful discussion of these distinctions in the context of business ethics (see French, 1979).[17]

iv. That the possibility of a body outliving the person does not reduce to the (rest of the) body outliving the brain is evinced by the grief, and the rupture in filial relations, that can ensue after a catastrophic loss of personal identity with advanced dementia.

v. For a similar breakdown of death (see Lustig, 2001).[18]

vi. Although certain philosophers[12] and philosophico–religious traditions (e.g., Buddhism) speak of nonsentient beings (roughly, beings that lack the capacity for sensation), my treatment precludes such an understanding of "being."

vii. That human embryos and fetuses lack a capacity for autonomous choice, complex thought, and self-awareness technically excludes them as candidates for personhood so understood here. Late-term fetuses, however, probably qualify as beings (i.e., human beings) so understood here.

viii. See the immediately preceding references.

REFERENCES

1. Shemie, S.D., Lazar, N., and Dickens, B.M. 2008. Brain death. In P.A. Singer, and A.M. Viens (Eds.), *The Cambridge textbook of bioethics*, pp. 85–91. New York: Cambridge University Press.
2. Pallis, C. (1982b). ABC of brain stem death. Reappraising death. *British Medical Journal* 285:1409–1412.
3. National Conference of Commissioners on Uniform State Laws. 1980. "Uniform Determination of Death Act." Retrieved October 29, 2009 from http://www.law.upenn.edu/bll/archives/ulc/fnact99/1980s/udda80.htm
4. President's Commission for the Study of Ethical Problems in Medicine and Biomedical and Behavioral Research. 1981. "Defining Death." Retrieved October 29, 2009 from http://www.bioethics.gov/reports/past_commissions/defining_death.pdf
5. Bernat, J.L. 2006. The whole-brain concept of death remains optimum public policy. *Journal of Law, Medicine and Ethics* 34(1): 35–43.
6. Ad Hoc Committee of the Harvard Medical School. 1968. A definition of irreversible coma. *Journal of the American Medical Association* 205(6): 85–88.
7. Koenig, B.A., and Marshall, P.A. 2004. Death. In S. Post (Ed.), *Encyclopedia of bioethics*, 3rd ed., pp. 546–560. New York: MacMillan Reference.

8. Shewmon, D.A. 2001. The brain and somatic integration: Insights into the standard biological rationale for equating "brain death" with death. *Journal of Medicine and Philosophy* 26(5): 457–478.

9. Anonymous. 2009. Delimiting death: Procuring organs for transplant demands a realistic definition of life's end. *Nature* 461: 570.

10. Döşemeci, L., Cengiz, M., Yilmaz, M., and Ramazano lu, A. 2004. Frequency of spinal reflex movements in brain-dead patients. *Transplantation Proceedings* 36: 17–19.

11. McMahan, J. 1998/2001. Brain death, cortical death and persistent vegetative state. In H. Kuhse, and P. Singer (Eds.), *A Companion to bioethics*, pp. 250–260. Malden, MA: Blackwell Publishing, 250–260.

12. DeGrazia, D. 2006. Moral status, human identity, and early embryos: A critique of the president's approach. *Journal of Law, Medicine and Ethics* 34.1: 49–57.

13. Tooley, M. 1998/2001. Personhood. In H. Kuhse, and P. Singer (Eds.), *A companion to bioethics*, pp. 117–126. Malden, MA: Blackwell Publishing.

14. Pallis, C. 1982a. From brain death to brain stem death. *British Medical Journal* 285: 1487–1490.

15. Jain, S., and DeGeorgia, M. 2005. Brain death-associated reflexes and automatisms. *Neurocritical Care* 3: 122–126.

16. Youngner, S.J., and Arnold, R.M. (1993). Ethical, psychosocial, and public policy implications of procuring organs from non-heart-beating cadaver donors. *Journal of the American Medical Association* 269(21): 2769–2774.

17. French, P.A. 1979. The corporation as a moral person. *American Philosophical Quarterly* 16(3): 207–215.

18. Lustig, B.A. 2001. Theoretical and clinical concerns about brain death: The debate continues. *Journal of Medicine and Philosophy* 26(5): 447–455.

3

care of the dying: *the barbarian invasions*

letícia ludwig möller

The Barbarian Invasions (2003). Rémy Girard, Stéphane Rousseau, Marie-Josée Croze, Dorothée Berryman, Dominique Michel. Directed by Denys Arcand. Duration: 99 minutes.

DVD Chapter 7 Scene 00.40.30 to 00.42.00

I N *THE BARBARIAN INVASIONS*, HISTORY professor Rémy (Rémy Girard) is admitted to a hospital in Québec, where he becomes aware of the inefficiency and chaos of a public health care system. Counting on the efficiency (and the money) of his son (Stéphane Rousseau), who he always thought was so different from him and with whom he has always had a difficult relationship, Rémy manages to feel more comfortable and relieve his pain. Also, he finds himself surrounded by his old friends, and can depart life in his own way, in the place and time he chooses.

In the referred scene, Rémy is still in the hospital. He learns he has an irreversible cancer but, being a convinced socialist, Rémy refuses his son's offer of transferring to a private clinic in the United States, where he would receive the best in terms of care. On the night before, he tried heroin for the first time (clandestinely introduced into the hospital by Nathalie [Marie-Josée Croze], a young drug addict) to relieve his pain. The next morning, a doctor followed by two young assistants, enters Rémy's room, and the patient awkwardly tries to disguise the lingering odor of the drug.

Rémy is still under the relaxing effect of the drug. Impatiently, the doctor begins to examine Rémy and asks him quickly and disinterestedly: "Any sleep problems? Take a deep breath. Is there any pain? Is it insufferable?" Addressing himself to the assistants, he concludes: "He looks relaxed, so he won't need to take any painkillers." It's obvious that the doctor has mistaken Rémy for another patient, because on his way out he says something like: "Good-bye, Mr. Parenteau." Rémy retorts: "Thank you, Dr. Dubé." The doctor then says to him: "But I am not Dr. Dubé." "And I am not Mr. Parenteau," replies Rémy. At the door, angry rather than disconcerted or embarrassed, the doctor asks his assistants: "Who is this guy?"

Although at first glance this scene may seem comical, it illustrates an unsatisfactory, although perhaps still dominant, medical attitude of lack of attention and concern for patient care. For that doctor, Rémy is just another patient to be seen for a few minutes, another hospital bed. Within the context of rapidly expanding scientific and biotechnological advancements, where new therapeutic options are constantly offered, the concern with care may be underestimated and relegated to a less prominent place by health care professionals. However, with the awareness of the excessive use of therapies, drugs, and medical procedures, particularly in terminal cases, the care of patient (and particularly the dying patient) is being perceived as an important theme that provides the opportunity to reflect on medical practice and patient's rights, as well as on the public health care system and the care it provides.

Reflecting on medical practice at the end of life, we can consider that the traditional medical paradigm of curing based on combatting disease, reiterated within medical schools and in deontological codes, should be gradually replaced by the paradigm of care: an attitude that favors the relief of pain and suffering, and which demands a good understanding of the different aspects (not only medical, but also psychological, social, cultural, and spiritual aspects) of dying. The so-called *palliative care*[i] given at the end of life, aimed to mitigate pain and suffering, is at the essence of an approach that seeks greater "humanization" of health care assistance.[1-4] Cicely Saunders and her proposal of the concept of "total pain," which considers pain not only in its physical dimension, but also in its mental, social, and spiritual dimensions, offered an important contribution to that issue.[5-7] In the film, the doctor is concerned with the patient's physical pain but does not seem to be interested in its other dimensions, which Rémy might be experiencing (as a matter of fact, he does not even appear to care much about the patient's physical pain).

Care of the dying is not merely a matter of deontological ethics, but also a philosophical and legal issue, for it involves the principles of autonomy and dignity. From a legal perspective, the terminally ill patient has the right to self-determination, which should involve the right to make clear and informed choices concerning the available therapies, as well as to decide to discontinue treatment that he may believe is no longer justified. Therefore, patient autonomy sets limits to so-called *medical paternalism*, in which the definition of what is "good" for the patient is exclusively based on medical criteria, excluding the patient's values, beliefs, and wishes. It's admitted that cultural elements affect the way an individual sees life and death, thus influencing his concept of a good or dignified death. The film stimulates this reflection when Rémy accepts his impending death and decides to leave the hospital in order to spend his last days in the company of old friends and his son in a lakeside house. Rémy wants his death to be consistent with his deepest beliefs and with the principles he has pursued all his life.[8-9,ii]

Beyond reflections on medical practice and the right to self-determination, *The Barbarian Invasions* provides another fundamental issue for reflection and discussion. The film depicts a chaotic public hospital in Canada, with crowded galleries and helpless patients, that offers a clear picture of a public health care system and concerns about its quality. In normative terms, Canada's health care system is directed to provide access to universal, comprehensive coverage for medically necessary hospital and physician services, with roles and responsibilities shared among the federal, provincial, and territorial governments. The principles of public administration, comprehensiveness (insurance plans must cover all insured health services provided by hospitals and physicians), universality (for all insured residents), portability (for residents moving from one province to another), and accessibility rule the Canadian health care system.[10] In Brazil, we have some important similarities with the Canadian health care system. Our Federal Constitution, in place since 1988, proclaims health care as a right of all Brazilian citizens and a government duty, and declares that the access to health assistance is universal and equal. For this purpose, the Constitution has introduced the Unified Health System (SUS; Sistema Único de Saúde), which aims to guarantee integral health assistance at no cost. Thus, the federal, regional, and municipal levels all share the in the administration and financing of the system.[11]

However, in spite of the democratic victory represented by the recognition of health care as a fundamental right and its fulfillment as a government obligation, the reality of public health care assistance (in Brazil and, according to the film, also in Canada) is far from fully accomplishing that normative goal. Widely available, high-quality health care remains a challenge and an ongoing problem. In that sense, one of the great values of the film is to stimulate reflection and public debate, leading us to face some questions: What would become of Rémy if he did not have a wealthy son? Under what circumstances would he have passed the last moments of his life? Is good care (in general cases, as well as at the end of life) to be available only to those who can afford it? Is dying with dignity a prerogative of the few or a common right?

NOTES

    i. According to the definition of the World Health Organization (2002), "Palliative care is an approach that improves the quality of life of patients and their families facing the problem associated with life-threatening illness, through the prevention and relief of suffering by means of early identification and impeccable assessment and treatment of pain and other problems, physical, psychosocial and spiritual."

    ii. Dworkin's view, according to which it matters how we die, illustrates this point: "There is no doubt that most people confer a special and symbolic significance to the way we die: whenever possible, they want their death to express and strongly confirm the most important values in their lives."

REFERENCES

1. Drane, J. 2003. Bioética e cuidados paliativos. In *Bioética: Poder e injustice,* pp. 415–426. São Paulo: Loyola.
2. Drane, J. 1994. *Clinical bioethics: Theory and practice in medical–ethical decision making.* Lanham, MD: Rowman & Littlefield.

3. Hill, T.P. 1996. Care of the dying: From an ethics perspective. In D. Thomasma, and T. Kushner (Eds.), *Birth to death: Science and bioethics,* pp. 218–226. New York: Cambridge University Press.

4. Pessini, L. 2001. *Distanásia: Até quando prolongar a vida?* São Paulo: Loyola. Pessini, L. 2005. Cuidados paliativos: Alguns aspectos conceituais, biográficos e éticos. *Prática hospitalar* 41. Retrieved from http://www.praticahospitalar.com.br/pratica%2041/pgs/materia%2021–41.html.

5. Saunders, C. 1959. *Care of the dying.* London, UK: Macmillan & Co.

6. Saunders, C., Baines, M., and Dunlop, R. 1995. *Living with dying: A guide for palliative care,* 3rd. ed. Oxford, UK: Oxford Medical Publications.

7. Saunders, C. 1996. Into the valley of the shadow of death. A personal therapeutic journey. *British Medical Journal* 313:1599–1601.

8. Dworkin, R. 1993. *Life's dominion.* New York: Vintage Books.

9. Möller, L.L. 2007. *Direito à morte com dignidade e autonomia.* Curitiba, BR: Juruá.

10. Canada Health Act. 1984. Retrieved from www.hc-sc.gc.ca.

11. Constituição da República Federativa do Brasil. 1988. Articles 196 to 200. Recently (September 2009), scattered documents on the functioning of SUS had been unified in a single regulation.

physician assisted suicide:
death on request

james w. green

Death on Request (1994). Documentary directed by
Maarten Nederhorst. Duration: 57 minutes.

DVD Chapter 2 Scene 1: 8:00–12:00

I N AMSTERDAM, DR. WILFRED SIDNEY van Oijen receives three to four
requests for aid in dying each year. One such patient is Kees de Joode, a 60-ish
man in the late stages of amyotrophic lateral sclerosis (ALS). Confined to a
wheelchair, his speech is so slurred that his wife must translate for the doctor. He
wants to die at home and that is his wife Antoinette's desire as well. Physician-aided
suicide has been practiced under regulation in Holland since the 1980s, and this
documentary film alternates between Dr. van Oijen's house visits and his private
ruminations on helping Kees peacefully end his life. It is a hard thing for this young
doctor to do, and he says it "leaves its mark on my whole body." But killing, he
insists, it is not. He wants only to relieve suffering, despite the anguish cases like
this bring him. Early in the film, he is shown discussing their options with Kees and
Antoinette. At these home consultations, he is frank, gentle, and deliberative; he is
not in a hurry.

Assisted dying is currently legal in Oregon and Washington State. I briefly
describe here the arguments, pro and con, and conclude by noting a procedure
advocated by some bioethicists for thinking through cases like Kees. Language is
part of the controversy. While "physician-assisted suicide" is the most familiar
term, it may not be the best. While suicide is generally illegal, physicians who
prescribe fatal medications under Oregon's 1994 Death With Dignity Act are not
legally involved in suicides. "Physician-assisted dying" is more descriptive.
Advocates prefer "aid in dying" and "death with dignity." I use these terms
interchangeably.

opposing arguments

Moral and theological objections were among the earliest responses to pathologist
Jack Kevorkian and his "suicide machine" in the 1990s. With nearly 130 assisted
suicides to his credit, he made the practice a controversial public issue. The phrase
"culture of life" was subsequently coined by Pope John Paul II as an expression of
his church's opposition to both euthanasia and abortion. Intense public scrutiny

and strong religious motivations were on display during the national television coverage of Terri Schiavo's death, clear evidence that, for many Americans, moral and theological principles are implicated in medical practices associated with the end of life. Physicians generally share that view. One study suggests that nationally 69% of physicians object to assisted suicide, often for religious reasons.[1]

A related argument is the "slippery slope" and its dangers, with the horrors of Nazi medical experiments commonly cited. If we start down this path, opponents ask, where does it end? Who next might be eligible for an early, perhaps unwanted, death? Those with disabilities remain particularly sensitive to these issues. Two advocacy groups, Not Dead Yet and the National Council on Disabilities, oppose assisted dying, the latter arguing that "the lives of people with any disability deemed too difficult to live with would be at risk, and persons with disabilities who are poor or members of racial minorities would likely be in the most jeopardy of all." Indeed, for some racial minorities, this is a sensitive issue as well. Many African Americans reject assisted suicide, a view reflecting their community's historic experience with discriminatory and poorly funded health care.[2]

A third position is that of the American Medical Association (AMA). In 1992, its Council on Ethical and Judicial Affairs issued Opinion 2.211 Physician-Assisted Suicide. It declares, "Physician-assisted suicide is fundamentally incompatible with the physician's role as healer, would be difficult or impossible to control, and would pose serious societal risks." The AMA recognizes personal autonomy in decisions about one's death, but argues it is limited in the instance of euthanasia by the principle of beneficence: medical skills should be used only to obtain beneficial results. Good pain management and hospice care should make assisted dying unnecessary. By "societal risks," the Council identified loss of public trust in the medical profession and pressure to reduce costs that would drive families and physicians to judge some lives less worthy of extending than others. While not all physicians, then or now, agree with the AMA prohibition, the organization's arguments recur in professional and public debates.

To protect public trust, Dutch law calls for "due care"—a request for assisted dying must be made by a competent patient without duress from others (three requests in Oregon, two oral and one written); an independent physician must examine the patient and concur with the primary physician's judgment of the situation; the fatal medications must be administered by the primary physician and no one else; and after death, a written report is required by a multidisciplinary review board that has the power to request additional information and a formal interview with the physician.[3] The Oregon law, however, has a subtle difference that some have questioned. In Holland, "unbearable suffering" is adequate to justify preparations for an assisted death. It is the patient who judges what is unbearable, while the physician must determine that no medical relief for that suffering is possible. For Kees, with his advanced ALS, that was the situation. Oregon law requires instead a prognosis of death within six months or less to start the process and that, say critics, is too open ended to guarantee public trust. In Oregon "the physician is immunized from civil and criminal liability for actions taken in 'good faith' in assisting a suicide," but prognoses made in "good faith" are too subjective to be a reliable standard.[4] These critics recommend that physicians treat instead the underlying fears of patients who seek aid in dying.

supporting arguments

A historically important article appearing in the *New England Journal of Medicine* in 1991 helped launch the current discussion. Dr. Timothy Quill described one of his patients, Diane, dying of leukemia. Familiar with the work of the Hemlock Society, she wanted to stockpile medications to induce death at a time of her choosing. Quill prescribed barbiturates for that purpose. Much troubled, he went public with his doubts and wrote, "She taught me that I can take small risks for people I really know and care about... . I wonder how many families and physicians secretly help patients over the edge into death in the face of such severe suffering."[5] Quill has since become one of medicine's prominent voices in this area.

Proponents commonly invoke several first principles in defense of their position. One is patient autonomy. An individual has a right to accept or reject life-saving procedures, a right that extends to choice in the timing of death. While the Supreme Court has ruled that no such right exists under the Constitution, it left it to the "laboratory of the states" to decide what rights they might recognize on other grounds. In the two states where assisted death is permitted, patient autonomy is treated as a "right" but only within a regulatory framework with specified guidelines.[6]

A second principle is quality of life. Terminal patients for whom pain control is not possible ought to be permitted to choose aid in dying since their remaining quality of life is severely compromised. That was Kees' situation. He hoped only to hold out until his birthday, several weeks away, followed by a quick end. At the bedside, after he died from a lethal injection, Antoinette and Dr. van Oijen agreed that ending his suffering when they did was the right thing. They are not alone in that. Interviews with survivors of Dutch patients who received aid in dying indicate general satisfaction with this proactive stance.[7]

A third argument, the desirability of controlled aid in dying through state regulation, is sometimes advanced to counter fears of the "slippery slope" and to make the point that implementation under the law is more nuanced than critics acknowledge. According to Oregon's Department of Human Services, between 1993 and 2007, a total of 341 state residents died from ingesting a prescribed medication, but many more who requested and received lethal drugs did not use them. In 2007, for example, 85 prescriptions were written, 46 patients died from the medication, 26 died from their underlying condition and, at the end of the year, 13 were still alive. The disparity between requests for a fatal drug and its use recurs yearly. From such data, proponents argue there is no slippery slope and, further, regulated aid in dying is preferable to "freelance" dying of the kind advocated by the Hemlock Society or quietly abetted *sub rosa*, which Quill feels some physicians allow. These numbers also reflect the fact that aided dying in Oregon is embedded in a distinctive social context, one that has grown up around the practice. That state has the highest rate of hospice referrals nationally, and most physicians participate in training courses on end of life care and decision making. No doctor is required to honor a patient request if he or she finds it personally unacceptable. There is also public support: Oregon voters have approved these arrangements not once but twice through the initiative process.

Who, then, is a typical Oregon patient seeking physician-aided dying? He is 70, married, has a high school education, and lives on the more urban west side of the state. His underlying illness is cancer, and his principle concerns are autonomy, dignity, and inability to engage in the things that once made life worthwhile. He is enrolled in hospice and will die at home. When that happens, his physician likely will not be there, but a caretaker will. He will use secobarbital, for which there is a minor risk of regurgitation, and will be unconscious in five minutes, dead in 25.

physician responses to patient requests

How does aid in dying affect physicians who, like Dr. van Oijen, are willing to accommodate patients like Kees? There is little qualitative data on this topic, but a 2004 study is suggestive.[8] Thirty five Oregon physicians who were interviewed said that requests for assisted dying were rare but always personally unsettling. Many felt they knew little of their patient's lives outside the patient encounter. They were surprised at the determination and insistence of these patients. Most were ambivalent about the Oregon law; they agreed with it, but preferred not to act on it. Their willingness to prescribe fatal drugs came at a cost. Some felt isolated, reluctant to talk with colleagues about it. Others, especially in rural areas, worried that rumors about them would spread, with negative consequences for their practice. All agreed that, while emotionally draining and time consuming, what they learned from the experience was valuable.

Given these ambiguities, how might a physician think through a request for aid in dying, and how might Dr. van Oijen have done so? One well-known model of bioethical reasoning divides the presenting problem into four parts.[9] First, medical indications. What is Kees' medical history, prognosis, the goals of treatment up to the present, and how has he benefitted? Second, patient preferences. Is Kees mentally competent and informed? Is he depressed, and is that what should be treated? Third, quality of life. What are his prospects, and what physical, mental, and social deficits does he face? Fourth, context. What are the relevant family and financial issues, provider concerns, and religious and cultural considerations?

Exploring each of these areas in frank and open conversation is difficult for most patients, families, and physicians as well, although guidelines for doing that are available in the medical literature.[10] Generous amounts of time and a gentle sense of presence are required. Dr. van Oijen had both, enabling Kees to hold on and meet his goal of dying on his birthday. The cost of error, a death that should not have happened as it did, is too high to do otherwise.

REFERENCES

1. Cullen, F.A., Nwodim, C., Vance, J.L., Chin, M.H., and Lantos, J.D. To die, to sleep: U.S. physicians' religious and other objections to physician-assisted suicide, terminal sedation, and withdrawal of life support. *Amererican Journal of Hospice and Palliative Care* 25: 112–120.

2. Crawley, L., Payne, R., Bolden, J., Payne, T., Washington, P., and Williams, S. 2000. Palliative and end-of-life care in the African American community. *Journal of the American Medical Association* 284: 2518–2521.

3. Buiting, H.M., Gevers, J.K.M., Rietjens, J.A.C., Onwuteaka, B.D., van der Maas, P.J., van der Heide, A., and van Delden, J.J.M. 2008. Dutch criteria for due care for physician assisted dying in medical practice: A physician perspective. *Journal of Medical Ethics* 34. e12.doi:10,436/jme. 2008. 024976.

4. Hendin, H., and Foley, K. 2008. Physician-assisted suicide in Oregon: A medical perspective. *Issues in Law and Medicine* 24(2): 121–125.

5. Quill, T.E. 1991. A case of individualized decision making. *New England Journal of Medicine* 324: 691–694.

6. Washington State Department of Health. "Oregon Death with Dignity Act." Retrieved July 15, 2009 from www.oregon.gov/DHS/ph/pas/index.shtml. See also Washington State Department of Health, www.doh.wa.gov/dwda.

7. Georges, J.J., Onwuteaka-Philipsen, B.D., Muller, M.T., and Van der Wal, G. 2007. Relatives' perspectives on terminally ill patients who died after euthanasia or physician-assisted suicide: A retrospective, cross-sectional interview study in the Netherlands. *Death Studies* 31: 1–15.

8. Dobscha, S.K., Heintz, R.T., Press, N., and Ganzini, L. 2004. Oregon physicians' responses to requests for physician assisted suicide: A qualitative study. *Journal of Palliative Medicine* 7: 469–471.

9. Jonsen, A.R., Siegler, M., and Winslade, W.J. 2006. *Clinical ethics: A practical approach to ethical decisions in clinical medicine.* New York: McGraw-Hill Professional.

10. Back, A.L., Arnold, R.M., and Quill, T.E. 2003. Hope for the best, and prepare for the worst. *Annals of Internal Medicine* 138: 439–443.

EDITOR'S NOTE

Readers may wish to view the 2010 HBO movie *You Don't Know Jack* (Director Barry Levinson, starring Al Pacino, Brenda Vaccaro, and John Goodman) depicting some of the life of right-to-die activist Dr. Jack Kevorkian.

5

do not resuscitate orders: *wit*

rené claxton and robert m. arnold

Wit (2001). Emma Thompson, Christopher Lloyd, Jonathan M. Woodward, Audra McDonald. Directed by Mike Nichols. Duration: 98 minutes. The teleplay by Nichols and Emma Thompson is based on the 1998 play of the same title by Margaret Edson.

DVD chapter 19 Scene 01.29:44 to 01.33:07

W IT, THE STORY OF AN English literature professor's struggle with metastatic ovarian cancer, is set against the backdrop of the modern academic health care system. The film opens with the patient, Vivian Bearing (Emma Thompson), matter-of-factly recalling her diagnosis: "I have stage four metastatic ovarian cancer. There is no stage five. Oh, and I have to be very tough. It appears to be a matter, as the saying goes, of life and death." The film negotiates the milestones of living and dying with metastatic cancer, including diagnosis, treatment, complications of treatment, and progressive disease. The cast of characters includes Jason (Jonathan M. Woodward), an oncology physician fellow eager to combat malignant cells but less eager to navigate the human experience; Susie (Audra McDonald), a nurse who crosses the divide between the impersonal health care system and the individual patient; Dr. Harvey Kelekian (Christopher Lloyd), the head doctor who cares more for his protocols than for his patients; and Dr. Bearing, a demanding poetry professor specializing in the Holy Sonnets of John Donne. In a series of flashbacks, the film compares and contrasts the behavior of Dr. Bearing, the uncompromising and demanding professor, with the hierarchical and impersonal medical staff. After confirmation that her disease has progressed despite chemotherapy, Dr. Bearing chooses to be a "no code," understanding that if her heart were to stop, doctors would not perform cardiopulmonary resuscitation (CPR). The movie ends with the oncology fellow calling the code team, despite the patient's documented wishes, when he finds her without a pulse.

Wit is not, at its core, really about the medical system. As Daniel Sulmasy points out in his extraordinary article describing the underlying themes of the movie, it is about forgiveness, relationship, and dignity.[1] Two things are striking in this essay. First, somewhat ironically, a play that seems to focus on end-of-life care is really about how to live and relate to each other more fully. To quote Sulmasy:

At its deepest level, it is not about health care professionals or the care of the dying. It is about "salvation anxiety": the question of whether we, as human beings, finally have any worth or value independent of how we appear to others or what we even think of ourselves; whether we can recognize this in each other; whether we can reconcile ourselves to each other for our individual and collective failures to treat each other with such dignity; whether we can allow ourselves, finally, to be loved and forgiven; and whether this, ultimately, in any way saves us.

Second, the ethical theory most appropriate for analyzing the play is not principle-based bioethics but a virtue-based theory. Virtue ethics focuses on virtue, or moral character, rather than rules (deontology) or consequences (consequentialism).[2,3] This approach argues that how one does something is as important as what one does. Some argue that being a good doctor requires the virtues of trust, care, and compassion in order to develop relationships with patients. Fidelity, courage, justice, and wisdom are required to deal with the health care system.[4] One question *Wit* raises, from this view, is how the health care system promotes or demeans the values that we hold as central to the caring endeavor.

This isn't to say that *Wit* cannot be used to illuminate certain bioethical practices. Two scenes in the movie exaggerate the unfortunate clinical reality of how health care professionals deal with decisions about resuscitation and death. First, in raising the issue, clinicians often focus on specific treatment decisions abruptly, without first determining patients' broader goals. Susie, for example, broaches the topic of a do not resuscitate order after Dr. Bearing asks, "My cancer is not being killed, is it?" Susie replies, "What you need to think about is your code status. What you want them to do if your heart stops beating." Second, physicians often focus more on curing the illness than caring for the person with the illness; that is, more weight is placed on specific medical interventions and technology rather than a therapeutic relationship. The interactions between Jason, the research-focused oncology fellow, and Dr. Bearing hyperbolize this tendency. As Dr. Bearing attempts to convey her apprehension and fear, Jason responds, "… cancer is the only thing I've ever wanted… cancer is awesome… it's immortality in culture." He is so enamored by the biology of malignancy that he fails to notice an opportunity for empathy that could help to reduce the professor's psychological suffering. In this way, the movie uses overstatement to illustrate ethical shortcomings in the medical system in the realm of end-of-life care.

When discussing goals for patients who are at the end of life, three ethical values should predominate: autonomy, beneficence, and nonmalfeasance. Autonomy refers to the patient's right to make decisions for him- or herself based on his best interest and to structure his life accordingly. This implies that health care providers should engage patients in discussions of their values and how these values inform treatment decisions. Health care providers also have a positive obligation to promote patients' good (beneficence) and avoid harm (nonmalfeasance).[2] As a patient's disease progresses, this means that health care providers should have a good understanding of what patients want to achieve and avoid. Data suggest that, rather than focusing on medical interventions, patients are concerned about social and spiritual issues.[5]

Practically speaking, actualizing the above principles means that end-of-life discussions should initially focus on the patient's goals, rather than isolated treatments such as cardiopulmonary resuscitation. After the health care provider understands the patient's hopes and concerns, she can make a recommendation to a patient about what *could be done* to achieve those goals and *what should not be done* as it will cause harm.[6] For example, a seriously ill patient may say that what is most important is to be at home with his family, given that current treatment is unlikely to prolong his life significantly. When asked about what worries him the most, he mentions being a burden to his wife and suffering a long extended death. Upon hearing this, the health care provider should offer to make a recommendation about what treatments will (and will not) achieve these goals. For example, one might say,

> "Given what you have told me, I want to suggest how we can help you achieve these goals. Would that be OK? I suggest that we focus on getting you home, so you can have time with your family. I also think we should consider getting some support at home—both physical support and psychological support. And if things get worse—that is, if you begin to get a lot sicker—I promise our goal will be to make sure you are comfortable. Given your illness, it would not make sense to do things that will only prolong your dying—things like being on machines or CPR. Does that make sense to you?"

Thus, the ethical tenets of autonomy, beneficence, and nonmalfeasance can be practically applied by discussing patients' goals and making recommendations to achieve those goals.

In *Wit*, Dr. Bearing's physicians and nurse fail to act on the principles of patient autonomy and beneficence. Her physicians marginalize her autonomy by not providing critical information regarding disease progression, treatment options, or end-of-life decisions, or by offering to include her in decision making. Susie should be commended for being willing to sit down with Dr. Bearing and talk honestly and compassionately about her illness. Still, she brings up the issue of resuscitation in isolation, assuming that the most important decision that the patient needs to consider is CPR. Moreover, the focus is on what should not be done (i.e., CPR), rather than what can be done to make Dr. Bearing's life better.

The final scene of the movie draws attention to the ethical issues of respect for dead persons and nonabandonment. When Jason mistakenly begins CPR on Dr. Bearing, despite her wishes otherwise, it appears that this action is based on the instinct of a young physician finding a patient without a pulse, rather than as a purposeful action aimed at overriding a patient's autonomy. Instead of allowing Dr. Bearing to die peacefully, the forceful resuscitation efforts of Jason and medical staff shatter the serenity of her death. Although Jason does not intend disrespect, the impact of his actions demonstrates disregard for the preferences of his patient. Susie clearly feels the impact and requests that Jason leave the room after the resuscitative efforts are discontinued, allowing her time alone with the body. The stark contrast between the chaos of the resuscitation effort and the gentle tranquility of the preparation of Dr. Bearing's body highlights the importance of respecting bodies even after death.

The movie also shows the importance of patient nonabandonment. As Dr. Bearing states,

> We are discussing life and death and not in the abstract, either; we are discussing *my* life and *my* death... Now is the time for, dare I say it, kindness.

The importance of health care provider nonabandonment (what Dr. Bearing calls kindness) cannot be overstated. Confronting decisions about death is frightening. Patients want to know that their doctors will be with them throughout their journey—regardless of what they choose. Should a patient choose not to be resuscitated, physicians should continue to offer interventions aimed at both disease and symptom management, as appropriate, given the patient's clinical situation and wishes. In addition to trying to promote patients' quality of life, doctors should not underestimate the positive impact of their presence. Just "being there" is a way to show patients that you care about them as a person worthy of your time and respect.[7] The final scene of *Wit* shows Susie caring for Dr. Bearing's body after the code team leaves the room. Once again, the doctors have left the room. While present to treat the cancer, they abandoned the patient when the cancer was not treatable. Viewing their role as treating the cancer, they were not psychologically willing to be present and listen to her as a person.

Wit portrays one woman's struggle with both metastatic cancer and the medical organization designed to help her. This struggle illustrates how one can use communication skills to promote the ethical principles of patient autonomy, beneficence, and nonmalfeasance. By referring back to these foundational principles, medical providers can provide ethical end-of-life care to patients. By individualizing care and eliciting patients' unique value systems, we can avoid seeing our patients as "just a specimen jar, just a dust jacket, just a white piece of paper."

REFERENCES

1. Sulmasy, D.P. 2001. At Wit's end: Forgiveness, dignity, and the care of the dying. *Journal of General Internal Medicine* 16: 335–338.
2. Beauchamp, T.L., and Childress, J.F. 2001. *Principles of biomedical ethics*, 5th ed. New York: Oxford University Press.
3. Hinman, L.M. 2005. Retrieved August 5, 2009 from http://ethics.sandiego.edu/presentations/Theory/virtue/index.asp

4. Hauerwas, S. 2004. Virtue and character. In S.G. Post (Ed.), *Encyclopedia of bioethics*, vol. 5, 3rd ed., pp. 2550–2556. New York: MacMillian Reference.
5. Singer, P.A., Douglas, M.K., and Kelner, M. 1999. Quality end-of-life care: Patients' perspectives. *Journal of the American Medical Association* 281: 163–168.
6. Back, A.L., Arnold, R.M., and Tulsky, J.A. 2009. *Mastering communication with seriously ill patients: Balancing honesty with empathy and hope.* Cambridge, UK: Cambridge University Press.
7. Quill, T.E., and Cassel, C.K. 1995. Non-abandonment: A central obligation for physicians. *Annals of Internal Medicine* 122: 368–374.

6

the rule of double effect: *two weeks*

lynette cederquist

Two Weeks (2006). Sally Field, Ben Chaplin, Tom Cavanagh, Julianne Nicholson, Glenn Howerton, and Clea Duvall. Written and Directed by Steve Stockman. Duration: 99 minutes.

DVD chapter 17 scene 1:01:14 to 1:02:52

THIS MOVIE TELLS THE STORY of four adult children who come home to care for their mother, Anita Bergman (Sally Field), who is in the terminal stage of metastatic cancer. Her only daughter, Emily (Julianne Nicholson), has been caring for her mother for some time when her three brothers arrive to help out. By then, their mother is essentially bedbound. Once all of the children are home, they enroll their mother in hospice. She has a bowel obstruction from the malignancy and is initially receiving total parenteral nutrition (nutrition from an IV). She is started on a morphine pump for control of pain. At one point, she asks her son to turn off the IV nutrition. One of her sons questions whether they are doing the right thing and whether their mother is dying from starvation and sedation from the morphine rather than from the underlying illness. His sister assures him that they are honoring their mother's wishes by focusing on comfort care, not pursuing any further aggressive treatment of the cancer. Their mother does die after two weeks of continuous care given by hospice, her four children, and her second husband. The movie gives a fairly realistic portrayal of the experience of families caring for a dying family member, including all of the family dynamics that may surface during that time. It also includes a special feature: a commentary on the entire movie, in which the writer and director, Steven Stockman, discusses the film with Dr. Ira Byock, a national leader in palliative and hospice care. Mr. Stockman discusses the fact that he wrote this story based on his experience of caring for his own mother.

In this particular scene, the mother appears to be sleeping, with her daughter sitting at her bedside. When her mother begins moaning, Emily picks up a book entitled "Caring for the Dying." She takes her mother's hand and tells her "It's OK to let go, Mom." Then, she calls the hospice nurse who comes out to the house. The following dialogue ensues:

HOSPICE NURSE: "We can increase the morphine dose and frequency."

DAUGHTER: "What happens if she gets too much?"

HOSPICE NURSE: "In hospitals, they tend to err on the side of a few more days of life, but in hospice, we leave that up to the patient and their families."

SON: "So, too much morphine?"

HOSPICE NURSE: "That's up to you and your mom."

SON: "Well she's not very responsive…"

There is a pause.

DAUGHTER: "Increase the dose."

This discussion illustrates the ethical rule of *double effect*. Bioethicists define the rule of double effect as an effect (such as hastening death) that would be morally wrong if caused intentionally, but if foreseen but unintended, is morally permissible when the intent of the action is to relieve suffering. Roman Catholic theologians developed the rule of double effect in the Middle Ages, as an ethical guide when a person faces a choice of actions in which it is impossible to avoid harm (allow suffering or shorten survival) in order to achieve good.[1] This dilemma can also be presented as a conflict between the basic ethical principles of benefi- cence versus nonmaleficence. When a physician must administer sedating medi- cations in order to achieve a benefit to the patient, but in order to do so risks potential harm (maleficence), which ethical value should take priority? When applied to provision of end-of-life care, the discussion is usually regarding the administration of analgesics and sedatives to control symptoms, which may also have the effect of suppressing respiration and shortening survival. When medica- tions are administered to a terminally ill patient and the patient stops breathing as a result, this may trigger a debate regarding whether this qualifies as an act of euthanasia. This debate is illustrated by the case of the physician and two nurses in New Orleans who were charged with murder after administering morphine and sedatives to four seriously ill patients in the hospital where they were trapped after Hurricane Katrina. Subsequent to the administration of the medications, the four seriously ill patients died. Did the doctor and nurses intentionally commit euthanasia (murder), or where they just trying to relieve the patients suffering? In this case, a grand jury refused to indict the physician or nurses. Although there have been other cases of physicians being charged with murder for administering high doses of morphine to terminally ill patients, none has been successfully convicted.[2]

Similarly, in the scene in which the mother dies in *Two Weeks*, her daughter and son try to play "catch up" with the morphine by administering several doses in succession. After they push the button several times, she stops breathing. As soon as they realize this, Emily and Keith exchange a look of alarm. Keith asks his sister, "What should we do?" After a pause, she replies, "Nothing." This scene certainly portrays the daughter and son's intent is to keep their mother comfortable when they administer the morphine, but when she stops breathing, they believe that they have just killed her. Should their actions be judged differently if they had administered the same doses of morphine with the intent of hastening their mother's death?

In clinical practice, the rule of double effect is intended to allow physicians to treat the pain and suffering of terminally ill patients by administering as much medication as necessary to get the patient comfortable, without fear of being charged with murder. Despite this acceptance both ethically and legally, physician fear of legal threat can still serve as a barrier to good end-of-life care.[3] Some argue that the rule of double effect exaggerates the potential for opioids to cause respiratory suppression beyond what is seen in clinical experience, thus exaggerating physician's fears of administering high doses of opioids. The data on the clinical importance of opioid-induced respiratory depression comes from three sources: opioid use by drug addicts, patients with acute postoperative pain, and volunteers without pain. Most of this data is likely not relevant to treatment of patients with chronic cancer-related pain. The largest source of information comes from the clinical experience of recognized experts in cancer pain, hospice, and palliative care. The overwhelming clinical experience is that respiratory depression in this setting is rarely seen.[4]

In addition, safeguards remain in place to protect the patient from inadvertently overdosing when using a morphine pump with patient-controlled analgesia. The physician's calculation of the appropriate dose programs the basal rate. The patient cannot change the continuous dose but can self-administer additional "as-needed" doses by pushing a button. These additional doses are controlled as well, usually limited to not more than every ten minutes in a quantity within safe dosing parameters relative to the basal rate. The scene in *Two Weeks*, in which the patient's children administer several doses from her morphine pump in rapid succession, is technically inaccurate because the pump does not allow one to administer doses that quickly.

The classical formulation of the rule of double effect mandates that four conditions must be satisfied: (a) The act must be good, or at least morally neutral; (b) the agent intends only the good effect; the bad effect may be foreseen but not intended; (c) the bad effect must not be a means to the good effect; and (d) the good effect must outweigh the bad effect.[5] A subject of controversy regarding the rule of double effect is that the physician's intent separates the action of administering morphine for purposes of relieving pain from euthanasia. The analysis of a person's intent is difficult to validate externally, so the agent's action must be judged based on their motives and character. Another conflict regarding the rule of double effect is that it prohibits shortening survival as an acceptable choice. Some argue that patients should be allowed to make that choice.[6] The rule of double effect does not address the debate regarding whether physician-assisted suicide or euthanasia is permissible. In applying the rule of double effect to the care of a dying person, it becomes clear why families caring for a dying loved one, such as the portrayal of the mother's death in *Two Weeks*, can create tremendous conflict for the family. Family members may disagree; they often feel conflicted and guilty about the care of the dying person. In order for physicians and other health professionals to be able to guide the care of dying patients, we must grapple with the ethics of our own actions and be able to educate our own patients and their families in order to effectively treat suffering at the end of life.

REFERENCES

1. Mangan, J.T. 1949. An historical analysis of the principle of double effect. *Theological Studies* 10: 41–61.
2. Alpers, A. 1998. Criminal act or palliative care? Prosecutions involving the care of the dying. *Journal of Law, Medicine & Ethics* 26: 308–331.
3. *Vacco v. Quill.* 1997. No. 117 S. Ct. 2293.
4. Fohr Anderson, S. 1998. The double effect of pain medication: Separating myth from reality. *Journal of Palliative Medicine* 1(4): 315–328.
5. Beauchamp, T.L., and Childress, J.F. *Principles of medical ethics*, 4th ed. New York: Oxford Press.
6. Quill, T., et al. 2007. The rule of double effect: A critique of its role in end-of-life decision making. *New England Journal of Medicine* 337: 1768–1771.

7

euthanasia: *the english patient*

marianne matzo and judith kennedy schwarz

The English Patient (1996). Ralph Fiennes, Kristin Scott Thomas, Juliette Binoche, Willem Dafoe. Directed by Anthony Minghella. Duration: 160 minutes.

DVD Chapter 29 Scene 02.28.58 to 02.33.44

THIS FILM DESCRIBES THE EXPERIENCES and memories of a Hungarian archeologist who participated with colleagues in a surveying expedition of Egypt and Libya during the late 1930s through the start of World War II. The early part of the movie describes the doomed but passionate love affair between Count Laszlo de Almásy (Ralph Fiennes) and the beautiful but married Katherine Clifton (Kristin Scott Thomas). Questions of national loyalty and personal fidelity provide a backdrop to the German advance. Count Laslo is horribly burned in a plane accident, and when he is eventually returned to the safety of a British camp in Italy, he pretends to suffer from amnesia rather than provide an account of his activities, which may have involved treason. The camp must be evacuated, and the count's suffering is heightened by the need to frequently stop and unload the patients so that mines and bombs left by the Germans can be defused. The count's medical care is overseen by a Canadian nurse, Hana (Juliette Binoche), who ultimately decides that she will stay and care for him alone in an abandoned villa. She believes he is dying, and that she will soon join her colleagues who have travelled ahead. She requests only that she be given lots of morphine— and a pistol.

The second half of the movie takes place in and around the villa. Hana has come to know her patient well as a result of their many conversations, and from seeing his one possession—a copy of Herodotus' *The Histories*, which has become a personal journal that contains his notes, photos, sketches, and letters from his lost love. Early in their relationship, he asks Hana for a cigarette. She responds "Absolutely not!" He asks, "Why are you so intent on keeping me alive?" She replies without reflection, "Because, I'm a nurse." A visitor to the villa, Caravaggio (Willem Dafoe) realizes that her patient is really Count Laszlo, whom he believes to be one of those responsible for his torture by the Nazis. Hana listens to Caravaggio and Count Laszlo recount the events of the last few years that have led to their current situation. Count Laszlo has lost the woman that he loved and feels responsible for her death. Caravaggio has been hunting down and killing those he believes responsible for his betrayal, and he intends to kill Count Laszlo. The count tells him, "You can't kill me, I died years ago."

In the final dramatic scene between Hana and the count, he is now actively dying; she feels great compassion for this person she has come to love. As she prepares to draw up his usual single vial of morphine, he silently pushes all the remaining morphine vials towards her. His plea that she help him to die is nonverbal but eloquent. She silently studies his face, reaches her decision, and draws up all the morphine into one large syringe. She sobs as she prepares the lethal dose. He says, simply, "Thank you." And then, following the injection, he asks her to "Read to me, will you... Read me to sleep." She sits next to him and reads the last words Katherine wrote to him as he peacefully dies. Hana administered the large dose of morphine with intention that the count would die; by ending his life, she ended his suffering in the only way she could.

Bioethicists define active voluntary euthanasia as an act performed by an agent with the intent to end the life of another who requests that assistance, typically as a means to escape suffering that cannot otherwise be relieved. It is sometimes known as *mercy killing*. The word *euthanasia* has Greek origins and originally meant only "good death," not the practice of killing a person for benevolent reasons. The term now has come to mean a peaceful death free of anxiety and pain, usually brought about by administering a lethal amount of medication. Is it ever morally or legally acceptable to intentionally and directly end the life of a suffering patient who makes a voluntary and informed request to be killed? These are two separate questions. From a legal perspective, in all of the United States, it is never acceptable for a clinician intentionally to kill a patient, regardless of the clinician's motives or the reasons for the patient's request. Euthanasia, in all states, is legally distinguished from assisting in a death. Outside of Oregon and Washington, the act of assisting, but not directly causing, death is generally considered a form of second-degree manslaughter. In contrast, euthanasia falls under the legal definition of second-degree murder because the defendant acts directly to intentionally cause the death of the "victim." Because consent of the victim is not a defense to murder, euthanasia is subject to prosecution as murder in the second degree, although legal experts note that in determining punishment, judges and juries often give great weight to both the consent of the victim and the motives of the defendant.

Well-established legal authority recognizes that competent adults have the right to determine what will happen to their bodies, including the right to refuse any and all medical treatment, even if that refusal means that they will die as a consequence. Outside of Oregon and Washington, the only legally recognized "right to die" in this country is the right to refuse unwanted life-prolonging treatment—no legal right to clinician-provided euthanasia exists. That being said...is there a moral justification for euthanasia? The ethical debate about euthanasia has on the "for" side, arguments that appeal to individual autonomy and relief of pain and suffering (mercy), while the "against" side argues the intrinsic wrongness of

killing, threats to the integrity of the medical and nursing professions, and potentially damaging social effects of such practices if legalized.[1]

Arguments for autonomy acknowledge a person's right to determine the course
of his or her own life, which includes the right to determine how long and under
what circumstance, and the course of his or her own dying. Foundational to this
argument is the notion that only the patient can determine whether the benefits of
life continue to outweigh the associated burdens of living with a terminal disease.
Autonomy requires both freedom from restriction (liberty) and the capacity to act
intentionally (agency). Within the context of end-of-life medical care, respect for
self-determination requires that clinician's honor their patients' informed and
voluntarily decision's about whether pursuit of continued life or comfort and
possibly hastening death shall be the central goal of care.

Somewhat related to the principle of autonomy, the principle of (medical)
mercy recognizes two professional obligations: the duty not to cause (unnecessary)
pain or suffering, and the duty to act to end existing pain and suffering. Under the
first of these is whether the expected benefits of the intervention can reasonably
be expected to outweigh the associated burdens of providing it. Thus, a painful
diagnostic procedure performed on a dying patient would be morally unjustified
unless the patient should choose treatment based on the results of the procedure.
The clinician's duty to relieve his or her patient's pain and suffering is a well-
recognized professional responsibility; the duty to relieve a dying patient's pain
and suffering is a moral imperative. Advances in symptom management, palliative care, and hospice support have greatly increased the likelihood that dying
patients will receive good end-of-life symptom management.

Arguments against euthanasia often feature the value of human life combined
with the intrinsic wrongness of killing. Opponents of euthanasia argue that those
who seek to end their lives contradict the value of autonomy, and as society limits
certain other "freedoms" like selling oneself into slavery, so too should the freedom
to end one's life be limited.[1] Similarly, many reject euthanasia because it violates
the fundamental prohibition against the killing of innocents. While certain
instances of killing are socially and legally accepted in America (in self-defense,
war, and capital punishment), the "victims" of those accepted killings are not
deemed "innocent" but are presumed to be guilty of some aggressive or immoral
acts.[2] Killing is understood as morally wrong in virtually all cultures and religious
systems.

Those who argue from the integrity of the medical and nursing professions
state simply that doctors and nurses should not kill. Health care professionals are
bound to save lives, not end them, and to permit or sanction clinician involvement
in killing patients would seriously undermine the patient's trust in his clinicians
and in his duty to treat disease and relieve suffering. Closely related to this
argument, the slippery slope argument concerns potential abuses that would arise
as a consequence of widespread clinician or social support for euthanasia. This
argument holds that, even if individual cases of assisted dying may be justified,

if such cases are permitted, it may happen that other unjustified situations might occur—therefore, all instances of the practice must be prohibited lest potential harms occur. When considering the possibility of slippery slopes and potential abuses, it is instructive to consider data from the Netherlands, a country with 30 years of experience with euthanasia, and one in which three separate studies of the incidence of euthanasia were completed in 1990, 1995, and 2001. While the incidence of euthanasia has remained relatively stable—1.8%, 2.4%, and 2.3%, respectively, in each of the studied years—so too has the incidence of "life-terminating acts without explicit request of the patient: 0.8%, 0.7%, and 0.7%, respectively.[3]

While it may be clear that Hana intended to cause her patient's death, other questions arising from this act may be more difficult to answer. Did Hana harm or benefit the count by intentionally causing him to die by administering a lethal dose of morphine? Is death always the worst thing that can happen to a competent person who wants to die? Are all intentionally caused deaths morally identical and equally impermissible, or are there circumstances in which death, all things considered, is the best outcome possible? Certainly those who believe in the sanctity of life will hold that it is always wrong to directly end the life of an innocent person, a position based in part upon the assertion that intentional killing is an intrinsic wrong and thus ethically unacceptable. Similarly, some moral theologians and clinicians view any act by a patient to intentionally hasten his death to be an equally unacceptable example of *self-killing*, or suicide. Other philosophers and clinicians maintain that killing per se is neither right nor wrong, and moral judgments about the rightness or wrongness of intentional killing depend upon the justification underlying the action. Attig argues that "some acts of self-killing also could be construed as justifiable—as acts of self-defense against intolerable life circumstances or irremediable suffering" (p. 179).[4]

Some who oppose clinician-aided death suggest that the issue is one of "life versus death." Battin and Quill[5] note that when terminally ill persons seek assistance in dying, the choice is not between death and an indefinitely prolonged life—instead, the difference is between an easier death now and a more difficult death in the not too distant future. Nurses and doctors often seek clear ethical and legal principles when determining when it is morally obligatory to save life, when one may be permitted to allow death to occur, and whether there is ever justification for causing death. A well-established legal and ethical consensus obliges clinicians to honor the informed request of a competent patient to withdraw or withhold life-sustaining treatments. The moral obligation to honor patients, treatment decisions based upon their right of autonomy and self-determination, ethical guidelines, judicial rulings, and professional policy statements combine to recognize and protect this right to refuse unwanted treatments regardless of the type of treatment, the extent of the disease, or the reason for the refusal—including a patient's desire to hasten or cause his or her own death.

Foregoing life-sustaining treatments, broadly known as *allowing to die*, is distinguished from unjustified killing by the valid authorization that an informed patient provides to the physician.[6] The moral question presented by this film was whether Hana was justified in killing her patient, all things considered—which includes the question of whether there were *any* practical alternatives. Nurses may turn to their Code of Ethics for guidance when faced with difficult choices among claims of beneficence and their duty to prevent or remove harm. The American Nurses Association Code of Ethics[7] encourages aggressive pain management and expects nurses to assume the potential risk of secondarily hastening death of dying patients when administering opiates, but proscribes acting with the sole intent of directly and intentionally ending a suffering patient's life. Physicians are similarly cautioned to, "First, do no harm." Challenges face those who seek clinical guidance from professional codes of ethics: How does one understand the meaning of "harm" or a clinician's "sole intent" when a hastened death might be the least bad option available to a suffering patient?

Count Laszlo's request to Hana came after they had developed a long and trusting relationship. Her decision to honor his wishes was not lightly made, but was consistent with the care that she had provided him all along. Hana is the embodiment of excellence in nursing practice. She nurtured his body by providing good nutrition, pain control, and excellent skin care; his mind by reading to him from his favorite book; his soul by taking him out to feel the rain; and, ultimately, his peace of mind by giving him control over the manner and timing of his death.

REFERENCES

1. Health Education Services. 1994. When death is sought: Assisted suicide and euthanasia in the medical context. Retrieved October 20, 2009 from http://www.health. state.ny.us/nysdoh/consumer/patient/aboutsui.htm
2. Battin, M.P. 2005. *Ending life: Ethics and the way we die*. New York: Oxford University Press.
3. van Delben, J., Visser, J., and Borst-Eilers, E. 2004. Thirty years' experience with euthanasia in the Netherlands. In physician-assisted dying. In T.E. Quill and M.P. Battin (Eds.), *The case for palliative care & patient choice*, pp. 202–216. Baltimore, MD: Johns Hopkins University Press.
4. Attig, T. 2005. Rational suicide in terminal illness: The ethics of intervention and assistance. In K.J. Doka, B. Jennings, and C.A. Corr (Eds.), *Living with grief: Ethical dilemmas at the end of life*, pp. 175–197. Washington, DC: Hospice Foundation of America.
5. Battin, M.P., and Quill, T.E. 2004. *Physician-assisted dying: The case for palliative care and patient choice Baltimore*. Baltimore, MD: Johns Hopkins University Press.
6. Beauchamp, T., and Childress, J. 2001. *Principles of biomedical ethics*, 5th ed. New York: Oxford University Press.
7. American Nurses Association. 1994. *Position statement on assisted suicide*. Washington, DC: American Nurses Association.

8

futility: *my life*

thomas wm. mayo

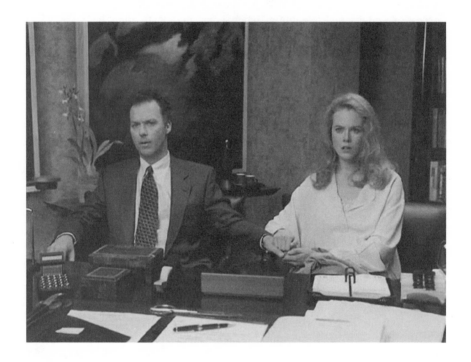

My Life (1993). Michael Keaton, Nicole Kidman, Bradley Whitford, Queen Latifah. Directed by Bruce Joel Rubin. Duration: 117 minutes.

DVD chapter 6 scene 00:20:00 to 00:22:53

PUBLIC RELATIONS SUPERSTAR BOB JONES (Michael Keaton) is described in an admiring *L.A. Magazine* piece as "one of the top ten most powerful men in the field," and a co-worker describes him as "charming, clever, funny, a real wheeler-dealer." He also has a terminal condition that started with kidney cancer and spread to his lungs. His wife, Gail (Nicole Kidman) is pregnant with their first child and—with the encouragement of a Chinese healer (Haing S. Ngor)—Jones sets out to record what he has learned about life for the benefit of a child he may not live to see.

In the selected scene, Dr. Joseph Califano (Kenneth Tigar) tells Bob that his tumors have not responded to interleukin therapy and that he "can't recommend further treatment." Bob appears stunned for a moment, and then challenges Dr. Califano: "What if I want to do the treatment? What if I want to do it? Are you going to stop me? Are you going to get a court order and stop me?" Dr. Califano advises Bob to not "make this any more painful than it has to be. You don't have a lot of time left. Don't waste it in futile searches. Medicine has got some terrible limitations." Bob and Gail leave the doctor's office, but once out on the street Bob suddenly turns back, races to the office, bursts into a room where Dr. Califano is examining an elderly patient, and dramatically exclaims, "Who the hell do you think you are? You think you can take away my hope like that? Let me tell you something. That's all I have. Got it? That's all I have!" The scene ends with Bob and Gail in bed. Bob: "I'm gonna beat this thing, yeah? I'll beat it." Gail, somewhat skeptically but trying to be comforting, responds, "I know."

In a "classic right-to-die" case (such as the *Quinlan* case[1]), a surrogate-decision maker seeks to end life-sustaining treatments on behalf of a patient (usually a family member) and is opposed by the treatment team, often out of a belief that to stop the treatments would constitute the tort of abandonment or even criminal homicide. A so-called "futility dispute" (such as the *Causey* case[2]) reverses those roles, with the surrogate asking for the continuation of life-sustaining treatment (often with the demand that "everything be done" to keep the patient alive) and the treatment team opposing the surrogate's request for treatment that it regards as nonbeneficial. The disagreement between Dr. Califano and Bob Jones is an example of the latter, although in most cases, the patient lacks decision-making capacity and the demand for continued treatment is made by a spouse, an adult child, or some other surrogate decision maker. Another distinction between Bob Jones' dispute and the typical "futility" case is that the latter usually involves a disagreement over end-of-life treatment in the setting of a critical-care unit, nursing home, or hospice, while Bob still has many months of relatively symptom-free existence ahead of him. The film is a good reminder, however, that disagreements over "futility" can arise in many different treatment situations.

Although competent patients (and, by implication, their surrogates) have a virtually unlimited ability to refuse treatments, including life-sustaining treatments, the right to demand a treatment—especially one that physicians regard as "futile"—is much more controversial. The American Medical Association has stated that physicians are not obligated to provide futile medical treatment,[3,4] a position concurred in by the 15 states that have adopted either the Uniform Health Care Decisions Act[5] or their own medical-futility law.[6] None of these sources, however, proposes a definition of "futile medical treatment" or similar phrases (e.g., "medically ineffective" or "medically inappropriate" treatment), which is one of the conceptual difficulties that afflicts any attempt to limit life-sustaining treatment on futility grounds.

Because unilateral decisions by physicians to withhold or withdraw life-sustaining treatment are still controversial, some have suggested the practice should be limited to the most narrowly circumscribed, objectively verifiable clinical situations, such as when it would be physiologically impossible for the treatment to achieve the goal for which it was designed. Other definitions have been proposed, such as probabilistic measures of success, benefit-to-burden ratio, and likelihood of producing an "acceptable quality of life," but none has been embraced by anything remotely resembling a consensus. Some bioethicists criticize such subjective definitions of futility as value-based rather than narrowly medical or scientific and, it is argued, not properly within the exclusive control of medical professionals.[7] Notwithstanding the definitional difficulty, patients eventually die, and prior to their death, patients cease to experience continued life-sustaining treatments as beneficial. The question, then, is how to balance the competing claims of surrogate decision-makers (for many of whom hope is in almost infinite supply) and treating physicians (whose prognostic abilities are not infallible). The search for an answer to this question properly begins with a search for the source of futility disagreements.

Most commentators focus upon poor communication between physicians and surrogate decision makers as a source of disagreement over end-of-life care. There is also a close connection between communication problems and the breakdown in what ought to be a trust relationship. The style of modern medical practice in tertiary care hospitals—with endlessly rotating teams of attending and consulting physicians, a focus upon organ systems and test results rather than overall goals of treatment, and highly technical aspects of care that isolate and alienate decision makers—undoubtedly makes effective communication even more difficult. Thus, taking the time to provide explanations and reasons for deeming life-sustaining treatment to be futile may help reduce the frequency of futility disputes. More time and more talk, however, do not always settle the disagreement. Resorting to an ethics consultant or ethics committee to provide mediation-type services may also be effective in addressing the concerns of surrogate decision makers, as well as in identifying cases in which the treating physician has improperly invoked "medical futility."[8]

It is in the very nature of futility disputes for disagreements to become entrenched. Some families may believe, for religious or other reasons, that all life is precious, regardless of the quality of that life. Most physicians claim a freedom of conscience that supports their right not to participate in the provision of treatments that violate their professional ethics. Unless a mutually acceptable middle ground can be found, disagreements over allegedly futile treatment can resemble the classic "immovable object" and "irresistible force." If an impasse between the surrogate decision maker and physician is irresolvable, most jurisdictions sort out the competing claims with some sort of a judicial process. Texas, almost alone in its adoption of a nonjudicial dispute-resolution mechanism, ties an ethics committee–based review of the dispute and an explicit "no duty to treat" rule to conditional immunity for the physicians, hospitals, and health care professionals involved in the dispute.[9] Although heavily criticized by some commentators, Texas' process-based approach has been praised for providing a practical and balanced approach to resolving treatment disputes that defy mutually acceptable resolution.[10]

As attention increasingly turns to evidence-based medicine, and as limitations on health care resources become more acute and widely recognized, disputes over claims that medical treatment is nonbeneficial will likely increase. Early discussions of treatment limits, family councils to discuss the patient's preferences and values, and sensitive discussions between physicians and patients (and their surrogates) may help avoid some futility disputes, but certainly not all of them.

In the film, Dr. Califano's brief discussion with Bob Jones encapsulates some important lessons about medical futility. He frankly acknowledges that medicine has "some terrible limitations." He attempts to establish some treatment limitations *before* Bob's condition worsens to avoid discussing limitations with Bob's surrogate decision maker for the first time when Bob is in an intensive care unit and unable to express his own treatment preferences. Dr. Califano also tries to turn Bob's attention to making the most of the limited time he has left. Implicit in his message is the promise that Dr. Califano will not abandon Bob and that comfort care will be there for him when and as needed. Often this is the message surrogate decision makers most want to hear in response to their demand that "everything be done" for their loved one.

REFERENCES

1. Matter of Quinlan, 70 N.J. 10, 355 A.2d 647 (1976).
2. *Causey v. St. Francis Medical Center*, 719 So. 2d 1072 (La. App. 1998).
3. American Medical Association. AMA Code of Ethics, Opinion 2.035, *Medical Futility.* Retrieved from http://www.ama-assn.org/ama/pub/physician-resources/medical-ethics/code-medical-ethics/opinion2035.shtml
4. Council on Ethical and Judicial Affairs, American Medical Association. 1999. Medical Futility in End-of-Life Care. *Journal of the American Medical Association* 281: 937–41. Retrieved from http://jama.ama-assn.org/cgi/reprint/281/10/937
5. National Conference of Commissioners on Uniform State Laws. 1973. "Uniform Health-Care Decisions Act." Retrieved from http://www.law.upenn.edu/bll/archives/ulc/fnact99/1990s/uhcda93.htm
6. Pope, T.M. 2007. Medical futility statutes: No safe harbor to unilaterally refuse life-sustaining treatment. *Tennessee Law Review* 75: 1–81.
7. Helft, P.R., et al. 2000. The rise and fall of the futility movement. *New England Journal of Medicine* 343: 293–296.
8. Meisel, A., and Cerminara, K. 2004. *The right to die: The law of end-of-life decision making* New York: Aspen.
9. Tex. Health & Safety Code §§ 166.044–.046. Retrieved from http://www.statutes.legis.state.tx.us/Docs/HS/htm/HS.166.htm
10. Paris, J.J., et al. 2006. *Howe v. MGH* and *Hudson v. Texas Children's Hospital*: Two approaches to resolving family–physician disputes in end-of-life care. *Journal of Perinatology* 26: 726–729.

9

professional roles and communication in end-of-life care: *magnolia*

david i. rosenthal and joshua hauser

Magnolia (1999). Julianne Moore, Tom Cruise, John C. Reilly, William H. Macy, Philip Seymour Hoffman. Directed by Paul Thomas Anderson. Duration: 188 minutes.

Scene: DVD chapter 9 Scene 02.17:44 to 02.19:0

P.T. ANDERSON COMPOSES HIS FILMS with many characters and narrative threads woven together in a multicolored, delicate tapestry. Throughout his career with films such as *Cigarettes & Coffee* (1993), *Hard Eight* (1996), *Boogie Nights* (1997), and *There Will Be Blood* (2007), Anderson has displayed his skills as a complex storyteller. In his film *Magnolia* (1999), Anderson tells the story of ten major characters, brought together in both mundane and fantastical ways. At the beginning of *Magnolia*, the narrator reveals how these seemingly coincidental and unconnected stories are, in fact, not due to chance, but that "these strange things happen all the time." *Magnolia* unveils a web of these strange stories to highlight the diversity of experiences and present them as life's oddities. Anderson's characters display a wide range of emotions, and his stories focus on tragedies not usually depicted realistically in cinema: death and dying, personal failures, extramarital affairs, estranged children, and drug use. This essay highlights a specific scene in *Magnolia* to provide a springboard for reviewing some ethical and communication issues surrounding end-of-life care.

The narrative tells the story of an elderly man, Earl Partridge (Jason Robards), who is dying of lung cancer, his young wife Linda (Julianne Moore), his home health aide Phil (Philip Seymour Hoffman), and his estranged son Frank T.J. Mackey (Tom Cruise). The film opens with Earl Partridge in bed wearing nasal cannula, then cuts to an animation of lung cancer, then to Partridge asking the home health aide for help, and then cuts to his wife Linda on the phone asking a doctor for more pills. In this brief moment, the director throws the audience into this social web that provides some context about the dying man and the connections around him. There is one patient, but a complex constellation of professional caregivers, family caregivers, and others surround him. They arrive at his bedside bearing their own relationships with him and with each other.

Later in the film, Linda visits his physician (Don McManus) to discuss her husband's care. This scene lasts only about three minutes but portrays a number of key aspects of physician encounters with patients and families at the end of life.

By analyzing this scene—both what it contains and what is absent—we will review some of the ethical issues touched upon, and present strategies for physicians as they approach family conversations about care at the end of life.

The scene begins with Linda Partridge standing anxiously in tears in the physician's office. Viewers can see grief in her face: it is drawn and pale. As the first step in moving the discussion forward, the physician asks Linda to sit down. Once seated, the encounter progresses. Linda expresses concern about her husband's symptoms, in particular, his pain, inability to swallow, and his moaning. The physician explains her husband's poor prognosis and tells her that his goal is "to make this experience as painless and easy for him [her husband] as possible." The physician goes on to recommend hospice and that "they will take care of all of the technical things… take care of the body…who you call when he dies." He then writes her husband a prescription for liquid morphine and tells her that it will diminish her husband's pain, but that he will drift in and out of consciousness. Linda's reaction is telling; fighting through her tears, she states, "I don't know what to [expletive] say to that."

In just three minutes, this scene touches upon many teaching points. The physician (1) communicated bad news, (2) set goals and expectations for the patient's death, (3) explained and made a referral to hospice, (4) discussed symptom palliation and possible side effects, and (5) exposed caregiver stress. We'll go through each of these items and briefly discuss the ethical issues inherent, along with their portrayal in *Magnolia*. We will end with ideas about how such a clip can be used in teaching situations.

communicating bad news

Many physicians consider communicating bad news to a patient or a patient's family to be both challenging and stressful.[1] A great deal of useful medical literature explores this subject as it relates to end-of-life care. Balaban, for example, constructed one framework for laying out the elements of such discussion using a four-step model: (1) initiating the discussion, (2) clarifying prognosis, (3) identifying end-of-life goals, and (4) developing a treatment plan. Another framework, developed by Buckman and later adapted by Buckman and Baile, is called SPIKES.[2] It consists of six steps and uses the acronym SPIKES to organize these into Setting up the interview, assessing the patient's Perception, obtaining the patient's Invitation, giving Knowledge to the patient, addressing the patient's Emotions, Strategy, and summary. Both of these frameworks offer helpful guides for physicians and others sharing bad news. Neither should be considered a script, but rather to act as landmarks in a conversation. The relative emphasis and time spent on each step will vary by clinician and patient and the context of the conversation. These approaches have been shown to be readily teachable and welcomed by patients and families.

Consider this scene through Balaban's lens. By asking Linda to sit down, the physician initiates a calming, conducive environment for shared conversation.

He uses clear, nontechnical language about the patient's prognosis, giving a time frame of weeks. The physician then identifies some goals: to make the process as painless and easy as possible. Last, he reveals his treatment plan consisting of symptom management and a referral to hospice.

However, what this scene in *Magnolia* reveals is that a mechanical recitation of these steps is not enough: Despite the fact that the physician went through these steps, Linda still appears stricken. And so, while an encounter can technically satisfy a checklist of requirements, other components play important roles in the process—tone, timbre, tenor, and timing—and require significantly more humanism from a health care provider. In the scene, the physician never elicited or considered Linda's reaction and coping. He also failed to offer any specific empathic statements about the emotions that she was going through. Students can see these difficult-to-characterize elements in a film but not in a textbook.

setting goals and expectations

Exploring goals of care is a core part of palliative care.[3] By necessity, it must be a negotiation between what is clinically or medically possible and the desires and values of a particular patient and family. Setting goals with patients and families is a vital part of the shared decision-making process.[4,5] Shared decision-making enacts three underlying ethical concepts: self-determination, patient autonomy, and beneficence.

In *Magnolia,* the physician stated his goal was "to make this experience as painless and easy as possible." While this comment was likely expressed to soothe Linda's fears and engender trust, it never explored the patient's goals or those of his family. It is important—and sometimes neglected—that physicians and other clinicians will frequently have their own objectives of care for patients. Yet, these must be balanced with the more important goals of patients and families. The one-sided conversation in *Magnolia* is less of a dialogue between physician and family member than a physician soliloquy.

One area where the physician does a better job is in setting expectations. He presents a clear prognosis and honest predictions of the side effects of pain medication. A number of studies have shown that physicians are at times reluctant to share prognostic information and estimates, while patients are often eager for such information.[6] *Magnolia* shows a model for clear prognostic disclosure with a family. Setting realistic expectations empowers patients, families, and caregivers with information and facilitates coping strategies. By doing so, it helps them to understand whether their goals are possible ones.

referral to hospice

Hospice care is focused on patient comfort and family support for patients whose life expectancy is less than six months.[7,8] In recent years, palliative care has risen as a medical specialty and an as approach to care often conceived of as broader than hospice; it can include symptom management of any type and care earlier in the illness trajectory focused on quality of life and support for patients and their families. The use of hospice, a leading model of palliative care for patients with life-threatening illnesses, has grown tremendously in the past 30 years. Since its beginnings in the United States in the mid-1970s, hospice use has expanded, such that in 2005, about 33% of all decedents had used hospice care.[9]

For many physicians, referral to hospice is a routine part of end-of-life care; however, issues can arise around the methods of referral, and in particular, surrounding the professional value of nonabandonment. Timothy Quill and Christine Cassel articulated this value in the following way: "Nonabandonment reflects a continuous caring partnership between physician and patient. ...It acknowledges and reinforces the centrality of an ongoing personal commitment to caring and problem-solving between physician and patient. It also captures the essential qualities whereby physicians and patients commit to mutual decision-making over time, even when the course is uncertain."[10] At the end of life, by providing a new team to help care for patients near the end of life, it has been a concern that hospice care may unintentionally promote abandonment. Recent empirical data consisting of interviews with patients and family members show that this does occur in some settings.[11] The physician in *Magnolia* does not provide reassurance that he will stay involved. Rather, it seems as if he is passing the patient along to hospice without the requisite follow-up. A clinician must strive to follow Balaban's succinct aphorism, "The first discussion should not be the last." This task of operationalizing is not seen in *Magnolia*, but is a key issue for clinicians: Will they, and how often might they, undertake a home visit? Will they see the patient in the hospital or in the nursing home when the patient is on "another doctor's team?" How will they coordinate and work with this new team of hospice clinicians? All of these are practical considerations that can impede the ethical principle of nonabandonment.

symptom palliation and side effects

The most common physical symptoms in terminally ill patients include pain, fatigue, insomnia, anorexia, dyspnea, delirium, depression, anxiety, and nausea and vomiting.[2] In *Magnolia*, Anderson highlights a few of these symptoms with Earl Partridge's experience of terminal lung cancer, as well as illustrates the decision-making process surrounding the alleviation of these symptoms. The physician addresses the patient's pain with a prescription for morphine and discusses the altered cognition and delirium he may experience with morphine. A critical goal of all health care providers, but especially those in palliative care, is patient comfort and ensuring that the dying have all of their physical, psychological, social, and existential needs met. Pain relief frequently involves medications, but also involves nonpharmacologic approaches, such as psychological and spiritual support of patients and their families. In *Magnolia,* the physician does not ascertain the wishes of the patient, and the risk versus benefit calculation of various treatment decisions is left to an uninformed, distraught family member. This reliance on family members is appropriate for a patient who no longer has the cognitive ability to speak on his own; but even then, the family member needs clear guidance and some effort from the physician because the heavy burden, all too often, is not only to know what the patient would have wanted, but to enact those wishes.

caregiver stress

One of the most powerful areas of expression in this scene is how caregiver stress is portrayed. As this is also one of the hardest to portray in writing, film provides an especially effective vehicle. Although this scene portrays Linda's interaction with the physician, other parts of the film allow us to see first-hand the effect of Earl Partridge's decline in three separate characters: his wife Linda Partridge, the home health aide Phil, and the estranged son T.J. Mackey. Their separate experiences serve to underline the fact that, while there may be only one patient in a particular patient–physician encounter, there are frequently many family members and other caregivers, each of whom present specific aspects of their relationship with the patient.

Particularly noteworthy is Linda's extreme emotional stress, characterized by her emotional outbursts and inability to respond to the physician's description of terminal delirium, even though she has full-time nursing support to address her husband's physical needs. It is ethically good care to address the needs of caregivers and medically important as well: Caregiver burden is well described in the medical literature, showing statistically significant elevated incidences of anxiety symptoms and anxiety disorders in caregivers.[12] As a physician, it is imperative not only to attend to the needs of the dying patient, but also to inquire about and support the needs of the caregiver. Assistance and support can often be provided via community groups, houses of worship, and other local or national resources.

conclusion

We have been able to highlight five different aspects of end-of-life care from a three-minute scene in *Magnolia* that can serve as fertile soil for discussion and for teaching end-of-life care strategies. Many resources and teaching materials concern the end-of-life care topics presented in *Magnolia.* The goal of a film clip is not to replace these materials but to distill them, to provoke discussion, and to give sound and depth to the written words. Seeing specific aspects of this interaction helps address two challenges found in teaching ethics and communication: having appropriate role models and having an ability to see an actual interaction. In *Magnolia,* a viewer can witness one example of a physician role model and react to it. The viewer can also watch one portrayal of a patient and his relatives and imagine how he or she might react to them during a clinical encounter. Few would argue this is as good as watching an actual physician and having the ability to reflect and react to that, but a film clip is readily available, portable, and probably more efficient.

Teaching with this type of video material, however, requires more than just showing it to students and, we would argue, is much different from seeing it as a form of entertainment. The skillful facilitator using *Magnolia* to teach about end-of-life care might therefore consider:

1. *Framing the exercise*: Many facilitators show a video clip and ask: "What did you think?" Although such an approach is a reasonable first step, it is only a first step. At a minimum, a facilitator needs to have clear objectives for the teaching session and an idea of the specific topics in end-of-life care that he or she wants to use the clip to portray (we have offered five different possibilities in this essay; depending on the time allotted for a teaching session, one or more of these will be addressed).

2. *Facilitating discussion*: Just as a good clinical history begins with open-ended questions and proceeds to more specific issues that physicians want to target, specific discussion questions keep students focused and move the discussion in the direction desired by the instructor.

3. *Relating the film* to materials from the arts, role-playing scenarios, and patient/family interview sessions in order to enhance the palliative care and ethics curriculum.

REFERENCES

1. Ptacek, J., and McIntosh, E. 2009. Physician challenges in communicating bad news. *Journal of Behavioral Medicine* 32(4): 380–387.
2. Baile, W.F., Buckman. R., Lenzi. R., Glober. G., Beale. E.A., and Kudelka, A.P, 2000. SPIKES—A six-step protocol for delivering bad news: Application to the patient with cancer. *The Oncologist* 5: 302–311.
3. Kaldjian, L.C., Curtis, A.E., Shinkunas, L.A., and Cannon, K.T. 2009. Review article: Goals of care toward the end of life: A structured literature review. *American Journal of Hospice and Palliative Medicine* 25: 501–511.
4. Hermsen, M., Ten Have, H. 2005. Decision-making in palliative care practice and the need for moral deliberation: A qualitative study *Patient Education and Counseling* 56: 268–275.
5. Charles, C., Gafni, A., and Whelan, T. 1997. Shared decision-making in the medical encounter: What does it mean? (Or it takes at least two to tango). *Social Science & Medicine* 44: 681–692.
6. Christakis, N. *Death Foretold*. Chicago, IL: University of Chicago Press.
7. National Hospice and Palliative Care Organization. "What is Hospice and Palliative Care?" Retrieved from http://www.nhpco.org/i4a/pages/index.cfm?pageid=4648.

8. Lynn, J. 2001. Serving patients who may die soon and their families: The role of hospice and other services. *Journal of the American Medical Association* 285: 925–932.

9. Emanuel, E.J., Hauser, J., Emanuel, L.L. 2008. Palliative and end-of-life care. In A.S. Fauci, E. Braunwald, D.L. Kasper, S.L. Hauser, D.L. Longo, J.L. Jameson, and J. Loscalzo (Eds.), *Harrison's Principles of Internal Medicine*, 17th ed., Chapter 11. New York: McGraw Hill.

10. Quill, T.E., and Cassel, C.K. 1995. Nonabandonment: A central obligation for physicians. *Annals of Internal Medicine* 122: 368–374.

11. Back, A.L., Young, J.P., McCown, E., et al. 2009. Abandonment at the end of life from patient, caregiver, nurse, and physician perspectives: Loss of continuity and lack of closure. *Archives of Internal Medicine* 169: 474–479.

12. Grov, E.K., Dahl, A.A., Moum, T., and Fossa, S.D. 2005. Anxiety, depression, and quality of life in caregivers of patients with cancer in late palliative phase. *Annals of Oncology* 16: 1185–1191.

suicide: *mar adentro (the sea inside)*

diana cohen agrest

Mar Adentro (*The Sea Inside*) (2004). Javier Bardem, Belén Rueda, Lola Dueñas, Mabel Rivera, Celso Bugallo, Clara Segura, Tamar Novas. Directed by Alejandro Amenábar. Duration: 125 minutes.

DVD chapter 14 Scene 01.50:35 to chapter 15 scene 01.57:11

MAR ADENTRO NARRATES THE LIFE of Ramón Sampedro (Javier Bardem). On a tragic summer day in 1968, 26-year-old Ramón went to a nearby cliff to take a bath in the sea, when he was distracted by the sudden appearance of his lover. Forgetting to estimate the ocean's depth, he dived carelessly and, in that moment, his life drastically changed forever. Ramón Sampedro became a quadriplegic for the rest of his life: 28 years and four months with just a slight movement of his mouth, during which his body was not a valuable resource but a burden that he no longer wanted to bear. The story describes Ramón's relationship with Julia (Belén Rueda), a lawyer who supports his right to die, and Rosa (Lola Dueñas), who tries to persuade him about the unconditional value of life.

In this touching scene, Rosa asks Ramón to send her "a sign of life after life." Distant from any eschatological meaning, Ramón tells her that he has a feeling: He will survive through her dreams and thoughts about him, reminding her that the accident had put an end to his worthy life many years ago. Concerning the fear of death, Ramon declares in a philosophical way that "it's just the same as it is before we are born. There is nothing."

Through his statement, Ramón alludes to a classical argument put forward by the Greek philosopher Epicurus (341–271 BC), who once faced to the question "Should we fear death?" He offered a very famous argument of why we should not, declaring, "So long as we exist death is not with us; but when death comes, then we do not exist. It does not then concern either the living or the dead, since for the former it is not, ante latter are no more."[1] Epicurus was followed by Lucretius (99–55 BC), the Roman poet who committed suicide at the age of 44 and exposed the asymmetrical human attitudes towards birth and death. Lucretius' thesis states that human beings are irrational because they are not sorry for their prenatal nonexistence, but they usually curse the future nonexistence. So, Lucretius recommends us to "Look back similarly at how the stretch of unending time before we are born has been nothing to us. Nature, therefore, offers this reflection *(speculum)* to us of the time to come after our eventual death."[2] Lucretius alerts us that no one claims to have been deprived of all the good things they might have experienced if they had been born earlier than they were. No one is aware that a long duration of past nonexistence is comparable to the period to come of one's future nonexistence. As a contemporary thinker interprets this view, "taking being dead to be nonexistence, Lucretius compared the nonexistence after death to that before conception, and apparently thought that since prenatal nonexistence is not bad for a person (and no one finds it distressing), then posthumous nonexistence is not bad either (though people *do* find it distressing). He seems to have thought that we should rectify our unjustifiably asymmetrical attitudes toward the two symmetrical states. The argument would be that if being dead (when one is nonexistent) is bad for one, then not having had life before one's conception (when one is also nonexistent) should be bad for one. Since the latter is not bad for one, then the former is not."[3]

In a similarly detached and fearless approach to death, the Roman Stoic philosopher Seneca (c. 4 BC–AD 65) considered self-killing an act of privilege "as soon as Fortune seems to be playing him false." The Stoics condemned frivolous suicide, but they admitted that a human being has a right to put an end to his life when its disadvantages outweigh its advantages, choosing the circumstances of one's own death, because "It is not a question of dying earlier or later, but of dying well or ill. Dying well means escape from the danger of living ill."[4] This was his own destiny: Seneca was caught up in the aftermath of the Pisonian conspiracy, a plot to kill Nero. Although it is unlikely that he conspired, he was ordered by Nero to kill himself. Following the tradition, Seneca severed several veins and bled to death.

Early Christians didn't hesitate to commit suicide; it was an act even celebrated amongst the Donatists, who believed that by killing themselves they could attain martyrdom and go to heaven. In the fifth century, when Alaric invaded the Roman Empire, his soldiers threatened to violate the Roman virgins, who preferred to kill themselves instead of being outraged. In order to stop this mass suicide, St. Augustine declared that although the virgins had been bodily violated, they need not declare their innocence through suicide, because they preserved their souls without sin. The biblical justification for this well-known Doctrine of the Sanctity of Human Life was the interpretation of the commandment, "thou shalt not kill." It was Christianity's first overall condemnation of suicide. Early theologians of the Catholic Church considered suicide as murder, and thus a mortal sin. This view was confirmed by Thomas Aquinas, who declared, first, that suicide is contrary to the inclination of nature and to charity, whereby every man should love himself; second, that as every man is part of the community, by killing himself he injures the community; third, that because life is God's gift to man, whoever takes his own life, sins against God.[5]

The expanded perception is that traditional Judaism also believes in the Doctrine of the Sanctity of Human Life. Furthermore, there is no passage in the

Old Testament that can be expressly understood as an explicit prohibition of suicide. Although the Mosaic Law in the Sixth Commandment forbids killing, it doesn't say that it is forbidden to kill oneself. In the Talmudic texts dated 6 AD, and probably under Christian influence, Judaism would express aversion toward suicide. Nevertheless, during the post-Talmudic period, some forms of suicide were more acceptable than others; suicide might be condemned in principle, but accepted in certain circumstances. Partly disagreeing with the idea that this putative universal prohibition of suicide was generally accepted within the Jewish community, scholars argued that Judaism is not committed to a belief in the sanctity of human life whenever it is faced with a residual life in pain.[6] In addition, suicide seemed to be even praiseworthy if it was a case of self-immolation or required by civil or military authorities. And, either individually or collectively (like that at Masada) suicide could be considered an act of heroism, the choosing of death over dishonor. Although the natural fortress of Masada, besieged by the Romans for a year, is just one example of the Jewish tradition of resistance, these exceptions were accepted by the three monotheistic religions.

Islam contains a very strong prohibition against suicide from its beginning, probably due, as in the Jewish tradition, to the Christian influence. Recently, some radical Islamic movements promote immolation, arguing that these acts are genuine operations of historical self-defense: If the suicide wants to sacrifice his life to strike a blow against the enemy, he will be rewarded by Allah; the individual is considered a martyr rather than a suicide. Thus, the martyr becomes a "human bomb" who blows up at a specific place and time, in the midst of the enemies of Allah. Contrary to the faithless individual who kills himself for his own benefit, the believer who commits voluntary martyrdom sacrifices himself for the sake of his religion and his nation.

Concerns about the moral permissibility of suicide usually appeal to a myriad of arguments that may be classified as religious or secular views. For the most part, these arguments aim to establish that God, and not human individuals, has the proper moral authority to determine the circumstances of human death. The first and basic religious argument is the just-mentioned suicide as violation of biblical commandment. The second general category of religious arguments rests on analogies concerning the relationship between God and humanity. One version declares that the human being is the servant of God and should do his master's bidding; a second version says that the human beings is stationed as a sentinel on earth by God, and should not desert his post. Another common analogy asserts that God bestows life upon us as a gift, and it would be a mark of ingratitude or neglect to reject that gift by taking our lives. In addition, it is said in another version, life is loaned or entrusted to the individual by God, and so should not be destroyed.[7]

These analogies are just few of several conceptual strategies. Another celebrated argument considers self-destruction as a violation of natural law or—in those cases in favor of suicidal acts—the opportunity for the reunion with the beloved deceased or even as a release of the soul.

Another moral principle associated with the biblical commandment, inaugurated by Augustine, and presented from then onwards in several versions was the Deontological Argument of the Sanctity of Life. It says that suicide is always wrong if the agent intends to take life, because the intentional killing of human life is always wrong. It may be expressed in a religious or secular background centered on the value of life. According to this secular "sanctity of life" view, human life is inherently valuable and precious, demanding respect from others and reverence for oneself. Today, in a secular world in which emotional links and family ties are so important, the impact of a suicidal act on friends and family is the argument most widely put forth.

Among secular views, social arguments against suicide center it as an offense or injury to the community (to family and friends, or as the deprivation of an individual's contribution to society). But self-killing has been considered also as a benefit to the community, as when suicide results in a removal of social burdens or bestows some benefit to society. In that case, appeals to community responsibility imply that the suicidal candidate should consider not only his or her interests, but also the interests of all affected. Hence, social cost-savings may favor some acts of self-destruction. For example, if a person cannot pay for his or her care, would not suicide be beneficial to his or her family and to society?

A moral principle highly praised today is self-determination, according to which the agent is free to take his or her life, as long as the action does not seriously limit the rights of others. Following this line of thought, the suicide debate reappeared in writings of later 20th-century existentialists, following World War II, when philosophers saw the choice to take one's life as a logical result of an individual's experience of the absurdity or meaninglessness of the world and of human endeavor. It was an important concern for Albert Camus, the famous novelist, who, in *The Myth of Sisyphus,* suggested that although suicide seems to promise an illusory freedom from the absurdity of our existence, it is in the end an abdication of our responsibility to confront that absurdity. In a similar line of thought, Jean-Paul Sartre was moved by the possibility of suicide as a sign of authentic human will in the face of absurdity. Suicide is, according to Sartre, an opportunity to affirm ourselves as individuals in a godless world. For the existentialists, suicide was not a choice shaped mainly by moral considerations but by concerns about the individual as the sole source of meaning in a meaningless universe.

Is suicide ever morally justified? The film portrays a circumstance that health care professionals may face during their lives; namely, the patient who wishes to put an end to his own life. Whenever they accept it, doctors typically conceal this practice. When, in spite of Lucretius' advice, they reject it, even they may argue that suicide is a foolish act. Confronted with a peaceful acceptance of death versus the right of self-determination, the psychiatric model, in particular, attributes to the potential suicidal a dual personality, one that ends up in a kind of Manichaean battle between Good and Evil in which "the suicidal action is a decision resulting from an internal debate of many voices, some for life and some for death."[8]

If good overcomes, then the potential suicide refrains from occurring. If evil does, then he succumbs,[9] and a suicide takes place.

What prejudices conditioned the Western view on suicide? Even today, some suicides seem to be more "morally acceptable" than others. Suicide is generally disapproved whenever the act of self-destruction is performed from the weariness of life or it is caused by shame (i.e., moved by loss of revenue or shame to family and loss of honor). Even today, suicide can be accompanied by substantial stigma: The family of the deceased feels embarrassment and blames itself for the death of the suicide. From a financial aspect, insurance companies are exempted from payment of benefits when a death is by suicide. In contrast, human attitudes toward suicide are different whenever it is committed in order to escape disease, disability, or another otherwise cruel fate.

The last decade has witnessed an increased rate of suicide attempts and suicides, figures that show the urgency for establishing sound politics of prevention for these kinds of behaviors. Suicide happens at an alarming rate among adolescents and old people, two life periods when people are very vulnerable. In addition, special conditions favor suicidal thinking: Research indicates that many newly disabled persons consider suicide in the course of their illness or in severe disability.

But suicide presents a number of theoretical problems as well. What exactly counts as a suicide? According to the *Oxford English Dictionary*, the word "suicide" is derived from the Latin word *"suicidium,"* meaning, "to kill oneself," and was first used in 1651. Several definitions of suicide, more or less broad, depend on the social attitudes toward suicide that influence its characterization and field where the definition is used. The most well-known definition of suicide is Emile Durkheim's, focused on the condition of the knowledge of the result: suicide is "death resulting directly or indirectly from a positive or negative act of the victim himself, which he knows will produce this result."[10] In the field of medicine, Tom Beauchamp's definition—"an act is a suicide if a person brings about his or her own death (1) in circumstances where others do not coerce him or her to the action, (2) except in those cases where death is caused by conditions not specifically arranged by the agent for the purpose of bringing about his or her own death"[11]—excludes death that results from a condition, such as a disease or a mortal injury, that the agent did not arrange as a means of death, and so he or she is not blameworthy.

There are not only numerous conceptual problems, but practical ones as well, condensed in moral views, psychological theories about the voluntariness and rationality of suicidal acts, and the role of depression in causing this kind of act. Suicidology is a new field of study that gathers a multidisciplinary scientific approach from sociology, anthropology, psychology, and psychiatry, each providing relevant insights into suicide. Among scientific views, theories consider the factors that influence people in their decision to commit suicide, offering psychoanalytic explanations or sociological influences. Another scientifically oriented view of suicide considers an attempt at suicide not as an action intended to result in death, but as a strategy for changing the agent's immediate social environment, an elaborate device to call for attention, and as a "cry for help." Particularly promising are the significant advances being made in our scientific understanding of the neurological basis of suicidal behavior and the mental conditions associated with it, in whose framework it is suggested that suicide results from a biochemical imbalance (low serotonin levels in individuals suffering from depression).

Opposing the current point of view, which focused on mental health, it is said that not all cases should be treated with the same theoretical and practical instruments. Although suicide is a major medical and social problem, the medical model doesn't consider the possibility that some suicides don't result from sudden emotions, but from rational decision. However, it is often argued that once prejudices that traditionally stigmatized voluntary death are put aside, and once the attention is turned to certain traits that make up human existence, it could be conceded that ending one's life is, in certain circumstances, a meaningful act. Facing the alternative of a purely biological life, without the possibility of deploying a biographical life and devoid of even minimal existential content, a rational decision to die can be taken. Some conditions exist under which suicide seems to be morally justified: The suicidal act may be exercised by a person capable of reasoning, who can process information properly and has a realistic vision of the world associated with a realistic assessment of his or her actual life situation and is capable of estimating the short- and long-term consequences of his or her actions. A suicidal act may also be based on adequate information about the condition or illness associated with what we might call a person's ground projects or basic interests, which arise from one's most fundamental values.[12]

When such conduct condenses autonomous attitudes that are consistent with personal integrity based on the independence of reasoning, suicide might acquire an undeniable value. A libertarian theorist such as H.T. Engelhardt thinks that, in a context defined by God's silence and the impotence of reason, a minimal ethics of postmodern societies does not imply, in any way, an unequivocal determination of how the lifestyle of its members should be; each and everyone is free to search for a good life in his or her own way, adopting a hierarchy of values according to his or her convenience. Basically, the values at stake are those involved in the moral and legal right to decide on the destiny of our own bodies and our own lives. In the same way that we can choose how to live according to our values, the right of others to live or die according to their own values should also be respected. Even though this hierarchy may be deviant, it should be respected as long as it does not imply violence against innocents. Arguments often invoked against suicide's legitimacy (for example, life's sacred status) are paternalistic ones, because they try to justify—making use of a particular conception of what is thought to be a good life—what, actually, is no more than a disguise of a private or public intrusion that has no justification. It is the individual who must choose her way to die, just as she chooses her lifestyle.[13]

The emergence of physician-assisted suicide is a practice more legally toler-
ated in some countries and regions of the Western world (Oregon in the United
States, and the Netherlands, Belgium, and Switzerland legalized this assistance).
The main arguments of the debate for physician-assisted suicide come are from
autonomy and mercy. According to the first, a person has the right to determine
the course of his or her dying. In particular, when a terminally ill person seeks
assistance in suicide from a physician, once the request is made freely and rationally, the doctor has the duty to provide this assistance. The objection raised to
this argument is that, in terminal illness, true autonomy is rare. Nevertheless,
everyone, even animals, seeks to maximize pleasure and minimize pain. Given
this characterization of sentient beings in general, it is clear that the aversion to
pain is a primitive, and apparently not learned, response of humans in general. If
an individual is suffering from intense pain, prolonged in time and without hope
of remission, the rational answer seems to be to seek an end to this pain. According
to the argument of mercy, the physician must relieve the patient's suffering. If the
only way to avoid such suffering is by death, the physician ought to assist in dying.
Objectors reply that palliative care may treat virtually all pain and relieve all
suffering, hence assisted suicide is not necessary.

The main arguments against physician-assisted suicide are from the wrongness of killing because of the doctrine of the sanctity of human life; the slippery
slope argument based on the risk for abuse, according to which permitting assistance in suicide in rational cases would lead to situations in which persons were
killed against their will; and the argument about the professional role of the physician, consecrated to save life and not to take it, associated with the potential for
loss of integrity of the health care profession if health care providers were to
support the use of suicide.

A view reflected in contemporary law dictates that obligations to prevent
suicide override a person's right to commit suicide. Fighting against the belief
that the state can justifiably protect persons against attempted suicide, Ramón
Sampedro had to violate the law: He had to commit suicide with friends' assistance
so as to put an end to a life he was obliged to live due to prejudices of a suspicious
social morality. As he says in this moving scene, his friends helped him with their
hands, but "the mastermind, the conscience was all" his. He recorded on video
his own death and sent the tape to the media. Its public broadcast caused a huge
impact both on a national and international scale. That led the Spanish Senate to
undertake a Special Commission on Euthanasia Studies, which was disbanded
before its analysis reached any valid conclusions or strong proposals. But the real
international impact would come six years later, hand in hand with the movie
Mar Adentro. This film brought back, once again, the controversy regarding the
right to die with dignity.

REFERENCES

1. Epicurus. 1994. The Pursuit of Pleasure. In P. Singer (Ed.), Ethics, pp. 188–189. Oxford, UK: Oxford University Press.

2. Lucretius. 2004. De Rerum Natura. In J. Warren (Trans.), *Facing death: Epicurus and his critics,* p. 58. Oxford, UK: Oxford University Press, 2004): 58.

3. Rosenbaum, S.E. 1993. How to be dead and not care: A defense of Epicurus. In J. Martin Fischer (Ed.), *The Metaphysics of Death,* p. 128. Stanford, CA: Stanford Series in Philosophy.

4. Seneca, 1920. *Epistulae Morales,* Vol. II, trans. R.M. Gummere. Cambridge, MA: Harvard University Press.

5. Aquinas, T. 1925. "Whether It is Lawful to Kill Oneself?" *Summa Theologica,* vol. 2, Part 2, Question 64, A5. New York: Benziger Brothers, Inc.; London: Burns & Oaks, Ltd.

6. Brody, B.A. 1989. A historical introduction to Jewish casuistry on suicide and euthanasia. In B.A. Brody (Ed.), *Suicide and euthanasia: Historical and contemporary themes,* pp. 39–75. Boston, MA: Kluwer Academic.

7. Pabst Battin, M. 1995. *Ethical issues in suicide,* pp. 36–37. New Jersey: Prentice Hall.

8. Shneidman, E.S. 1990. Preventing suicide. In J. Conelly (Ed.), *Suicide. Right or wrong?* p. 116. New York: Prometheus Books.

9. Cohen Agrest, D. 2007. *Por mano propia: Estudios sobre las prácticas suicidas.* Buenos Aires, AR: Fondo de Cultura Económica.

10. Durkheim, E. *Suicide: A study in sociology,* trans. J.A. Spaulding, and G. Simpson, New York: The Free Press, 1951.

11. Beauchamp, T. 1980. Suicide. In T. Regan (Ed.), *Matters of life and death,* p. 77. New York: Random House.

12. See M. Pabst Battin (1995).

13. Engelhardt, T.H. 1995. *The foundations of bioethics.* New York: Oxford University Press.

part nine

other ethical issues in medical specialities

medicine and religion:
wild strawberries

keith g. meador

Wild Strawberries (1957). Victor Sjostrom, Ingrid Thulin, Bibi Anderson. Directed by Ingmar Bergman, Duration: 90 minutes.

DVD Chapter 12 Scene 00: 43:01 to 00:45:02

WILD STRAWBERRIES FOLLOWS THE ROAD journey taken by 76-year-old Professor Izak Borg (Victor Sjostrom), from Stockholm to Lund to receive an honorary degree, during which he reviews his life via a series of dreams and relationships. Accompanied by his initially estranged daughter-in-law, Marianne (Ingrid Thulin), he encounters a group of young travelers and a middle-aged married couple in some distress. These encounters provide stimuli to generate the dream material and set the contexts to challenge Professor Borg with his own mortality. Ultimately, this self-examination leads the professor to consider essential conflicts in his life: the problematic marriage to his long-deceased wife, the loss of a young true love to his brother, his lack of genuine concern and engagement, and redemptive possibilities with his housekeeper and his son (who is struggling with his own marriage). The search for "wild straw-berries" in his youth conveys a symbolic hope for finding crucial emotions lost through experiences of suffering and trauma, and thereby redeeming the inevita-bility of decline and mortality. Engagement of this redemptive hope culminates in the fresh possibilities embodied within the tenderness and warmth for an old man with his housekeeper, the reminder of young love in the good wishes of his fellow travelers, and the anticipation of a child within the newly reunited marriage of his son and daughter-in-law. These hopes allow Professor Borg to find sleep and rest.

The essay focuses on the scene that occurs during a lunch along the road journey. Professor Borg, his daughter-in-law, and the three young fellow travelers catching a ride—Sara, Viktor, and Anders—are having lunch, when Anders initiates a conversation regarding the beauty of creation and the "radiance of its source." Anders, who is studying for the ministry, is chided by Viktor, who is studying medicine, for bringing up God, which he says breaks a promise not to speak of God or science during this trip. Viktor takes pride in being a "modern man" who "believes only in himself" and "biological death," and cannot understand how "anyone can study to be a minister" in these "modern" times. Anders responds with disdain for Viktor's cold "rationalism" and accuses him of having "no imagination," while being as dry as "dust and ashes" and viewing "death as horror."

When Sara, to whom they are both a suitor, responds that she always believes whoever "spoke last," the young men ask Professor Borg whether he is a religious person. The professor initially avoids directly responding, deflecting their question, but then pensively reciting the following poem:

Where is the friend I seek at break of day?
When night falls I still have not found Him.
My burning heart shows me His traces
I see His traces wherever flowers bloom
His love is mingled with every air.

Professor Borg leaves this as his final response to their inquiry about his religiousness. Intriguingly, he needs Marianne's assistance to recall the poem during the second line when speaking of nightfall, but then regaining his recall as they share the further recitation. All parties accept this resolution at the time, although the two young men regress to petulant fisticuffs as they argue about God later in the trip, only to be greeted by young Sara pointing to the futility of their pursuit of God proofs and reflecting the wisdom of Professor Borg's poetic response.

This scene offers a window on the context in which we can consider some of the basic issues facing the current engagement of religion and spirituality in medicine and health care. The young men's argument regarding the existence of God and the relevance of such concerns for "modern man" is a frequently engaged discussion in science and religion; but, it may lack as much significance as it frequently receives, especially with the religion and health conversation. While an inherently important philosophical question for many individuals, the more important question with regard to religion and health may be the patient's perception of relationship, sense of support, and purpose derived in relation to God or their understanding of a "higher power." When focusing on the ethical implications for religion and spirituality in health care, the more crucial issue is the faith constructs of the patient and the narrative by which he or she would describe the importance of religion and spirituality in personal meaning-making and in forming daily practices and health behaviors.[1]

One distortion of the current spirituality and health movement is the presumption that some specific religious or spiritual belief or practice in and of itself can serve as an efficacious technique for facilitating health. In actuality, the only consistently significant finding regarding this relationship is an association between attendance in worship services and health,[2] and there is no firm proof of causality even for that finding. The limitations of the evidence to date does not diminish the potential significance for gaining a fuller understanding of the relationship, but it does necessitate that care be taken regarding making inferences as to religious or spiritual interventions. Even if particular spiritual or religious interventions were found to have medical efficacy, the necessity of honoring the particular traditions and narrative of the patient as he or she presents in the context of illness and vulnerability remains crucial and merits a consistent and sustained position as an ethical priority.

The dialogue between Viktor and Anders also points to the issue of religion and death. Anders describes "modern man" with his focus on science as being only concerned with "biological death" and consequently viewing "death as horror," implying that the more religious or spiritual person sees death differently, with an understanding of human existence in a more multidimensional fashion both temporally and spatially. The degree to which death is approached and negotiated differentially according to religious or spiritual commitments is considered within the contemporary appropriation of religion as a coping mechanism. Phelps and colleagues found that persons using a higher level of positive religious coping were more likely to desire mechanical ventilation and more intensive life-prolonging care in the last week of life than others.[3] While there are a number of possible critiques of this finding, including the coping measure used and the lack of comprehensiveness in knowledge of the religiosity and personality constructs of the subjects, one possible interpretation reflects a prevalent trait of "modern" religiosity and spirituality as frequently reflected in the current spirituality and health movement. The tendency to assume that God can be domesticated to serve our expectations—as if health were a commodity for negotiated exchange with God—has permeated modernity's engagement of faith in relationship to health in general and particularly death. The modern appropriation of religion and spirituality as a commodity upon which to trade as a quasi-technological intervention in order to gain health or extend one's life distorts both religion and health.

Wild Strawberries offers an opportunity to share in the life review and self-examination of a distinguished physician as the surrounding world honors him. Such accolades challenge him to scrutinize his interior sense of self more circumspectly than in the past while managing a busy career. In the context of this journey, symbolized by his road journey from Stockholm to Lund, the debate of two young men regarding religion and science in the "modern" world frames a recurrent issue that arises for the physician with respect to religion and the practice of medicine. Some patients of particular religious traditions will inquire of physicians as to their own faith commitments. Although a fair question of some increasingly evident significance,[4] Professor Borg's response to the young men when they inquire as to whether he is "a religious man" is instructive. At first he demurs, as if his beliefs are not that important, but he then offers the poem stated earlier. Rather than engage the debate as to the existence of God in the "modern" era with the young men, he pensively reflects through poetry an experiential awareness of God noting "His traces" in "my burning heart" and "wherever flowers bloom." Perhaps Professor Borg has much to teach all of us as we struggle with our rationalistic tendency to overly objectify and domesticate that which is frequently ineffable and is a poetically beautiful mystery waiting to aid us in healing suffering, embodied souls.

REFERENCES

1. Shuman, J., and Meador, K. 2003. *Heal thyself: Spirituality, medicine and the distortion of Christianity*. New York: Oxford University Press.
2. Koenig, H.G., McCullough, M.E., and Larson, D.B. 2001. *Handbook of religion and health*. New York, NY: Oxford University Press.
3. Phelps, A., Maciejewski, P., Nilsson, M., et al. 2009. Religious coping and use of intensive life-prolonging care near death in patients with advanced cancer. *Journal of the American Medical Association* 301(11): 1140–1147.
4. Curlin, F., Lawrence, R., Chin, M., and Lantos, J. 2007. Religion, conscience, and controversial clinical practices. *New England Journal of Medicine* 356(6): 593–600.

teenage sexuality, ethics, and law: *kids*

jerome singh

Kids (1995). Leo Fitzpatrick, Sara Henderson, Justin Pierce, Chloe Sevigny, Rosario Dawson. Director: Larry Clark. Duration: 91 minutes.

DVD chapter 7 Scene 00: 25: 46 to 00:26: 51

KIDS CENTERS AROUND THE LIVES of teenagers living in New York City in the mid 1990s and is shot in semi-documentary style. The movie is characterized by graphic scenes of teenage sex, violence, and substance abuse. The main character, Telly (Leo Fitzpatrick), is a 15-year-old whose goal is to have sex with as many young virgins as possible. The movie opens with Telly seducing a 12-year-old girl. In the next scene, Telly meets up with his friend, Casper (Justin Pierce), and explains that he loves to convince young virgins to sleep with him, believing that sleeping with virgins will prevent him from acquiring sexually transmitted infections (STIs). *Kids* also focuses on the lives of Jennie (Chloe Sevingny) and Ruby (Rosario Dawson). We are introduced to these characters, gathered with a group of other teenage girls, discussing sex. Thereafter, Jennie accompanies Ruby to a public health clinic for STI testing. Ruby, who has been sexually active on many occasions, sometimes without the use of protection, is found to be HIV negative. Jennie, on the other hand, who has had sex on only one occasion, with Telly, is diagnosed with HIV. In breaking the news to Jennie, the physician simply says, "I am sorry." A shocked Jennie spends the rest of the movie trying to find Telly to reveal the news to him. She sees him later that evening at a party, seducing another young girl. Before she has a chance to speak to Telly, she passes out intoxicated on a couch at the party and is raped by Casper.

Kids highlights that teenage sexuality raises numerous moral, ethical, and legal challenges for those involved in their treatment and care. For the health professional, such challenges typically present in the context of solicitation of informed consent, communicating emotionally distressing health results to the child and, possibly, also to his or her parents, confidentiality dilemmas, disclosure obligations to third parties at risk, and termination of pregnancy. Before some of these contexts can be explored, it is important to outline what is traditionally meant by the terms "adolescent," "teenager," "child," and "minor" as they are not necessarily synonymous with each other and sometimes carry specific legal connotations in certain settings.

The term "adolescent" is generally ascribed to a child at the stage of life between puberty and adulthood. This period generally corresponds with the years of the child's life ending with "teen" (namely, the ages 13–19), during which time the child is referred to as a "teenager." However, the end of adolescence and the beginning of adulthood (the age when the child is no longer regarded as a "minor") varies from country to country. In some settings, a "child" is defined as someone under the age of 18. Upon attaining this age, the law classifies the child as an adult, regardless of his or her maturity level. In such settings, a 19-year-old is legally an adult but still a teenager. The term "minor" similarly varies in meaning from country to country. In some settings, a minor denotes a child under the age of 18, while in other countries that term applies to those under the age of 21. Even more confusingly, in some settings, a "child" denotes someone under the age of 18 while a "minor" is defined as someone under the age of 21. In such settings, not all minors are children. Put differently, those aged 19–20 in such settings are no longer regarded as children but still as minors.

In most settings, the age of autonomous consent for treatment and diagnostic testing is lower than the age of autonomous consent for surgery. Depending on the relevant local laws applicable, the former types of procedures are generally accessible autonomously from the age range 12–16, while surgery is typically accessible autonomously from the age range 16–18. In addition, some countries have different ages of autonomous consent for procedures such as termination of pregnancy, sterilization, access to contraception, dispensing of medication, and participation in research. Some of these ages of consent must also be borne in mind in relation to the minimum age of consent for sexual intercourse. For example, if a child is deemed incapable of giving consent for sexual intercourse until he or she is 16 years of age, the health professional may face a dilemma if a child aged 14 years of age presents at a clinic seeking contraceptive services. Those involved in the care of children must also consider the mental status of the youth they encounter as, even if a child is above the legal age of consent for sexual intercourse, their apparent consent to intercourse may be vitiated if they are classified as mentally incompetent. In such instances, their sexual activities could be deemed nonconsensual and their sexual partner could be charged with rape. Although familiarizing oneself with the various ages of consent and laws applicable in a local setting can be intimidating, doing so is crucial as specific laws may govern important issues such as whether the child may consent autonomously to treatment or a diagnostic test, or is eligible to access contraception, or a termination of pregnancy. Aside from the legal dimensions implicit in managing child patients, health workers must also be sensitive to the cultural and social milieus at hand too.

In some settings, even though a child may have the right to seek treatment or undergo a diagnostic test autonomously, from a social and cultural perspective, the parent or caregivers (or in some cases, even community elders) may regard it as their right or duty to accompany the child to the health facility concerned, or to give their prior approval for the child to access such services. Given that premarital sex is frowned upon in many settings, respecting such a cultural norm would not be in the child's best interest, as requiring a child to present at the clinic with their parent or guardian would likely deter them from seeking sexuality-related health services. Conversely, health workers may face instances in which patients legally below the age of consent for treatment but who urgently require access to health services, present at their facilities (for example, if the patient has an STI). If the health worker were to follow the law, he or she would have to deny treatment to the child unless they presented with their parent or guardian. A child may be deterred from doing so as this would expose their sexually active status to their parents/guardians. Such a child would likely not return to the health facility. This, in turn, could result in the health condition of the child worsening, and the untreated disease spreading to other children the infected child comes into sexual contact with. In some developing countries, high HIV prevalence and associated mortality has resulted in many child-headed households. Obtaining parental or guardian consent in such settings is impossible. In either of the above instances, health professionals may opt to treat a child on ethics grounds, in disregard of the law, as doing so would be in the best interests of the child. Such an action, although ethically laudable, could have legal consequences for the health professional, should it come to light.

Such scenarios also raise disclosure obligations and confidentiality dilemmas. Should the health worker disclose the HIV status of the child to other identifiable parties (for example, to an identified and traceable at-risk girlfriend or boyfriend), if the patient unreasonably refuses to do so? Should the health worker inform the parent or guardian of the child's test results if the required treatment involves potentially serious side-effects (for example, some antiretroviral HIV drugs precipitate severe side effects), or should the condition be deemed life-threatening if left untreated (in which case the parent or guardian may have to monitor treatment adherence)? In such instances, the involvement of the parent in the diagnosis or treatment of the child may be crucial to the child's best interest. This may be best illustrated in *Kids*.

In *Kids*, Jennie underwent a HIV test, seemingly without her parent's knowledge, as she was legally entitled to do so. However, inadequate empathy on the part of the diagnosing physician coupled with the absence of social support mechanisms such as post-test counseling services, left Jennie emotionally unprepared to cope with her test result and made her vulnerable to becoming intoxicated and later being raped. Assuming Jennie's parents were loving and supportive, it could be argued that, were they to have accompanied her to the clinic, she would have had access to immediate emotional support and may not have found her way to a party where she was raped while in an intoxicated state.

Kids also raises the issue of whether children, like the character Jennie, could prevent themselves becoming HIV infected by insisting that their sexual partners wear condoms. In reality, a lack of, or inadequate, sex education in schools in some settings, coupled with systemic male domination and/or violence against females, and peer pressure, leaves young women unable to negotiate condom use with their male sexual partners. *Kids* illustrates this power imbalance in the scenes where Telly seduces young pubescent virginal girls (for example, in the opening scene of the movie, where Telly seduces a girl who is barely a teenager, and later in the movie, when he seduces the young character, Darcy, at the party). In some settings, condoms are not freely available to children in schools, either because doing so is culturally frowned-upon, or not legally permissible. The end result is that those most at risk of STIs are unable to protect themselves against infection. In some settings, condoms are accessible at schools but gatekeepers deter access (for example, condoms have to be sought from an authority figure such as teacher, guidance counselor, or principal). Such practices deter children from seeking condoms and leave them vulnerable to STI infections and pregnancies. On the other hand, the provision of condoms to school children, particularly to those under the legal age of consent for sexual intercourse, raises disclosure obligations for the individual dispensing the condoms. For example, if a 13-year-old student solicits a condom from an educator, it would imply the student is probably sexually active. However, if the child is not legally entitled to have sex until, for example, 16 years of age, it would imply that any penetrative sexual activities he or she engages in with others could constitute rape or sexual assault. In some settings, disclosure laws aimed at protecting the interests of the young would require the educator to inform relevant authorities. This could conflict with the student's right to confidentiality.

As is evident, those involved in the treatment and care of teenagers face many ethical and legal dilemmas, as epitomized in *Kids*. While we never learn the fate of Telly, Jennie, Casper, Ruby, and Telly's numerous young sexual conquests, we all have a duty to ensure that we anticipate and handle the needs of vulnerable children, like these characters, sensitively and ethically.

REFERENCES

1. Singh, J.A., Abdool Karim, S.S., Abdool Karim, Q., Mlisana, K., Williamson, C., Gray, C., et al. 2006. Enrolling adolescents in research on HIV and other sensitive issues: Lessons from South Africa. *Public Library of Science Medicine* 3(7): e180.
2. Lyon, M.E., and D'Angelo, L.J. (Eds.), *Teenagers, HIV, AIDS: Insights from youth living with the virus*. Westport, CT: Praeger Publishers.
3. Neinstein, L.S., and Gordon, C.M. 2008. *Handbook of adolescent health care*. Philadelphia, PA: Lippincott Williams & Wilkins.

3

personhood and the ethics
of dementia: *iris*

solomon liao

Iris (2001). Kate Winslet, Hugh Bonneville, Judi Dench, Jim Broadbent, Eleanor Bron. Directed by Richard Eyre. Duration: 91 minutes.

DVD chapter 4 scene 00:17:02 to 00:19:12

RIS TELLS THE STORY OF Dame Iris Murdoch (Judi Dench), a successful English philosopher and author who develops dementia. The story chronicles the progression of her dementing illness as she progresses from a brilliant and dominating personality to a confused and dependent adult. Intermittent and frequent flashbacks to her as a younger woman contrast her past vibrant energy with her current decline as dementia begins to rob her of her mind. When she becomes more and more child-like, her relationship with her husband, John (Jim Broadbent), changes. Whereas she was once the organizer who kept order in the house and gave direction to their relationship, he must now become her caregiver and deal with her worsening behavioral problems. Her dementia places a strain on their relationship, leading to angry outbursts from both of them. At the funeral of her best friend, he begins to feel lonely and questions if her love for him has faded. On their way home, she confesses her love to him, allowing him to let go and place her in a nursing home. The movie ends with John at her death bed and then crying as he cleans out her things.

In this scene, Iris begins to show early signs of her dementia as she struggles to find the words for the book she is writing. She then becomes agitated by a cat fighting with a fox outside her window. She wonders out loud if she is "going mad" and asks, "How would we know, those of us who live in our minds anyway?" She tries to reassure herself by saying, "Other people would tell us." But then doubt arises, and she turns to her husband and asks, "Would they, John?"

This movie asks the fundamental philosophical question, "What makes us human?" The constellation of illnesses we call dementia, challenges and heightens this question. We find the main character, Iris, defining herself by her ability to shape the world through words. She constructs her own world through her words. As her husband, John, says later on in the movie, Iris has always lived in her own world. At the beginning of their relationship, John asks her, "You love words, don't you?" She replies, "If one doesn't have words, how does one think?" Her reply triggers us to recall Rene Descartes' famous proof of human existence, "I think therefore I am."[1] However, John replies that language is "not the only way of understanding each other." As the movie progresses, we find love and relationships more powerful than words and the mind. As she loses her mind and her ability to use words, her relationship with her husband and the love that they share gives her value as a human being. Ultimately, the movie answers the question, "What makes us human?" as our ability to engage in relationships, to love and be loved.

Several years ago, the daughter of a patient with advanced dementia told me, "That's not my dad. It's just a shell, his body. The man I knew is long gone." Yet, she became angry when nursing staff placed restraints on the patient when he got agitated. She demanded that the nurse remove the restraints, saying, "Why are you tying my dad down like a dog?" These seemingly paradoxical comments reflect the conflict we feel about personhood in individuals who no longer have the higher cognitive abilities we associate with being a fully functioning human. At what point of brain damage do we say the person is no longer a human being? The answer has implications for how we define brain death and how we treat comatose patient and babies born with no brain cortex.

The fear is that patients with neurological impairments will be treated as subhuman or less than human, that they will be given less dignity than what they deserve. Yet, how do we protect them from harming themselves? The tension and ethical struggle is finding the balance between respecting their rights (autonomy) and protecting their welfare (beneficence or nonmaleficence). When should the car keys be taken away or their driver's license revoked? When should a guardian or conservator be appointed to make all their legal decisions for them, thus taking away all their constitutional rights? When should they be locked away in a care facility? As in this movie, John struggled with placing Iris in nursing care facility and resisted even when he clearly was unable to care for her and their primary care physician prompted him to do so. Families of dementia patients struggle every day with such decisions. This challenge constantly changes as the patient's disease progresses, leading to caregiver fatigue. At one point in the movie, John turns to Iris and says, "nobody wants you... I don't want you." People with dementia are therefore at high risk of being abused and neglected.[2]

Iris' second question to John hints at the concern that most individuals with mild cognitive impairment have: that is, the social stigmata of dementia. A discussion with 301 individuals with mild dementia across the United States performed by the Alzheimer's Association revealed that a major concern was the societal stigmata associated with the label of dementia.[3] These individuals were fearful of discrimination. Indeed, studies show that health care disparities exist for people with dementia.[4] One reason cited for this health care inequality is the lack of education and training of physicians on the topic of dementia.[5] Near the end of this scene in the movie, Iris's primary care physician confesses that her condition ranges "beyond my competence."

In the biomedical model, the loss of cognitive functioning is linked with the notion that the "inner person" vanishes.[6] Popular images reflect this concept of dementia patients as "the living dead" or "a vacant house" in this process of "the loss of self."[7] Opponents to this notion have tried to rescue this "inner person" by providing counter-notions of personhood.[8] One such effort returns to the concept of the human soul. Personhood may reside in the organic brain or body, but the physical brain and body are not what defines the person. A richer (fuller and more in-depth) view of personhood is integration of the psychosocial with the physical.[9] The movie hints at this kind of approach. Throughout the movie, the theme that love, not one's intellectual abilities, is what is important, recurs. Ultimately, when all else is stripped away, the ability to love and receive love is what makes us human. Our ability to engage in relationships is what gives us value and is at the core of personhood. Thus, the wife of my advanced dementia patient still found value in her interactions with him even in the last two weeks of his life as she sat at his bedside. The implication for this type of holistic approach demands the need for interdisciplinary care. To meet the needs of the patient and his or her family requires the skills of multiple professionals. Indeed, dementia affects the family as much as it does the patient. The treatment unit, therefore, needs to be both the patient and the family.

In conclusion, dementia challenges our perception of personhood by slowly and inevitably robbing the individual of his or her cognitive abilities. Individuals like Iris, who define themselves by their intellectual accomplishments, suffer existential struggles in their self-identification. Persons with dementia fear being devalued or discriminated against. Yet, as their functional abilities decline, a balance must be struck between their capacity to make decisions and their protection. What this movie and dementia itself teach us is that personhood is about relationships and the ability to love. The answer then to dementia is to increase relationships (not decrease them), to increase human contact, and to increase our expressions of love.

REFERENCES

1. Rene Descartes. 1637. *Discourse on Method*.
2. Cooper, C., Selwood, A., Blanchard, M., Walker, Z., Blizard, R., and Livingston, G. 2009. Abuse of people with dementia by family carers: Representative cross-sectional survey. *British Medical Journal* 338: b155.
3. Voices of Alzheimer's disease: A summary report on the nationwide town hall meeting for people with early stage dementia. Released August 2008. Retrieved August 27, 2009 from http://www.alz.org/townhall.
4. Murray, L.M., and Boyd, S. 2009. Protecting personhood and achieving quality of life for older adults with dementia in the U.S. health care system. *Journal of Aging Health* 21: 350–373.
5. Turner, S., Iliffe, S., Downs, M., Wilcock, J., Bryans, M., Levin, E., et al. 2004. General practitioners' knowledge, confidence and attitudes in the diagnosis and management of dementia. *Age and Ageing* 33: 461–467.

6. Novas, C., and Rose, N. 2000. Genetic risk and the birth of the somatic individual. *Economy and Society* 29: 483–513.

7. Gubrium, J. 1986. *Oldtimers and Alzheimer's: The descriptive organization of senility.* Greenwich, CT: JAI Press.

8. Leibing, A. 2006. *Divided gazes: Alzheimer's disease, the person within, and death in life.* In A. Leibing, and L. Cohens (Eds.), *Thinking about dementia—Culture, loss, and the anthropology of senility*, pp. 240–268. New York: Rutgers University Press.

9. Leibing, A. 2008. Entangled matters—Alzheimer's, interiority, and the 'unflattening' of the world. *Culture, Medicine and Psychiatry* 32: 177–193.

4

the patient-physician journey
to diagnosis: *go now*

timothy krahn

Go Now (1995). Robert Carlyle, Juliet Aubrey, James Nesbitt, Sophie Okonedo, Berwick Kaler. Directed by Michael Winterbottom. Duration: 81 minutes.

DVD chapter 04, Scene 00.32.30 to 00.33.32

GO *NOW* TELLS THE STORY of Nick Cameron (Robert Carlyle) who, with the care of his devoted girlfriend Karen (Juliet Aubrey), endures the somewhat confusing process of being diagnosed with multiple sclerosis (MS). Nick first experiences numbness in his hands. Next, he starts seeing double. Nick's family doctor conducts some tests, asks leading questions (that later reveal his prior suspicion of MS), and prescribes eyeglasses, claiming that the problem is likely caused by what he terms a *trapped nerve*. Nick's continuing symptoms provoke Karen to seek answers on her own. In a private visit, she confronts Nick's doctor, accusing him of withholding Nick's real diagnosis of what she suspects is MS. The doctor acknowledges this as a "possibility," but justifies his paternalist approach by maintaining that the symptoms of MS may "come and go" or "disappear altogether" and may amount to "no more than a tingle in the arms." Karen retorts: "If [Nick's] got it, he's got a right to know he's got it." The doctor counsels Karen that if she so wishes she can tell Nick her suspicions, but that he himself (for now) will do "nothing."[i]

Admittedly, diagnosing MS is extremely complicated: as no etiological agent for the disease has been identified, diagnosis is reached through a process of elimination. Making a determination of MS is initially tentative and only increases in probability over an extended period of time.[1,2] Moreover, the prognosis of MS is always uncertain, ranging from "the near trivial to the severely disabling, or fatal (p. 1308)."[3] There is, as yet, no cure and only partial medical therapies available.[1] Even so, the doctor's response in the above scene is problematic on several levels,[ii] not the least of which is a failure to properly communicate with Nick and Karen.

While a doctor's professional role as diagnostician and expert adviser always involves the exercise of discernment as to what information is relevant to communicate to the patient, this does not include (except in extenuating cases) a duty to protect the patient from receiving information, even if this means "bad news."[4] This chapter uses the narrative case study of MS diagnosis and disclosure in *Go Now* as a springboard to discuss (a) the main reasons why physicians should follow a policy of open disclosure; (b) what exceptions to such a policy are permissible; and finally (c) some basic guidelines for physicians to negotiate relationships with patients who undergo the process of MS diagnosis.

the importance of open disclosure

Communication of specific information to the patient is an important duty of physicians.[5] Not providing it violates the patient's autonomy and right to self-determination, thereby depriving the patient of an important means by which to live and shape her life as she sees fit.[6] Significantly, this also allows patients to incorporate knowledge into their resultant choices of diagnostic and treatment options, thus taking joint responsibility for the management of their health outcomes.[7] Even in cases like MS, where reaching a diagnosis can be an involving, protracted process, telling patients about the clinical uncertainties of their health situation and the range of interventions available to them allows them to appreciate the complexities and limitations of modern medicine.[4]

Open and clear disclosure, as well as transparent decision-making, is critical to maintaining and fostering trust and respect in relationships with patients.[4,iii] In general, such an approach to communication increases patient compliance with appropriate care and reduces patient morbidities during medical interventions.[6] Due care may require a physician perceiving symptoms of abnormality to alert the patient to the condition and to instruct "the patient to any limitations recently observed for [her] own welfare, and as to any precautionary therapy [s]he should seek in the future."[5]

disclosing a diagnosis of ms

On both a practical and an ethical level, MS disclosure is not a question of whether to disclose or not, but rather what, when, and how to disclose. Trying to predict what information patients will find upsetting (let alone the degree of personal impact) is difficult and highly speculative.[4] In the case of MS, personal testimonials and studies (especially in the past) show that attending physicians not uncommonly delay communicating the diagnosis,[7] disregarding or misjudging the fact that, as a rule, most patients clearly prefer immediate disclosure of diagnosis.[3,8,iv] MS patients have also complained of being harmed by the way doctors who use unclear, nonspecific language—e.g. "chronic virus infection," "inflammation of the nervous system," "neuritis," etc.—to avoid the true diagnosis. As a result, some MS patients have had to seek translation of these euphemisms elsewhere or been forced to diagnose themselves, sometimes leading to wrongful or unnecessary treatments.[7]

After seeing a specialist, Nick finally receives word of his diagnosis over the telephone, a communication format woefully inadequate to his needs as a patient. Experience shows that it is often useful for close family members or intimate relations to be present to provide support to the patient and to assist the patient in remembering the facts of the diagnosis. Patients should always be offered ample time to hear, discuss, and ask questions about their diagnosis in person.[8] It is also important after the initial disclosure for the responsible physician to offer further opportunities to discuss concerns with the doctor or other relevant health care professionals after taking some time to reflect upon and to "digest" this news.

variability among patients' informational needs and preferences

In sum, making and communicating a diagnosis is often not an act, but a process. The scope and manner of the physician's communications with the patient must be adjusted to the patient's needs.[5] To make communication meaningful for the patient requires the physician to see her as a person—it requires tact, timing, and the practice of flexible, caring responsibility in relation to the particular needs of *this* patient in *her own* situational context. Doing so increases the likelihood that the "journey to MS diagnosis" becomes understandable for the patient. Moreover, it is the responsibility of the doctor to initiate communication,[4,5] not to simply answer if the patient has questions.

To repeat, the "truth" of an MS diagnosis is rarely, if ever, "naked" at presentation.[v] Although the literature on MS diagnosis shows that a strong majority of patients wish to know once an MS diagnosis is certain, not all prefer to be apprised of the different levels of (un)certainty during the various stages of testing that precede such a determination. Respect for patient autonomy also means that a patient's wishes, in this case not to be informed, must be respected.[8] As Hébert advises:

> [D]octors can best establish what their patients want to know by specifically asking them what they want to know and ensuring these information needs are met. It is as simple as engaging patients in conversation, albeit conversation that emphasizes a doctor's responsibility to ensure dialogue.[4]

Freedman concurs, arguing that in those situations where families or physicians may want to protect the patient by withholding information about a diagnosis, the truth is never to be imposed on the patient, but at the very least, respect requires that the patient be "offered" the opportunity to learn the truth about his or her diagnosis.[9] As Freedman further points out: "Concretely the offering of truth is about [the patient's] diagnosis; symbolically, it is a process that allows her to declare her own preference regarding which [cultural, familial, or other] norms shall be respected and how (p. 576)."[9] It stands to reason that "the truth" to be offered should include not only being informed once a diagnosis is reached, but also the relevant details of the steps of the process leading up to such a determination, at whatever level of detail the patient wishes. After all, medical testing under normal circumstances requires consent from the patient, and for consent to be valid, the patient must be informed of the reasons for this testing.

exceptions to the duty to disclose

Exceptions to the duty to disclose would include the following cases: a patient's waiver expressing a will not to have certain information revealed; incompetence, when a patient is not capable of receiving and processing the relevant information; and emergency situations in which a patient's medical condition is so unstable or compromised that ordinary disclosure is considered unsafe. For each case, evidence (as opposed to assumption or presumption) is required to warrant the exception.[4,vi]

guidelines for negotiating the ms patient–physician relationship

To repeat: The duty to disclose is part of the physician's duty of due care, and the courts have ruled that "[p]hysicians cannot substitute their judgment about what is important for patients to know for the patients' own judgment (p. 2107)."[4] Indeed, the matter of open disclosure should be seen as part of a wider move to invite the patient to consider, and in turn demonstrate to the patient, the multiple layerings of responsibility involved if care is to be achieved.[4] For example, Nick first finds out that he might have MS by happening upon an MS self-help guide (in his own apartment) that presumably Karen had kept hidden from him out of paternalistic (albeit care-motivated) sentiments. He confronts Karen who, when pressed, admits not only to her private conversation with the family doctor, but that she also has shared facts about Nick's prospective diagnosis with her boss to be excused from work to care for Nick. In this regard, Nick feels wronged by Karen: He is hurt by the breach of trust implied in all this talk about him "behind his back"; he is angered by the violation of his privacy, that others have been given confidential information about him without his consent. That the family doctor agreed to engage in a discussion with Karen about Nick's health condition without Nick's knowledge or consent is also ethically suspect. Furthermore, it is evidence of a missed opportunity to entreat Nick to take more of an active role himself in devising his plan of care. If the doctor had taken a more proactive approach to communication, perhaps encouraging Karen to come back with Nick to discuss the possibility of an MS diagnosis, he might have enabled Nick to feel more in control of his situation, rather than leaving him to feel ignorant, powerless, and resentful of his state of ever-increasing dependence on Karen.[2]

At this stage, medical science has rather limited treatments and no cure to offer persons with MS. But this itself cannot be sufficient reason either to delay or hide a diagnosis. Moreover, a commitment to good communication and trust as a basis for the patient–physician relationship also requires, at the very least, a certain amount of transparency and honesty concerning the uncertainty that goes with the process of trying to *reach* a diagnosis. Roger Higgs has usefully distinguished truth from truth-telling, as follows:

> It is easier to decide what to do when the ultimate outcome is clear. It may be much more difficult to know what to say when the future is less certain, such as in the first episode of what is probably multiple sclerosis (p. 90).... . The whole truth may be impossible to attain, but truthfulness is not. "I do not know" can be a major piece of honesty.[8]

As *Go Now* dramatizes so well, for physicians facing a prospective case of MS, there can only be informed guesses in charting the route to diagnosis in areas where uncertainty is difficult to bear.[8] In the opinion of Judge Robinson: "The patient's reliance upon the physician is a trust of the kind which traditionally has exacted obligations beyond those associated with arms-length transactions."[5] Accordingly, the doctor–patient relationship can be usefully viewed as being situated in a negotiated space. The metaphor of negotiation is appropriate, in this regard, because it emphasizes respect for autonomy of both parties, and it suggests a process that occurs over time, as opposed to an event occurring at a particular moment.[10] Appreciating MS diagnosis and disclosure as a process (not an event) requiring open and ongoing communication is necessary for the health of the patient–physician relationship; in turn, the health of this relationship is critical to the successful care of the patient through the various stages of the mutually challenging experience of arriving at a differential diagnosis. As such, MS researchers have found over time that despite the limits of MS treatments, "the single most important therapeutic tool may be the relationship developed between the patient and his or her physician. It can enable the patient to participate actively and fruitfully in the frustrating but important process of disease management."[3,7] And, making sure the patient–physician journey to diagnosis follows a path of respectful, open communication can also set the stage for continuity of care, which is all-important for satisfactory, if not good, health outcomes for patients.

ACKNOWLEDGMENTS

Thanks to Nuala Kenny, Letitia Meynell, Sheri Alpert, Michael Hadskis, Françoise Baylis, Simon Outram, and Andrew Fenton for feedback on previous drafts of this paper. Research for this project has been funded by the Canadian Institutes of Health Research, MOP 77670, *Therapeutic Hopes and ethical concerns: Clinical research in the neurosciences* and Canadian Institutes of Health Research, NNF 80045, *States of Mind: Emerging Issues in Neuroethics.*

NOTES

i. The doctor further explains that MS is stress related and that disclosure of an indefinite diagnosis might only aggravate Nick's condition or "induce an attack." In the literature, the impact of emotional stress on MS exacerbation is "probably minimal and remains controversial."[1]

ii. There is not much evidence shown in the film that the doctor performs an adequate history for Nick. The "trapped nerve" diagnosis is quite implausible. If the doctor did truly suspect MS, it was irresponsible of him not to alert Nick to the gravity of the situation, given that MS is potentially quite debilitating. Faced with an uncertain diagnosis, the doctor should have initiated procedures aimed at establishing a definitive diagnosis. This could have included more investigative testing. At the very least, it should have included counseling Nick on what symptoms to look for and to report back on to the doctor. A follow-up appointment was also in order. By "shielding" his patient, Nick's doctor inadvertently put him in danger: Shortly following the appointment, Nick loses control of his vehicle (presumably caused by further sensation loss in his limbs) while driving and crashes into another vehicle. By not taking appropriate measures, the doctor also inadvertently compromised public safety in this instance.

iii. This is also critical for upholding confidence in physicians, the medical profession, and public trust in health care systems writ large.

iv. *The National [UK] Collaborating Centre for Chronic Conditions* states that: "Although making and telling the diagnosis is a process that may extend over some time" it is recommended that "an individual should be informed of the potential diagnosis of MS, as soon as it is considered reasonably likely (unless there are overwhelming patient-centred reasons for not doing so)."[2]

v. Attending physicians might expect some variability among MS patients, their families, and cultures concerning informational preferences and expectations.[6] Thus far, there is little evidence gathered on this in the English-speaking medical literature.

vi. Another, but very controversial, exception to the rule of open disclosure is *therapeutic privilege,* whereby the physician, for therapeutic purposes, judges it to be in the patient's best interest to withhold information from the patient. North American courts, for several years now, have ruled against invocations of therapeutic privilege. As Judge Robinson has pointed out: "The physician's privilege to withhold information for therapeutic reasons must be carefully circumscribed... for otherwise, it might devour the disclosure rule itself."[5]

REFERENCES

1. Dangond, F. 2009. *Multiple Sclerosis.* 2009. Retrieved from http://emedicine.medscape.com/article/1146199-overview
2. Stirrat, G.M. 2007. Truth-telling, autonomy and paternalism in healthcare: A commentary on the case of *Gary Dimmock v. East Sussex NHS Trust. Clinical Risk* 13: 226–228.
3. Papathanasopoulos, P.G., Nikolakopoulou, A., and Scolding, N.J. 2005. Disclosing the diagnosis of multiple sclerosis. *Journal of Neurology* 252(11): 1307–1309.

4. Hébert, P.C. 1994. Truth-telling in clinical-practice. *Canadian Family Physician* 40: 2105–2113.

5. Robinson III (Circuit Judge), S.W. 464 F2d 772 *Canterbury v. Spence,* 150 U.S.App.D.C.263. Canterbury v. Spence. [22099]. 12–18–1969. United States Court of Appeals, District of Columbia Circuit. 5–19–1972. Ref Type: Case.

6. Tuckett, A.G. 2004. Truth-telling in clinical practice and the arguments for and against: A review of the literature. *Nursing Ethics* 11(5): 500–513.

7. Levine, C. 1983. Delaying the diagnosis: Truth-telling and multiple sclerosis. *The Hastings Center Report* 13(3): 2–3.

8. Higgs, R. 2006. On telling patients the truth. In T.A. Mappes, and D. DeGrazia (Eds.), *Biomedical ethics,* pp. 90–95 xviii. Oxford, UK: Oxford University Press.

9. Freedman, B. 1993. Offering truth: One ethical approach to the uninformed cancer patient. *Archives of Internal Medicine* 153: 572–576.

10. Childress, J.F., and Siegler, M. 1984. Metaphors and models of doctor-patient relationships: Their implications for autonomy. *Theoretical Medicine* 5(1): 17–30.

5

futility of care: *my life without me*

marina boykova

My Life Without Me (2003). Actors: Sarah Polley, Amanda Plummer,
Scott Speedman, Julian Richings. Directed by Isabel Coixet.
Duration: 106 minutes.

DVD chapter 21 scene 01:10:50 to 01:14:20

MY LIFE WITHOUT ME TELLS the life story of Ann (Sarah Polley), a young woman rendered a diagnosis of a terminal illness. Ann, married and with two young children, knows she will die soon and decides to live her last days differently; she will do what she had wanted to do before but had not had the courage to try. In her last days, she strives to make peace with those she previously fought. She reconciles with her parents, rekindles her love with her husband, makes birthday greetings for her two girls, and tries to find something of value in new friends. One of Ann's friends (a nurse) tells her a story that influenced her nursing career. It happened when she was a nursing student in a neonatal unit and cared for Siamese or *conjoined* twins. Having no chance for survival, the twins were left to die. The parents even refused to see them. Ann held and cuddled them during their last hours. These hours wore on her, as she could not reverse their fate. This event changed her life forever. She turned to comforting geriatric patients at the end of their lives.

This scenario describes the ethical dilemma often faced by nurses: What is ethically and morally right or wrong, and according to whom—the nurse, patient, or family? Let them die, or provide all the technologically supportive care possible? Even if the treatment is futile, as in the exemplar of the twins, should life be preserved at all costs? Who decides? In the example of Ann, she determined her quality of life and she lived her life as if she was going to die at any time. She cherished the moment. Ann could speak for herself and decide her fate. Ann's friend accepted that for Ann, but when it came to providing nursing care, she suffered a moral dilemma, feeling an obligation to help the doomed babies. She failed to carry out her nursing obligation to try to save them, and yet forgot the obligation to "first do no harm." The parents made the decision to let them die, but this determination is hard to accept because babies should not die; they are the celebration of a new beginning. Yet, for these babies, their beginning was also their end. When someone dies too young, the moral and ethical dilemmas loom large, often creating a cognitive dissonance between what is known from science and what the heart feels.

Futility of care is an issue of everyday neonatal practice. A concept of futile care refers to "medical care that either prolongs suffering, does not improve the quality of life, or fails to achieve a good outcome for the patient."[1] Sometimes babies are born prematurely or with congenital anomalies incompatible with life. Preterm babies often suffer from blindness, hearing loss, neurodevelopmental delays, cerebral palsy, and lifelong disabilities that lead to a very low quality of life. The prognosis for some in the neonatal intensive care unit (NICU) can be gloomy. However, because no one can exactly predict the future, despite existing research, treatment can become aggressive and extraordinary. Health professionals often question the appropriateness of treatment or if it should be withheld. Beneficence ("doing good") and nonmaleficence ("not doing harm") are very important issues in the NICU, where technology can save lives. Ironically, great success in reducing mortality has created unforeseen ethical dilemmas in dealing with issues such as the quality of life and the futility of care.

Ethics is rooted in morality, values, and cultural and social norms. Ethics and morals are interwoven and related, but should be distinguished. Morals refer to an individual's code of acceptable behavior, influenced by culture and shaped by societal values; ethics is a more organized system of beliefs that focuses on the rightness or wrongness of behaviors, and it very often acts as a standardized guide to professional behavior.[2] Depending on societal values, care of these twins might be rendered in one setting, while they might be only supported without aggressive treatment in another setting. The Westernized, biomedical approach to acceptable and appropriate behaviors can be different from the standard behavior of Eastern cultures. Cultural norms vary widely when neonatal care is considered.

What constitutes an ethical dilemma in neonatal care ranges from clear utilitarian to strict deontological views, from a paternalistic approach to full parental autonomy. Newborn infants have no way of representing themselves and are unable to express their wish or will. Often, health professionals have to make decisions and guide parents and relatives. Surrogate decision-making is often used, and the best-interest standard is considered most appropriate for neonatal practice, but the outcomes of decisions made during the critical stage of neonatal illness may not be seen until years later, making the ethical dilemmas in neonatal care even more difficult.[3] Do health professionals or parents always act in the best interests of their baby? Obviously, all are concerned about the baby's future and possible handicaps; consideration must be given to burdens for the baby, the mother, family; and the baby's suffering must be diminished. If the burden is too great, then beneficence dictates nontreatment, and ordinary care should be provided. This case can be considered as passive involuntary euthanasia, which "means that a person who seems to be suffering or living 'senseless' life in coma or other vegetative state is not treated any further in crucial situations."[4]

Sometimes conflicts occur between parental and a health professional's views. Accepted professional ethical norms and principles can also come into conflict with personal morals and values. Moreover, ethical decision-making and futility are related to legal issues. Parents are legal decision-makers. However, it may be illegal not to treat, even with a parental request in the case of incurable disease. For instance, in Russia, treatment cannot be withdrawn even if there are clear estimates of a persistent vegetative state. Euthanasia is prohibited. But, "what is legal can be immoral, and vice versa" and "what is legal and what moral are not necessary related."[5] The case of the conjoined twins increases moral distress in health professionals, and this moral distress may lead to impaired ethical reasoning and decision-making. In part this is because it might be seen as legal yet immoral to treat the twins, and simultaneously viewed as illegal yet moral to not treat them. Some regulations can be culturally unacceptable, such as the *Baby Doe* regulations promulgated in 1984 in the United States, which proscribed withholding treatment based on an actual or potential handicap.[1]

Whether countries use medical paternalism as an acceptable method of decision-making—for instance, in France—or patient autonomy as the prevailing model, medical authority is still a key issue in ethics.[6] Some doctors and nurses believe that the final decision is too burdensome for families, and this decision should not be left up to them.[7] Depending upon the country, there are three approaches to neonatal care: (a) the "treat until certainty" approach, whereby each infant is treated until death or discharge; (b) the "statistical" approach, whereby treatment is withheld from infants defined as underweight and/or immature; and (c) the "initiate and re-evaluate" approach, whereby aggressive treatment is begun and then reevaluated relative to the infant's progress and parents' wishes.[8,9] In Russia, a fourth approach can be seen: "Provide treatment in any case." These different approaches are understandable as countries view ethical dimensions differently in accordance with cultural values and beliefs. Each approach has its own advantages and disadvantages, and money plays a role that is beyond the scope of this chapter.

The principle-based approach of contemporary biomedical ethics is widely used. This approach obviously helps nurses and physicians come to ethically appropriate decisions. However, the universality of the four principles of autonomy, beneficence, nonmaleficence, and justice does not imply that their application should lead to an absolute ethical decision. The principle-based approach is criticized for its predetermined balance of ethical principles in favor of respect for autonomy and does not necessary guide ethical decisions that are aimed at promoting good for the individual.[10] Overemphasizing respect for autonomy and the stigma of paternalism may lead to suppression of beneficence and nonmaleficence.[10] Many other situations exist in which parents' autonomy can be overridden if their decision brings more harm than good for a child. At the time of hospitalization, the parents' rationality and moral integrity may be impaired related to overwhelming stress, anger, or fear of having a disabled child; however, health professionals should not impose their own values on parents. The four principles have special considerations in the NICU and should be applied as much as possible in contextual situation. Ethical decision-making is one of the most difficult parts of the NICU job, as it carries many controversial and emotional issues. Neonatal care is a very specialized practice, in which the four core ethical principles can be modified to examine dilemmas. In neonatal care, when making decisions concerning extraordinary care, we should use the infant's potential quality of life and suffering, as well as the family's and society's opinions, as determining factors in assessing the infant's best interests. In each case, futility of care should be evaluated on an individual basis by incorporating patient and family desires, and opinions from the interdisciplinary health team within the context of professional ethical guidelines and policies. Different ethical approaches should be taught, and appropriate guidelines should be developed that could improve ethical decision-making. Open and ongoing discussion between health professionals and consensual agreement are vital. As in this movie, there is no right answer— only questions.

REFERENCES

1. Romesberg, T.L. 2003. Futile care and the neonate. *Advances in Neonatal Care* 3(5): 213–219.
2. Finkelman, A., and Kenner, C. 2010. *Professional nursing concepts: Competencies for quality leadership.* Sudbury, MA: Jones and Bartlett Publishers.
3. Spence, K. The best interest principle as a standard for decision making in the care of neonates. *Journal of Advanced Nursing* 31(6): 1286–1292.
4. Tschudin, V. 1993. *Ethics: Aspects of nursing care*, p. 113. London, UK: Scutari Press.
5. Seedhouse, D. 1998. *Ethics: The heart of health care*, p. 93. Chichester, UK: Wiley.
6. Orfali, K. 2004. Parental role in medical decision-making: Fact or fiction? A comparative study of ethical dilemmas in french and American neonatal intensive care units. *Social Science and Medicine* 58(10): 2009–2022.
7. McHaffie, H.E., Laing, I.A., Parker, M., and McMillan, J. 2001. Deciding for imperiled newborns: Medical authority or parental autonomy? *Journal of Medical Ethics* 27(2): 104–109.
8. Gross, M.L. 2000. Avoiding anomalous newborns: Preemptive abortion, treatment thresholds and the case of baby Messenger. *Journal of Medical Ethics* 26(4): 242–248.
9. Lorenz, J.M. 2001. The outcome of extreme prematurity. *Seminal Perinatology* 25(5): 348–359.
10. Woodward, V.M. 1998. Caring, patient autonomy and the stigma of paternalism. *Journal of Advanced Nursing* 28(5): 1046–1052.

6

futility in the nicu: *my life without me*

sadath a. sayeed

My Life without Me (2003). Sarah Polley, Amanda Plummer, Scott Speedman, Julian Richings. Directed by Isabel Coixet. Duration: 106 minutes.

DVD chapter 21 scene 01:10:50 to 01:14:20

N THE FILM, *MY LIFE Without Me*, a 23-year-old woman, Ann (Sarah Polley), is diagnosed with terminal ovarian cancer that leaves her with only a few months to live. Ann is married to Don, with whom she has had two daughters, and they live in a trailer behind her mother's house. After receiving her diagnosis, Ann chooses to keep the condition secret from her loved ones, believing that this is the one gift she can leave her family—a few parting memories of daily happiness rather than memories of her death in a hospital. The remainder of the film turns into her intense meditation on extracting the most out of what time she has left to live. Ann's sentimental epiphany takes form in a short handwritten list of "things to do before I die" and includes items such as: "making someone fall in love with me" and "drink and smoke as much as I want."

In the scene chosen for this chapter, Ann has coffee with a neighbor (a nurse also named Ann), who is similarly aged and who shows heartfelt affection for her girls. Ann asks her neighbor about having children and bluntly quizzes her if she hasn't found the right man yet, or whether she is incapable. The other Ann hesitates, then shares the following story: she loves children but she hasn't gotten over a prior deeply upsetting and transformative experience as a nurse. She was assigned to the maternal–newborn unit, and was involved in caring for a woman who unexpectedly gave birth to conjoined twins. Doctors told the parents nothing could be done to save the twins. The father then insisted they did not want to see them prior to their demise. Ann volunteers to hold them until they die. She recollects how she held the babies for some 30 hours, watching as one child died a few hours before the other. This is why, she concludes, she has been a geriatric nurse ever since and, presumably, why she has not sought to have children of her own.

In this dramatic, short narrative between two women chatting over a cup of coffee, a broad range of tense emotional and moral concerns emerge from the world of modern neonatal medical care. Here are just a few: How should parents handle unexpected and devastating news about the health and welfare of their newborns? How do medical providers manage such tragic situations? What are minimally acceptable ways of demonstrating compassion for a dying child? Whose lives are impacted most by neonatal death? What makes a medical condition futile? Who should decide?

Newborns occupy a unique "human life" position. They have not yet begun a personal biographical story beyond that which their parents may have imagined, but nevertheless have begun to possess an independent biological existence. Whatever early senses and experiences babies have, they are undeniably their own; yet, it is a nonsensical task to try and estimate the value of life from the perspective of a newborn. Informed preferences, desires, or values are built upon interaction with others and the environment; the ideal of autonomy or self-governance is decades in the making. It is also harder to calculate the value of what is lost when babies die early in life. Certainly, there is the loss of others' expectations and individual potential, but genuine disagreement exists among reasonable people about the depth and quality of these kinds of moral losses.[1]

Many people intuit, for example, that the death of a 13-year-old is a far worse thing than the death of a 2-month-old.[2] A philosophical adage that captures this intuition goes as follows: an acorn isn't the same as a tree. One plausible explanation for this perception involves a natural human tendency to suffer the loss of another more substantially when there exists greater emotional and social attachment (to follow the tree analogy, when the roots are deeper). On a charitable interpretation, something like this sentiment may motivate the film's fictional father to avoid any contact with his doomed twin newborns. He may be worried about his own ability to let go if he comes to love them. It is also possible that he is (less admirably) repulsed by their reported physical deformity. Regardless, we ought not to confuse what is perhaps an adequate psychological explanation for predictably different feelings of loss at different epochs of human death with satisfactory moral justification. Just because we might be predisposed to lament a baby's death less does not mean that the *intrinsic* value of human newborn life is by necessity different from that of older children or adults.

Following from such abstract debate, disagreement also occurs about how to ethically frame medical treatment decision-making for gravely ill neonates. Most agree that the interests of the newborn must be prioritized, but calculating a baby's interest in, say for example, surviving without serious disability, might be notoriously dependent on the person asked to do the arithmetic.[3] There is hardly a consensus (even among health care providers) about what kinds of human lives are worth living. Also, there is something inherently risky about asking another person, often from the vantage of relative physiological normalcy, to project what it must "be like" to live with limited mental and physical capacities.[4] Yet, we have, as a practical matter, little choice. Almost every day in neonatal intensive care units, difficult decisions are made about whether to try to keep alive some critically ill and permanently injured newborn. In the United States, we typically start with a presumption that parents are entitled to make these decisions.[5] However, in other countries, a form of "benign paternalism" often supplants this ethical approach, where a counter-argument prevails: Parents faced with such unexpected and personal crises often cannot make life-ending decisions that are in their child's (and their own) best interests.[6] In effect, the bioethical claim is that they should not be asked to feel responsible for the final decision to let their child die, and so providers must take the responsibility.

It is important to note that, in the United States, newborns and infants have for some time received special attention in law. One historical impetus for this protection stems from the political fallout that followed national publicity of a death of a neonate born with trisomy 21 (Down syndrome) in Indiana in the early 1980s. The baby had a surgically correctable condition. However, upon the advice of the medical provider, and largely because the baby was known to be permanently mentally disabled, the parents opted against intervention, resulting in her death. Many vilified this decision as an egregious example of discrimination against the handicapped, and the federal government responded by adopting the so-called "Baby Doe rules." These regulations, which emanate from amendments to the federal Child Abuse Prevention and Treatment Act (CAPTA), have been interpreted by many authorities (but not all) to severely circumscribe the situations in which life-sustaining treatment can be withheld or withdrawn from children under one year of age.[7]

Under CAPTA, one of the primary criterions for permitting the discontinuance of life-extending medical interventions is a finding of futility. Unfortunately, in practice, it is quite often unclear why medical interventions are regarded as futile. Especially in neonatology, this loaded term lends itself to a multiplicity of meanings. Sometimes it conveys the message that no available therapy will stave off a near and proximate death; this seems to be the interpretation favored by the original conservative crafters of the Baby Doe rules. This stands in distinction to so-called "qualitative" futility, where a decision to end life-sustaining treatments might be made based on physicians' or parents' concerns about the infant's ability to enjoy a reasonable future quality of life.[8]

Despite this long-standing regulatory presence, today, many U.S.-based neonatal practitioners feel ethically compelled to consider quality-of-survival judgments in discussing treatment options for critically ill newborns who depend for some period of time on intensive care. Physicians often strongly encourage removal of life support for babies with birth asphyxia when the neurological injury is thought to be overwhelmingly severe. They make this recommendation even though it is, strictly speaking, rarely physiologically futile to provide intensive care in the form of mechanical ventilation and/or intravenous nutrition. With such therapies, these babies can transition to long-term rehabilitation facilities where they might live with minimal cognitive capacities for years or even decades. Arguably, strong professional affirmation of allowing quality-of-life judgments in such cases acts as a complex gesture of social empathy. Pediatric health care providers are often acutely aware of the minimally existent community support for families with neurologically devastated children, and are at least anecdotally aware of the tremendous burden suddenly levied upon even the most compassionate parents.[9] As such, there is an understandable reluctance to force parents to bear this uninvited, unanticipated, and possibly life-long cost when there is an opportunity at an early stage to allow more comforting and peaceful closure—precisely because of the relative absence of entrenched emotional and social attachments.

In the NICU, where uncertainty blunts much of our diagnostic and prognostic precision, and lack of patient autonomy forecloses our preferred source for decision-making, we often struggle mightily to craft ethically elegant decisions. In the film, Nurse Ann implied that medical treatment for the conjoined twins was futile. When such a claim is noncontroversially accurate, all stakeholders' tasks are ideally a little simpler. Providers are left with an obligation to provide a dignified and respectful death. Kudos to Nurse Ann for recognizing this! Parents are left to handle and, eventually, come to terms with personal grief. While there ought to be a clear standard for professionals in all cases when babies die in our hands, there can never be a straightforward prescription for parents in learning to cope with the premature loss of their child.

REFERENCES

1. Harris, J. 1999. The concept of the person and the value of life. *Kennedy Institute of Ethics Journal* 293–308.
2. Persad, G., Wertheimer, A., and Emanuel, E. 2009. Principles for allocation of scarce medical interventions. *The Lancet* 373: 423–431.
3. President's Commission for the Study of Ethical Problems in Medicine and Biomedical and Behavioral Research, *Deciding to forego life-sustaining treatment: A report on the ethical, medical, and legal issues in treatment decisions*, 1983. Library of Congress 218–222.
4. Saigal, S., et al. 2006. Self-perceived health-related quality of life of former extremely low birth weight infants at young adulthood. *Pediatrics* 118: 1140–1148.
5. AAP Committee on Fetus and Newborn. 2007. Noninitiation or withdrawal of intensive care for high-risk newborns. *Pediatrics* 119: 401–403.
6. Orfali, K., and Gordon, E. 2004. Autonomy gone awry: A cross-cultural study of parents' experiences in neonatal intensive care units. *Theoretical Medicine* 25: 329–365.
7. Sayeed, S. Baby Doe redux? The department of health and human services and the born-alive infants protection act of 2002: A cautionary note on normative neonatal practice. *Pediatrics* 116: e576–e585.
8. McCullough, L. 2005. Neonatal ethics at the limits of viability. *Pediatrics* 116: 1019–1021.
9. Drotar, D., et al. The impact of extremely low birth weight on the families of school-aged children. *Pediatrics* 117: 2006–2013.

organ trafficking and happiness: *dirty pretty things*

richard a. demme

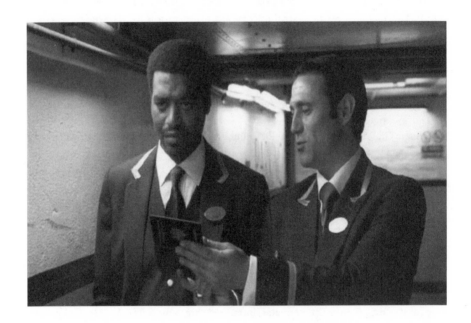

Dirty Pretty Things (2002). Chiwetel Ejiofor, Audrey Tautou, Benedict Wong. Sergi Lopez. Directed by Stephen Frears. Duration: 97 minutes.

Scene: DVD chapter 10 Scene 00:49:33 to 00:50:50

THE HOTEL BUSINESS IS ABOUT strangers... and strangers will always surprise you. They come to hotels in the night to do dirty things. And in the morning, it's our job to make things look pretty again." This is the advice that Sneaky (Senor Juan), the hotel manager, gives to Okwe (Chiwetel Ejiofor), the night receptionist, after Okwe distressingly discovers one of the hotel room toilets plugged up with a human heart. *Dirty Pretty Things* portrays the adventures of Okwe, a Nigerian physician who is an undocumented alien in London, and Senay (Audrey Tautou), a Turkish woman seeking asylum, when they encounter an organ trafficking ring that operates out of the hotel where they are employed.

In this scene, Sneaky discusses how organ trafficking is beneficial. He has discovered that Okwe is a physician, and wants to lure him into the organ trafficking ring. Sneaky shows Okwe a well-made falsified passport, and tells him:

If you were just some African, the deal would be simple. You give me your kidney, I give you a new identity. I sell the kidney for ten grand [pounds], so I'm happy. The person who needs the kidney gets cured, so he's happy. The person who sold his kidney gets to stay in this beautiful country, so he's happy. My whole business is based on happiness.

The sale of human organs is illegal in most countries, including the United States and the United Kingdom. Iran is a notable exception, where kidney sales are regulated. Despite being illegal, the sale of human kidneys flourishes in many countries. The pressure for the legalization of organ sales mounts every year, as the waiting list for transplants grows. As of December 20, 2009, over 83,000 people are on the U.S. waiting list for kidneys.[1] Only 16,518 kidney transplants were performed in the US in 2008. The National Organ Transplant Act of 1984 (NOTA) prohibits the transfer of "any human organ for valuable consideration."[2] Violators of NOTA may be fined up to $50,000 or imprisoned up to five years, or both, although I am not aware of anyone having been convicted (yet) in the United States for such a crime.

In organ trafficking, most often kidneys are sold for money, but in *Dirty Pretty Things*, kidneys are sold for false papers and new identities. Since the wait for a deceased donor kidney can be several years, some U.S. insurance programs have actually promoted "transplant tourism," encouraging waiting patients to find kidney donors overseas.[3]

The ethical question is whether human organs *should* be bought and sold like other commodities. In many countries, kidney dialysis is not available to all, as it is in the United States. In places where dialysis is not readily available, the wealthy and powerful have found opportunities to buy kidneys, usually from poor or desperate people. This has been called the Indian question, or, "To buy or let die." When a wealthy person buys a kidney, it keeps him alive, and the donor gets paid so he can support his family; this appears to be a win–win situation in which both parties benefit.[4] How can it be unethical if everyone benefits? In the movie scenario, as described above, the broker benefits as well, so everyone's happy. Or are they?

Okwe discovers a Somalian kidney donor in Sneaky's office seriously ill from an infection at the site of his kidney removal and is pressured into stealing antibiotics from a hospital to treat him. The donor and his family do not want to go to the hospital because they are undocumented aliens. Okwe laments "He swapped his insides for a passport." But, perhaps this scene was only used for dramatic effect. How do paid kidney donors fare? Studies from India, Pakistan, Egypt, and Iran have demonstrated that a majority of paid donors, sometimes called vendors, report a decline in their health status after kidney removal. Furthermore, a majority of such vendors report no significant economic improvement in their lives. Many regret their decision, and a majority of those who have sold a kidney would not recommend that others sell a kidney.[5]

Illegal organ sales even occur in the United States. In July 2009, a "matchmaker" broker was arrested for paying an Israeli donor $10,000 for a kidney planned to be sold to an American for approximately $160,000.[6] Even more distressing are reports in 2008 about an Indian organ trafficking ring that lured men with promises of work, and then abducted them. Some "donors" were forced onto the operating table to have a kidney removed at gunpoint.[7] I suspect none of those "donors" were happy. But, let the buyer beware as well. Those who have traveled abroad for kidney transplant experienced higher rates of organ rejection than in most U.S. transplant centers, as well as higher rates of infections transmitted with their kidneys, including hepatitis, HIV, tuberculosis, and schistosomiasis.

Beyond questions of risk to donor and risk to recipient is the issue of autonomy.

Why should individuals be prohibited from selling their organs? Who "owns" your insides? Is someone who has been economically coerced truly making an autonomous donation? These questions typically arise early in seminars about ethics and transplantation.

Another common analogy is made between selling organs and reproductive transactions. An obvious and significant difference exists between the sale of human sperm and eggs from solid organs. Such human "products" are regenerative or may be replenished and are not necessary for daily function; their loss puts donors at minimal risk. While kidney donation is generally safe, over the years there have been dozens of donor deaths, and over 100 living kidney donors are themselves now awaiting kidney transplants.[8] This is not meant to discourage kidney donation, but to point out that kidney donation is a serious matter, and donors may suffer serious harm with no benefit to themselves. Physicians, who have sworn to "do no harm" are necessary for transplantation to safely occur, and should take care to ensure that living organ donors undergo safe procedures, and are not coerced.

Is it "just" when the rich are able to purchase body parts from the poor? Living organ donors may benefit psychologically from donation, and are looked upon with favor by their communities. As noted above, a majority of people who sold a kidney out of economic pressure do not receive the financial benefits they had hoped for, or any psychological benefit. Many develop depression, and do not wish the sale of their organs to be known by others. We cannot pretend that such vendors benefit. Such practices foist the desperation of those on dialysis (who can afford to buy a kidney) to those already economically desperate.

A meeting of more than 150 representatives of scientific and medical bodies from around the world convened an International Summit on Transplant Tourism and Organ Trafficking in Istanbul, Turkey in 2008. The summit resulted in a declaration.

The Declaration of Istanbul on Organ Trafficking and Transplant Tourism defined organ trafficking as "the recruitment, transport, transfer, harboring, or receipt of living or deceased persons or their organs by means of threat or use of force or other forms of coercion, of abduction, of fraud, of deception, of the abuse of power or of a position of vulnerability, or of the giving to, or the receiving by, a third party of payments, or benefits to achieve the transfer of control over the potential donor for the purpose of exploitation by the removal of organs for transplantation." The assembly agreed "Organ trafficking and transplant tourism violate the principles of equity, justice, and respect for human dignity and should be prohibited. Because transplant commercialism targets impoverished and otherwise vulnerable donors, it leads inexorably to inequity and injustice and should be prohibited…. Practices that induce vulnerable individuals or groups such as illiterate and impoverished persons, undocumented immigrants, prisoners, and political or economic refugees to become living donors are incompatible with the aim of combating organ trafficking, transplant tourism, and transplant commercialism."[9]

The current pope, Benedict XVI recently wrote: "With regard to the practice of human transplants, it means that someone can give only if he/she is not placing his/her own health and identity in serious danger, and only for morally valid and proportional reason. The possibility of organ sales, as well as the adoption of discriminatory and utilitarian criteria, would greatly clash with the meaning of the gift that would place it out of consideration, qualifying it as a morally illicit act."[10] So, while organ sales may result in some benefit to recipients, they are considered by many to be unethical. In *Dirty Pretty Things*, Sneaky leaves Okwe the picture of an 8-year-old girl for whom he is trying to obtain a kidney. Sneaky tells Okwe: "Her family brought her over from Saudi, hoping for a miracle. If she doesn't get the new kidney in the next few weeks, she's going to die…So, I'm an evil man, but I'm trying to save her life. That's weird, huh? Kind of thing that keeps you awake at night."

Indeed.

REFERENCES

1. Waiting list candidates. Retrieved December 20, 2009 from http:www.unos.org/data.
2. National Organ Transplantation Act. Pub. L. 98–507, 98th Congress.
3. Bramstedt, K.A., and Xu, J. 2007. Checklist: Passport, plane ticket, organ transplant. *American Journal of Transplantation* 7(7): 1698–1701.
4. Reddy, K.C., Thiagarjan, C.M., Shunmugasundaram, D., et al. 1990. Unconventional renal transplantation in India. *Transplantation Proceedings* 22(3): 910–911.
5. Budiani-Saberi, D.A., and Delmonico, F.L. 2008. Organ trafficking and transplant tourism: A commentary on the global realities. *American Journal of Transplantation* 39(3): 29–44.
6. *United States of America v. Levy Izhak Rosenbaum.* United States District Court, District of New Jersey, July, 2009.
7. Dolrick, S. 2008. Kidney Ring Uncovered in India. *Democrat and Chronicle,* January 31.
8. Demme, R.A. 2010. Ethical concerns about an organ market. *Journal of the National Medical Association* 102: 46–50.
9. The Declaration of Istanbul on organ trafficking and transplant tourism. 2008. *Kidney International* 74: 854–859.
10. Pope Benedict XVI. 2009. A message from the Holy Father Pope Benedict XVI. *Transplantation* 88(7S): S96–S97.

8

organ transplantation and health disparities: *john q*

jeffrey m. ring

John Q (2002). Denzel Washington, Robert Duvall, James Woods, Anne Heche, Eddie Griffin, Kimberly Elise, and Ray Liotta. Directed by Nick Cassavetes. Duration: 118 minutes.

DVD Chapter 5 Scene 00:21:07 to 00:23:31

THE CENTRAL CHARACTER IN THIS film, John Q. Archibald, is an African American factory worker, husband, and devoted father. As the story unfolds, John and Denise's young son collapses during a baseball game and is rushed to the hospital. The physician informs the parents that their boy has an enlarged heart and will require transplantation surgery. Upon discovering that their insurance will not cover the surgery, and even after convincing the surgeon to waive his customary fees, the couple realizes that they still lack sufficient funds to pay the hospital for the surgery. Growing desperate, John holds the patients and staff of the hospital emergency room as hostages, demanding surgery for his son, while police negotiators and media attention gather and grow outside the walls of the hospital.

This particular scene, from early on in the film, might be referred to as "the delivery of bad news." In this case, however, the bad news is both diagnosis/prognosis, as well as the intervention price tag of $250,000 with a required $75,000 down payment. A rather compassionate physician delivers the diagnostic news, but a cold-as-ice hospital administrator reveals the financial details. She also, and not so subtly, encourages the parents to forego the surgery and instead consider hospice care for their young son. In this scene, we witness the great tragedy and psychological trauma for these parents, and watch John Q slowly cut through his misinformation and denial to face the real limitations of his insurance coverage. We hear John Q's anger as he lashes out at the hospital administrator, "...our son is dying and you are talking about money..." This film clip serves as a rich and provocative introduction to larger discussions of the ethics of health disparities and economic health policy.

health disparities

Health care providers must understand the nature and causes of health disparities in the United States as part of their education toward the provision of culturally responsive health care.[1] Health disparities in the United States have been well documented for over two centuries and defined as "the disproportionate burden of poor health status and premature mortality."[2] Epidemiological data indicate health care disparities vary by race/ethnicity, gender, income and educational levels, and sexual orientation. For African American patients, in particular, the disturbing health disparities in the area of transplantation and organ donation have been extensively documented.[3] These inequalities exist in the (a) magnitude of need for organ and tissue transplantation, (b) within the organ transplantation infrastructure, (c) in the epidemiological data regarding prevalence and incidence rates (particularly for kidney failure) in the African American community, and (d) in treatment adherence. For example, Callendar and colleagues underscore, "African Americans are referred later for kidney transplants, are wait-listed later, and are transplanted later than the majority population regardless of financial status. (p. 219)."

How ethnic and racial health disparities originate and are maintained remains a very complex question. The Institute of Medicine Report (2003) suggested that health disparities arise from the contributions of patient factors (such as genetics and risk behaviors), provider factors (such as biases and stereotypes), health care system factors (such as access to care and profit motive) and society factors (such as poverty, racism and resource distribution).[4] In the case of John Q, it would be productive for learners to articulate the degree to which each of these factors may have contributed to the lack of seamless and timely intervention with this young patient.

provider bias

Ayanian and colleagues[5,6] documented the contribution of provider bias to health disproportions among renal failure patients, highlighting the differences between physician beliefs and actual research data. For example, surveyed physicians believed that African American patients did not want to have renal transplantation at rates similar to white patients, while the data showed similar rates of desire for the intervention in African American and white women. Similarly, surveyed physicians believed that there was less availability of living donors for African Americans as compared to white patients, while research data indicated no such gap in the real world. Finally, while physicians believed that African American patients were less likely to complete the rigorous work-up for transplantation, African American patients indicated full ability to do so. Physicians and students should be encouraged to self-reflect on their own potential blind spots and biases as part of ethical self-monitoring and quality improvement. Fortunately for John Q, the white surgeon in the film is optimistic and hopeful about the potential benefits of transplantation surgery for this young African American boy, yet this film portrayal does not often bear out in real life medical practice.

ethics and economic health policy

As this is being written, the United States government is embroiled in heated debate and town hall meetings to discuss health care reform in this country. The media is filled with personal case examples, not unlike that presented in John Q, of patients unable to access needed medical intervention without significant financial sacrifice. Himmelstein and colleagues[7] conducted a national survey to explore links between medical expenditures and bankruptcy rates. The authors found that (a) 62.1% of all bankruptcies had a medical cause, (b) most medical debtors were well educated and middle class and had medical insurance, and (c) that the share of bankruptcies attributable to medical problems rose by 50% between 2001 and 2007. These findings result from a complicated weave of education, poverty, and racism variables in the realm of employment, insurance benefits, and access to adequate health care coverage for oneself and ones' family.

After watching the John Q film clip, learners should be instructed to consider the ethics of insurance denials, alternative systems of payment for care versus the value of human life, and of life-saving procedures such as heart transplant in a young child. Moreover, it is worth exploring how true financial realities, insurance company denials, and withholding of care are best and ethically communicated to patients within the greater context of informed consent. Learners are encouraged to share cases in which they had to make difficult decisions, and how they communicated these to the patient, while brainstorming alternative strategies together in the group. With trained facilitators, learners must deepen their understanding of power dynamics in the doctor–patient relationship, how these are managed, and the potential implications of abused power in the health care arena in terms of racism, sexism, and the resultant health disparities that can arise. This scene from John Q is especially rich in tracking who is holding the power, how each character demonstrates their power differences, and the impact of the power differences on patient and physician/administrator alike.

Finally, the film clip raises the issue of patient anger and desperation. Health care in emergency situations may be a matter of basic survival, and as such, is linked to strong emotions. John Q sees no other alternative than forcibly to take hostages in the hospital emergency room as a way of making his needs known and seeking resolution. Learners may have strong feelings about John Q's choice of fighting for his son's transplant, in either agreement or disagreement. The ethical implications of his actions, potentially placing other patients, their family members, and hospital medical staff in danger is also worth discussing, to enhance the learner's sense of empathy for the patient experience of illness, blocked access to health care, the great cost of medical care, and insurance company denials.

This is an excellent opportunity to work with learners on enhancing their communication with patients in situations of strong emotions. The skills of listening, empathy, honest communication, and respectful dialogue are essential for satisfactory outcomes, as are the skills of negotiating a treatment plan, with the patient's fully informed consent, that is mutually agreeable and one to which the patient is more likely to adhere.

The elimination of health disparities in this country will likely depend on health reform, equalization of educational and economic opportunities, and a shifting of physician attitudes, awareness, knowledge and skills toward the provision of culturally responsive care. Through focused educational intervention,[1] we must train physicians to increase their own capacity for self-reflection and awareness of their biases, stereotypes, and blind spots. While health providers clearly cannot know everything about all the varied cultural backgrounds of the patients they see, they can certainly become familiar with the sociocultural realities of the patients they most commonly see. Moreover, they can grow comfortable navigating websites and resources that can facilitate the provision of excellent care across linguistic and cultural barriers (for example, see www. ethnomed.org).

The skills of culturally responsive care can be developed through observation, practice, and precepting. The skills of working effectively with an interpreter can be readily taught and can greatly assist the physician with his or her patient flow, and decrease medical errors. As such, physicians can return to the ethical principle of "do no harm," even when practicing beyond their cultural and linguistic comfort zone. The devastating health disparity data in this country indicates, in fact, that much harm is indeed being done to patients, whether or not the health care providers are aware of their contributions to the problem. The hospital administrator in *John Q*, for example, would certainly be a good candidate for a refresher course in medical ethics, respectful communication, and the etiology of health disparities. Learners should be invited to consider how they would provide feedback to her about her power, decision-making, and communication style, and as such, will be engaged in important self-assessment as they develop their own unique ways of working with patients.

REFERENCES

1. Ring, J., Nyquist, J., Mitchell, S., Flores, H., and Samaniego, L. 2008. *Curriculum for culturally responsive health care: The step-by-step guide to cultural competence training.* Oxford, UK: Radcliffe Publishing.

2. Atrash, H., and Hunter, M. 2006. *Health disparities in the United States: A continuing challenge.* In D. Satcher, and Pamies, R. 2006. *Multicultural medicine and health disparities.* New York: McGraw Hill.

3. Callendar, C., Maddox, G., and Patrice. 2006. Transplantation and organ donation. In D. Satcher, and R. Pamies (Eds.), *Multicultural medicine and health disparities.* New York: McGraw Hill.

4. Smedley, B.D., Stith, A.Y., and Nelson, A.R. 2003. *Unequal treatment: Confronting racial and ethnic disparities in health care*. Washington: National Academy Press.
5. Ayanian, J.Z., Cleary, P.D., Keogh, J.H., Noonan, S.J., David-Kasdan, J.A., and Epstein, A.M. 2004. Physicans' beliefs about racial differences in referral for renal transplantation. *American Journal of Kidney Diseases* 43: 350–357.
6. Ayanian, J.Z., Cleary, P.D., Weissman, J.S., and Epstein, A.M. 1999. The effect of patients' preferences on racial differences in access to renal transplantation. *New England Journal of Medicine* 341: 1661–1669.
7. Himmelstein, D.U., Thorne, D., Warren, E., and Woolhandler, S. 2009. Medical bankruptcy in the United States, 2007: Results of a national study. *The American Journal of Medicine* 122: 741–746.

life-prolonging treatment in minors: *lorenzo's oil*

mark s. pian

Lorenzo's Oil (1993). Nick Nolte, Susan Sarandon, Peter Ustinov.
Directed by George Miller. Duration: 129 minutes.

DVD Chapter 8 Scene 01:01:22 to 01:02

L*ORENZO'S OIL* IS A DRAMATIZATION of the true story of Lorenzo Odone and the struggle of his parents, Augusto (Nolte) and Michaela (Sarandon), to find an effective treatment for his progressive neurological decline due to adrenoleukodystrophy (ALD). The movie depicts Lorenzo as an apparently healthy and gifted child until he begins to suffer first emotional outbursts, and then a series of falls a few months before he is diagnosed with ALD at age six. Lorenzo's parents are told "All boys with ALD die, usually within two years of diagnosis." Thus begins an inspirational story of courage and determination as Lorenzo's parents learn of the apparent helplessness of physicians to save their son and systematically attempt to find a cure for him themselves. The real Lorenzo Odone did not, in fact, die in childhood, but survived to the beginning of his fourth decade.[1]

This unprecedented feat certainly resulted from the remarkably attentive care delivered by his parents, perhaps aided by the therapy (a mixture of monounsaturated oleic acid and erucic acid) they pioneered. The degree to which the actual "Lorenzo's Oil" arrests or reverses neurological decline in ALD appears quite limited, although data suggest its efficacy if begun before imaging or symptomatic evidence of ALD appears in at least a subset of patients.[2,3] Against this background, it should be noted that the movie *Lorenzo's Oil* is not a documentary and, as noted unobtrusively after the movie credits, "... is a true story although certain characters and incidents are fictional." Without attempting to distinguish the actual from the fictional aspects of the story, my remarks here should be taken as pertaining solely to characters and events as depicted in the movie.

> And I am not a scientist, I am a father. And nobody can tell me what dressing I put on my kid's salad, OK?

In this scene, Augusto has just told Lorenzo's ALD specialist, Dr. Nikolais, about his plan to feed Lorenzo an industrial triglyceride preparation of oleic acid in hopes that it will reverse or slow the progression of his disease. Augusto's line is delivered as a retort to Nikolais' statement that, as Lorenzo's doctor and a scientist, his duty is to maintain his objectivity and to oppose what amounts to an uncontrolled experiment with unknown but real potential for doing harm. At the close of the scene, Nikolais, previously introduced as "the so-called 'world expert' on the leukodystrophies," acknowledges that this position "can appear heartless." He goes on to violate the duty he cites by offering an "unofficial" collaboration and suggesting an initial dose for the oil.

This powerful scene illustrates the conflict that can arise between parents and caregivers when conventional therapies are ineffective, and raises questions regarding not only parental autonomy pertaining to medical decision-making for minor children, but also physicians' professional responsibilities concerning beneficence and nonmaleficence. What authority do parents have in such situations? What, if any, are the limits to parental authority? What is the physician's professional responsibility to provide the greatest benefit with the least harm to a child in their care, as informed by their own expertise and judgment?

Historically, parents are looked to as autonomous decision makers regarding medical treatment for children who are too young to decide for themselves. However, the standards that parents are to use, and the criteria by which the appropriateness of their decisions are to be gauged, continue to be debated. It is often argued that parents exercise "consent by proxy" and as surrogate decision-makers can, except under limited circumstances, be relied upon to make choices intended to safeguard the welfare and "best interest" of their children. However, what constitutes "best interest" can be difficult to define, and although a parent's opinion is privileged in this regard, it is not absolutely binding. There is now increasing recognition of the child as a patient in his own right, and that treatment decisions must be made with regard to what is best for the child rather than what treatment the parent or the physician wants.[4]

In Lorenzo's case, his parents chose to go against medical advice and to embark on an unproven and potentially dangerous course of treatment. If this novel treatment is regarded as experimental, as the movie often describes it, what does this say about the defensibility of the parent's actions? How would we feel about their actions if they further harmed their son? If it were Nikolais, the physician–scientist, who suggested such experimental therapy in the absence of institutional review, safety data from animal experimentation, and preliminary evidence of efficacy, he would rightfully be accused of violating important standards of medical and scientific ethics. It might well be inferred that he is pursuing his own interest over that of his patient. Despite the movie's depiction of medical scientists' adherence to strict standards regulating the ethical conduct of clinical research as slavish, "heartless," and even exploitative, these standards were developed in response to the shocking excesses of the not-so-distant past.[5] What then, distinguishes unregulated research conducted by a physician–scientist from experimental treatment administered by a parent? Parents are widely assumed to be more likely to act in a child's best interest than a physician would be, particularly a physician who depends upon scientific publication to ensure grant support and professional advancement. Although this assumption is defensible in a general sense, the concept that parental conflict of interest does not also drive decisions away from the welfare of the child is open to challenge.

A career in subspecialty pediatric practice exposes one to extreme examples of such conflict of interest. Instances in which an abusive parent insists that his or her child, neurologically devastated by nonaccidental trauma, be subjected to life-sustaining treatment in order to avoid a murder charge, or parents who make their severely disabled and permanently dependent child the family bread winner by living off the child's disability payments are, thankfully, unusual. More subtle conflicts driving parents to acts of therapeutic desperation, however, are not uncommon; a parent's need to assuage his or her own feelings of guilt remains among the most important of these.[6] Numerous scenes in *Lorenzo's Oil* suggest guilt as an important factor in the parents' medical decision-making. In the clearest of these, Michaela first learns that ALD is an X-linked disorder, occurring only in males whose mothers are carriers of the defective gene. Intense pain is evident on her face and mirrored to some degree in every subsequent scene touching on the inherited nature of the disease.

Another common source of conflict is the parents' desire not to "give up" on their child. Lorenzo's mother ostracizes anyone, including her own sister, who expresses doubts about the suffering Lorenzo is forced to endure, suffering worsened by the parents' refusal of sedative and pain-relieving medication. Lorenzo's father states that hospice "would not do honor to Lorenzo" and that they persist because "he expects it of us." But how carefully do they consider whether this is true? The movie is prefaced by a heroic quote attributed to a Swahili warrior song: "Life has meaning only in the struggle. Triumph or defeat is in the hands of the gods... So let us celebrate the struggle." While the parents may view their own struggle this way, by what indication are they certain that Lorenzo does also, or even comprehends that there is a choice? How likely is it that he would ever have the opportunity to celebrate their struggle or his? Physically restrained, with a feeding tube in his stomach, how would he exercise the permission Michaela gave him to "fly to baby Jesus" if the suffering became too much?

Finally, there are limits to the treatments parents can demand of physicians on behalf of their children. Parents have a responsibility to make medical decisions to enhance the well-being of their children. However, the ethical principles of beneficence and nonmaleficence, as well as their own clinical judgment, must guide physicians in constructing a range of choices that do not include unproven therapies outside the context of an approved clinical trial.[7] Subjecting a child to significant risk without a compensatory likelihood of significant benefit is unethical, even when parents demand it. This includes denying pain medication to a suffering child. These same principles also proscribe the use of life-prolonging therapies that, within the context of an individual child's condition, provide more risk and burden than benefit.[8]

Lorenzo's physician, as portrayed in the film, fails in his duty to his patient by assisting his parents in using him as a subject in a poorly constructed and dangerous experiment. As our choice of treatments available to prolong the life of children with terminal diseases grows, so does our responsibility to ensure that research to develop those treatments is conducted in a manner that respects the rights of the children who participate. Equally important is a commitment to guarantee that those entrusted with making medical decisions on behalf of children are given the tools necessary to make choices which benefit the individual child and to identify factors such as desperation, guilt, and pride, both of physicians and parents, which might confound those decisions.

REFERENCES

1. Staff Writer. Lorenzo Odone: Obituary. *Telegraph Media Group Limited*. Retrieved January 18, 2010 from http://www.telegraph.co.uk/news/obituaries/2062622/Obituary-Lorenzo-Odone.html

2. Moser, H.W., et al. 2005. Follow-up of 89 asymptomatic patients with adrenoleukodystrophy treated with Lorenzo's oil. *Archives of Neurology* 62(7): 1073–1080. Retrieved July 2009 from http://www.ncbi.nlm.nih.gov/entrez/query.fcgi?cmd=Retrieve&db=PubMed&dopt=Citation&list_uids=16009761

3. Costello, D.J., Eichler, A.F., and Eichler, F.S. 2009. Leukodystrophies: Classification, diagnosis, and treatment. *Neurologist* 15(6): 319–328. Retrieved November 2009 from http://www.ncbi.nlm.nih.gov/entrez/query.fcgi?cmd=Retrieve&db=PubMed&dopt=Citation&list_uids=19901710

4. American Academy of Pediatrics Committee on Bioethics. Informed consent, parental permission, and assent in pediatric practice. *Pediatrics* 95(2): 314–317.

5. Beecher, H.K. 1966. Ethics and clinical research. *The New England Journal of Medicine* 274(24): 1354–1360.

6. Paris, J.J., Schreiber, M.D., and Reardon, F.E. 2003. Hyperbaric oxygen therapy for a neurologically devastated child: Whose decision is it? *Journal of Perinatology* 23: 250–253.

7. Moore, F.D. 1989. The desperate case: Care (costs, applicability, research, ethics). *Journal of the American Medical Association* 261(10): 1483–1484. Retrieved March 10, 2009 from http://www.ncbi.nlm.nih.gov/entrez/query.fcgi?cmd=Retrieve&db=PubMed&dopt=Citation&list_uids=2918643

8. Schneiderman, L.J., and Silbergeld Jecker, N.A. 1995. *Wrong medicine: Doctors, patients, and futile treatment*. Baltimore, MD: Johns Hopkins University Press.

10

family care-giving and the ethics of responsibility: *marvin's room*

carol schilling

Marvin's Room (1996). Diane Keaton, Leonardo di Caprio, Meryl Streep, Robert DeNiro, Hume Cronyn, Gwen Verdon, Hal Scardino. Directed by Jerry Zaks. Duration: 98 minutes.

DVD Chapter 11 Scene 00:54:30 to 00:57:26

MARVIN'S ROOM DRAMATIZES THE CONFLICT between two siblings over responsibilities to care for two disabled family members. Bessie (Diane Keaton) has fully dedicated the past two decades of her life to caring for her father Marvin (Hume Cronyn), mute and bed-bound by multiple strokes, and her dotty Aunt Ruth (Gwen Verdon), who suffers from back pain and does little more than watch soap operas. Bessie's estranged sister Lee (Meryl Streep) is the exasperated single mother of two sons: emotionally volatile teen-aged Hank (Leonardo di Caprio) and ten-year-old Charlie (Hal Scardino). When Bessie calls to reveal that she's been diagnosed with leukemia and to request bone marrow donors, mother and sons reluctantly drive from Ohio to the Florida home where Bessie and Lee grew up and where Marvin and Ruth still live. There the sisters confront their estrangement, their family's medical needs, and each other's life choices.

In this scene, Bessie's physician Dr. Wally (Robert DeNiro) explains to Lee that if she or her sons do not provide bone marrow, her sister's prognosis is grim. He matter-of-factly describes how Bessie will become "bedridden, totally dependent, and hopelessly depressed." He believes that he's offering compassion when he suggests that, when the time comes, Lee should hire a nurse to help her care for Bessie. However, Lee snaps that she plans to return to Ohio, receive her cosmetology certification, and find work there. Startled, the doctor replies, "I assume...," leaving the implied end of his sentence—*that you'd stay to care for your sister*—hanging in the air.

While this scene opens up ethical questions about the responsibilities of a patient's family to provide organs, tissue, or marrow for a relative in need, Dr. Wally's assumption incites a less frequently asked question needing clinical and ethical attention: Is it right to assume that family members should provide sustained or intensive care for chronically ill or disabled relatives? At first, this question might seem audacious. Certainly, we recognize a general duty to care for the vulnerable, no less the particular responsibilities arising from parenthood, marriage, and other special relationships. Like Bessie, many people find deep satisfaction, despite frustrations, performing familial caregiving—sometimes called informal caregiving—and would be pained to surrender a loved one to institutional care. But are responsibilities for such caregiving unconditional? Which family members can be assumed responsible, under what circumstances, for what duration? Who decides? How do we simultaneously acknowledge the moral value of placing another's needs above one's own and avoid exploitation?

Such questions urgently need attention in the context of recent medical advances and cultural circumstances. Today, medical conditions that were once fatal are now survivable. As a result, more people at all stages of the life cycle are living longer with chronic illness and disability, including dementia. At the same time, the pool of potential adult caregivers is shrinking with the increase of two-earner, blended, geographically scattered, and single-parent families. In the United States in 2007, an estimated 34 million adults provided about $375 billion in significant unpaid, hands-on, and administrative services to sick or disabled relatives. This figure, which does not include lost income or opportunity costs, amounts to more than federal and state Medicare spending combined.[1] In addition, an estimated 1.4 million children and youth ages 8 to 18 provide relatives with companionship, medications, injections, assistance communicating with professional health care providers, and all levels of assistance with daily living from mobility, dressing, bathing, and feeding to diapering.[2] Many caregivers—often women, but increasingly men—are sick or feeble or, like Bessie, become ill or die during the course of intensive caregiving.[3] Many lose life savings, employment, or whole careers. The Family Leave Act, while helpful, hardly addresses the risks that make long-term caregivers vulnerable persons.[4] Some interpretations of The Health Insurance Portability and Accountability Act (HIPAA) Privacy Rule can place families in a marginal relationship to health care information and decisions regarding a patient for whom they take responsibility at home.

Despite these circumstances, family caregiving has eluded bioethics for historical and philosophical reasons. Historically, bioethicists have inhabited academic medicine, the clinic, and sites producing complex medical technologies, where questions of doing no harm and patient autonomy prevail.[5] As a discipline, bioethics has mirrored medicine's interest in acute care and decisions about the beginning and end of life.[5] Intrigued by solving exotic problems, the field considers the daily concerns entailed in providing chronic care intellectually uninteresting. Philosophically, the physician–patient relationship is regarded as the basic ethical unit of medical practice, leaving family caregivers no clear or central moral standing in medical encounters.[6] From the discipline of philosophy, bioethics has inherited a lexicon pertaining to individual rights and a rationalistic model of decision-making. Neither field engages a rich vocabulary for describing human relationships or their accompanying values of dependency, particularity, and passionate partiality that comprise the ethics of care.[7] As a result, when families surface in bioethics, problems are typically defined as conflicts of interest, rather than as networks of shifting dependencies, responsibilities, and values.[6-9]

Furthermore, while recognizing the patient as an undeniably vulnerable person, bioethics can disregard the myriad ways that caregivers are also vulnerable.[3] Ironically, such inattention can cause harm to the patient who depends on a physically or psychologically exhausted caregiver, possibly a child, to carry out medical protocols that can demand hourly vigilance and the ability to follow complicated instructions, to manage medical services, to provide transportation, and to operate, monitor, and often repair complex machines.[1-3] Immersed in the clinic, bioethics hardly considers ways that homes become virtual hospitals managed by a non-professional staff providing services that even certified home health aides are prohibited from performing.[1]

By representing the moral good and the spiritual richness of caring for others, *Marvin's Room* counters the American cultural emphasis on independence and self-expression that the field of bioethics has absorbed. The film especially dignifies the ethic of caring for others traditionally valorized in women's lives. Yet, by representing saintly Bessie as the sole solution to the problem of how to care for Marvin and Ruth—and a reformed version of Lee as the solution to caring for everyone as Bessie declines—the film reinstates the cultural value of rugged independence and the belief that chronic illness and disability are personal tragedies. Health care systems and medical insurance providers depend on such a framing to deflect the responsibility to care for the chronically ill away from these institutions or social structures and onto families.[7] So, while Bessie enacts the ethics of care toward her vulnerable family, for 20 years she has not been the beneficiary of those same ethical values. Such lack of reciprocity creates a startling moral asymmetry.[7]

While the respected theorist of care ethics and dependency relationships, Eva Feder Kittay, has observed that the "the source of moral claims in an ethic of care has not been made sufficiently explicit" (p. 54), she unambiguously asserts that the "proscription against coercion and domination inheres in the moral vision that begins with relationships no less than one that begins with individuals" (p. 73).[7] However, this proscription raises practical ethical questions. How do we limit care obligations to prevent coercion and exploitation? How do we avoid cultural stereotyping in determining who will provide care? How do we ensure reciprocity for caregivers and recognize their vulnerabilities? Kittay argues that dependency work ultimately requires structures of social justice because "the obligation to redress the 'cost' that duties of dependency work exact from the dependency worker must fall to those outside the relationship itself" (p. 54).[7]

While social policy offers one solution beyond the relationship itself, bioethics can provide another. To do so, the field would need to include duties beyond the physician and patient relationship when defining the ethical practice of medicine. *Marvin's Room* can promote conversations about those practices, especially the family caregivers' vulnerability and susceptibility to coercion.

Such practices would, undoubtedly, place physicians in an unfamiliar sphere, where their moral duties extend to the patients' families.[6] This shift could incorporate, for instance, protocols that require home visits to understand the effects of the doctor's orders on patients and caregivers alike. Such visits could determine whether caregivers have the necessary education and training, emotional support, and resources to carry out their responsibilities. Interpretative models of decision-making, which have been employed in relation to caring for a patient[6] can be called upon, and regularly renewed, to negotiate the responsibilities of a family caregiver. Such processes of mediation could protect informal caregivers against coercion much as consent does. As the long-term caregiver Carol Levine has remarked, no consent process exists for caregivers.[10] Yet, isn't that lack morally unsettling when we agree that consent is mandated for donating a body part while, at the same time, medical and social systems assume that caregivers will donate long-term physical and mental labor—in essence give their whole bodies—for the good of another?

REFERENCES

1. AARP Public Policy Institute. Washington, D.C. 2008. *Valuing the invaluable: The economic value of family caregiving* [8 screens]. Retrieved July 20, 2009 from http://assets.aarp.org/rgcenter/il/i13_caregiving.pdf For the full report of April 2004, see http://assets.aarp.org/rgcenter/il/us_caregiving.pdf.

2. National Alliance for Caregiving. Bethesda, MD. 2005. *Young caregivers in the U.S.: Findings from a national survey* [66 screens]. Retrieved July 20, 2009 from http://www.caregiving.org/data/youngcaregivers.pdf.

3. Navaie-Waliser M., Feldman, P. H., Gould, D.A., Levine, C., Kuerbis, A.N., and Donelan, K. 2002. When the caregiver needs care: The plight of vulnerable caregivers. *American Journal of Public Health* 92(3): 409–413.

4. U.S. Department of Labor, Wage and Hour Division. Washington, D.C. 2008. *The family and medical leave act of 1993; Final rule. Federal register* [201 pages]. Retrieved July 20, 2009 from http://www.dol.gov/federalregister/pdfDisplay.aspx?DocId=1763.

5. Rosenberg, C.E. 1999. Meanings, policies, and medicine: On the bioethical enterprise and history. *Daedalus* 128(4): 27–46.

6. Kuczewski, M.G. 1996. Reconceiving the family: The process of consent in medical decisionmaking. *Hastings Center Report* 26(2): 30–37.

7. Kittay, E.F. 1999. *Love's labor: Essays on women, equality, and dependency*. New York and London: Routledge.

8. Levine, C., and Murray, T.H. (Eds.) 2004. *The cultures of caregiving: Conflict and common ground among families, health professionals, and policy makers*. Baltimore, MD and London, UK: The John Hopkins University Press.

9. Nelson, H.L., and Nelson, J.L. 1995. *The patient in the family: An ethics of medicine and families*. New York: Routledge.

10. Levine, C. 1999. The loneliness of the long-term care giver. *New England Journal of Medicine* 340(20): 1587–1590.

filmography

While not an exclusive collection of medical movies, the following list contains 140 films not used in *The Picture of Health: Movies and Medical Ethics*. These films also raise various bioethical issues that can be addressed in classroom settings. Many more of course exist. If you have ideas and suggestions, please do not hesitate to contact Dr. Colt at hcolt@uci.edu.

'night, Mother (1986)

Accused, The (1988)

Alfie (1966)

Alice (1990)

Angels in America (2003)

Any Given Sunday (1999)

Arrowsmith (1931)

Awake (2007)

Away from Her (2006)

Babel (2006)

Bella (2006)

Beyond Rangoon (1995)

Beyond Torture (2007)

Big Fish (2003)

Bird Flu (2006)

Blade Runner (1982)

Bobbie's Girl (2002)

Bone Collector, The (1999)

Boys from Brazil, The (1978)

Breakfast on Pluto (2005)

Charley (1968)

Chattahochee (1989)

Children of a Lesser God (1986)

Children of Mme (2006)

The Citadel, The (1938)

Citizen Ruth (1996)

Color of Paradise, The (1999)

Coma (1978)

Coming Home (1978)

Critical Care (1997)

Darius Gone West (2007)

Dead Ringers (1988)

Death and the Maiden (1994)

District 9 (2009)

Doc Hollywood (1991)

Doctor and the Devils, The (1985)

Doctor in the House (1954)

Doctor, The (1991)

Down Came a Blackbird (1995)

Dr. Akagi (1998)

Dying Young (1991)

English Surgeon, The (2007)

Eternal Sunshine of the Spotless Mind (2004)

Every Girl Should Be Married (1948)

Existenz (1999)

Exit, the Right to Die (2005)

Eyes Wide Shut (1999)

Flatliners (1990)

Florence Nightingale (1985)

Freaks (1932)

Generation RX (2008)

Ghost in the Shell (1995)

Girl Interrupted (1999)

Godsend (2004)

Goodbye Lenin (2003)

Grey Zone, The (2001)

Gross Anatomy (1989)

Hanoi Hilton, The (1987)

Hard Pill (2009)

Heart Condition (1990)

High Anxiety (1977)

Honey and Ashes (1996)

House of God (1984)

I, Robot (2004)

I've Loved You So Long (2008)

Ikuru (1952)

In the Name of the Father (1993)

Inherit the Wind (1960)

Interns, The (1062)

Intoxicating (2003)

Island of Dr. Moreau, The (1996)

Island, The (2005)

Juno (2007)

Killing Field, The (1984)

Knocked Up (2007)

K-Pax (2001)

Kung Fu Panda (2008)

Lady with the Lamp, The (1951)

Last Angry Man, The (1959)

Life Before Her Eyes, The (2007)

Live and Become (2005)

Lost Weekend, The (1955)

Love Story (1970)

Love with a Proper Stranger (1964)

M. A. S. H. (1970)

Madame Curie (1943)

Madness of King George, The (1994)

Man Facing Southeast (1986)

Manic (2001)

Mary Stevens MD (1933)

Mask (1995)

Men in White (1934)

Minority Report (2002)

Motorcycle Diaries (2004)

Murderball (2005)

My Brother's Keeper (1995)

My Left Foot (1989)

My Sister's Keeper (2010)

Nell (1994)

No Way Out (1950)

Nun's Story, The (1959)

Nuremberg (2000)

One True Thing (1998)

Out of Ashes (2003)

Paper Mask (1990)

Parenthood (1989)

Patch Adams (1998)

Pianist, The (2002)

Playing God (1997)

Precious (2009)

Pressure Point (1962)

Prince of Tides, The (1991)

Promises in the Dark (1979)

Proof (1991)

Repo Man (1984)

Requiem for a Dream (2000)

Serpents Egg, The (1977)

Sicko (2007)

Snake Pit, The (1948)

Soloist, The (2009)

Something the Lord Made (2004)

Son of the Bride (2001)

Sophie Scholl (2005)

Spellbound (1945)

Splice (2010)

Startrek V: The Final Frontier (1989)

State of Emergency (1993)

Station Agent, The (2003)

Step Mom (1998)

Stop-Loss (2008)

Story of Louis Pasteur, The (1935)

Stuck on You (2003)

Talk to Her (2002)

Terms of Endearment (1983)

Thin (2006)

Tsotsi (2005)

Turistas (2006)

Vanishing Line, The (1998)

Voices from the Front (1992)

What About Bob (1991)

index